Veterinary Medical Education: Challenges and Perspectives

Veterinary Medical Education: Challenges and Perspectives

Editors

Simona Sacchini
Ayoze Castro-Alonso

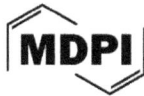

Basel • Beijing • Wuhan • Barcelona • Belgrade • Novi Sad • Cluj • Manchester

Editors
Simona Sacchini
Department of Morphology
University of Las Palmas de Gran Canaria
Las Palmas de Gran Canaria
Spain

Ayoze Castro-Alonso
Instituto Universitario de Sanidad Animal y Seguridad Alimentaria (IUSA)
University of Las Pamas de Gran Canaria
Las Pamas de Gran Canaria
Spain

Editorial Office
MDPI
St. Alban-Anlage 66
4052 Basel, Switzerland

This is a reprint of articles from the Special Issue published online in the open access journal *Veterinary Sciences* (ISSN 2306-7381) (available at: https://www.mdpi.com/journal/vetsci/special_issues/Veterinaryl_Medica).

For citation purposes, cite each article independently as indicated on the article page online and as indicated below:

Lastname, A.A.; Lastname, B.B. Article Title. *Journal Name* **Year**, *Volume Number*, Page Range.

ISBN 978-3-7258-1400-8 (Hbk)
ISBN 978-3-7258-1399-5 (PDF)
doi.org/10.3390/books978-3-7258-1399-5

© 2024 by the authors. Articles in this book are Open Access and distributed under the Creative Commons Attribution (CC BY) license. The book as a whole is distributed by MDPI under the terms and conditions of the Creative Commons Attribution-NonCommercial-NoDerivs (CC BY-NC-ND) license.

Contents

About the Editors vii

Preface ix

Roberto Bava, Fabio Castagna, Vincenzo Musella, Carmine Lupia, Ernesto Palma and Domenico Britti
Therapeutic Use of Bee Venom and Potential Applications in Veterinary Medicine
Reprinted from: *Vet. Sci.* **2023**, *10*, 119, doi:10.3390/vetsci10020119 1

Zih-Fang Chen, Yi-Hsin Elsa Hsu, Jih-Jong Lee and Chung-Hsi Chou
Perceptions of Veterinarians and Veterinary Students on What Risk Factors Constitute Medical Disputes and Comparisons between 2014 and 2022
Reprinted from: *Vet. Sci.* **2023**, *10*, 200, doi:10.3390/vetsci10030200 25

Zih-Fang Chen, Yi-Hsin Elsa Hsu, Jih-Jong Lee and Chung-Hsi Chou
Are They Thinking Differently? The Perceptions and Differences in Medical Disputes between Veterinarians and Clients
Reprinted from: *Vet. Sci.* **2023**, *10*, 367, doi:10.3390/vetsci10050367 38

David C. Dorman, Robert H. Poppenga and Regina M. Schoenfeld-Tacher
The Current State of Veterinary Toxicology Education at AAVMC Member Veterinary Schools
Reprinted from: *Vet. Sci.* **2022**, *9*, 652, doi:10.3390/vetsci9120652 53

James Fairs, Anne Conan, Kathleen Yvorchuk-St. Jean, Wade Gingerich, Nicole Abramo, Diane Stahl, et al.
The Evaluation of a High-Fidelity Simulation Model and Video Instruction Used to Teach Canine Dental Skills to Pre-Clinical Veterinary Students
Reprinted from: *Vet. Sci.* **2023**, *10*, 526, doi:10.3390/vetsci10080526 69

Holger Fischer, Petra Heidler, Lisa Coco and Valeria Albanese
Leadership Theories and the Veterinary Health Care System
Reprinted from: *Vet. Sci.* **2022**, *9*, 538, doi:10.3390/vetsci9100538 91

Sandra Foltin and Lisa Maria Glenk
Current Perspectives on the Challenges of Implementing Assistance Dogs in Human Mental Health Care
Reprinted from: *Vet. Sci.* **2023**, *10*, 62, doi:10.3390/vetsci10010062 106

Jaime Espinosa García-San Román, Óscar Quesada-Canales, Manuel Arbelo Hernández, Soraya Déniz Suárez and Ayoze Castro-Alonso
Veterinary Education and Training on Non-Traditional Companion Animals, Exotic, Zoo, and Wild Animals: Concepts Review and Challenging Perspective on Zoological Medicine
Reprinted from: *Vet. Sci.* **2023**, *10*, 357, doi:10.3390/vetsci10050357 126

Sarah E. Hooper, Kent G. Hecker and Elpida Artemiou
Using Machine Learning in Veterinary Medical Education: An Introduction for Veterinary Medicine Educators
Reprinted from: *Vet. Sci.* **2023**, *10*, 537, doi:10.3390/vetsci10090537 140

Ricardo Marcos, Sónia Macedo, Macamen de Vega and Pablo Payo-Puente
The Use of Simulation Models and Student-Owned Animals for Teaching Clinical Examination Procedures in Veterinary Medicine
Reprinted from: *Vet. Sci.* **2023**, *10*, 193, doi:10.3390/vetsci10030193 165

María del Pino Palacios-Díaz and Vanessa Mendoza-Grimón
Environment in Veterinary Education
Reprinted from: *Vet. Sci.* **2023**, *10*, 146, doi:10.3390/vetsci10020146 . . . . **177**

Kirsten Persson, Wiebke-Rebekka Gerdts, Sonja Hartnack and Peter Kunzmann
"What If It Was Your Dog?" Resource Shortages and Decision-Making in Veterinary
Medicine—A Vignette Study with German Veterinary Students
Reprinted from: *Vet. Sci.* **2023**, *10*, 161, doi:10.3390/vetsci10020161 . . . . **188**

**Ana S. Ramírez, José Raduan Jaber, Rubén S. Rosales, Magnolia Conde-Felipe,
Francisco Rodríguez, Juan Alberto Corbera, et al.**
Nurturing a Respectful Connection: Exploring the Relationship between University Educators
and Students in a Spanish Veterinary Faculty
Reprinted from: *Vet. Sci.* **2023**, *10*, 538, doi:10.3390/vetsci10090538 . . . . **201**

About the Editors

Simona Sacchini

Prof. Dr. Simona Sacchini (DVM, M.Sc., Ph.D.) is professor and vice dean at the Faculty of Health Sciences of the University of Las Palmas de Gran Canaria (ULPGC), where she teaches in the area of human anatomy and embryology. She had her veterinary degree at the University of Milan, Italy (2007). She was a resident veterinarian at the Clinical Hospital for Small Animals, Faculty of Veterinary, ULPGC (2007–2008). Then, she spent 10 years as a pre- and post-doctoral researcher at the University Institute of Animal Health (IUSA), Faculty of Veterinary, ULPGC, where she developed her expertise area in comparative neuroanatomy and neuropathology, focusing on neurodegenerative diseases in marine mammals. She collaborated on five different national research projects and published and contributed to congresses on marine mammals, neuroscience, and comparative anatomy and pathology. She is a member of societies on neuroscience and comparative anatomy.

Ayoze Castro-Alonso

Dr. Ayoze Castro Alonso (DVM, M.Sc., Ph.D.) is a full-time lecturer at the Morphology Department of the University of Las Palmas de Gran Canaria and develops his research activity at the Institute of Animal Health and Food Safety (IUSA). During the past ten years, he has been the innovation manager at the Oceanic Platform of the Canary Islands (PLOCAN). His research lines include veterinary pathology and applied marine sciences and technologies for the sustainable use of marine space. He has been the project coordinator of several European projects (FLOTANT, INTERTAGUA, EO MAMMALS, and SUSME) and has participated, as a researcher, in many other projects of the FP7, H2020, or INTERREG programs (TROPOS, NEXOS, ATLANTOS, MARCET, etc.). In addition, together with research activity, he has robust experience in the direction and management of research and innovation activities and is certified as a practitioner in the well-known international methodology "Project In Controlled Environment (PRINCE2T M)".

Preface

Veterinarians are valued and respected professional figures. Veterinary research transcends species boundaries and includes the study of both spontaneously occurring and experimentally induced models of both human and animal diseases. In fact, the health of humans, animals, and ecosystems is interdependent, and this is materialized in the concepts of "One Health" and "Planetary Health". Scenarios such as the COVID-19 pandemic have generated new challenges, and adaptation has been essential to the field of veterinary medicine and science. The COVID-19 pandemic has highlighted the importance of the One Health program, and this adaptive and responsive approach should be implemented in veterinary medical education. These fundamental changes in the roles, responsibilities, and spectrum of activities of veterinary professionals require equal changes, improvements, and adaptations to veterinary science and medical education training programs. These modifications may include, for instance, increasing the participation of veterinary professionals in multidisciplinary human medicine teaching, training, and research teams (i.e., human anatomy, physiology, or biology, among others). Significantly, recent scientific and technological breakthroughs (i.e., RNA-based vaccines, improved molecular diagnostic tools (PCRs), innovative ICTs applied to health assessment and research, etc.) have been seen to influence current teaching and training programs in key, modern, and innovative veterinary colleges and universities. Ultimately, the main goal of these centers is to provide high-quality and cutting-edge knowledge and skills to their students, which is essential for the development of their future careers. Technical advances can—and should—influence teaching and learning in different veterinary fields.

Simona Sacchini and Ayoze Castro-Alonso
Editors

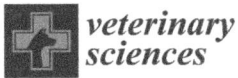

Review

Therapeutic Use of Bee Venom and Potential Applications in Veterinary Medicine

Roberto Bava [1,2,†], Fabio Castagna [1,2,†], Vincenzo Musella [1,2], Carmine Lupia [1,3], Ernesto Palma [1,4,5,*] and Domenico Britti [1,2]

1. Department of Health Sciences, University of Catanzaro Magna Græcia, 88100 Catanzaro, Italy
2. Interdepartmental Center Veterinary Service for Human and Animal Health, CISVetSUA, University of Catanzaro Magna Græcia, 88100 Catanzaro, Italy
3. Mediterranean Ethnobotanical Conservatory, Sersale (CZ), 88054 Catanzaro, Italy
4. Nutramed S.c.a.r.l. Complesso Ninì Barbieri, Roccelletta di Borgia, 88021 Catanzaro, Italy
5. Department of Health Sciences, Institute of Research for Food Safety & Health (IRC-FISH), University of Catanzaro Magna Græcia, 88100 Catanzaro, Italy

* Correspondence: palma@unicz.it
† These authors contributed equally to this work.

Simple Summary: Bee products consist of many substances that have long been known for their medicinal and health-beneficial properties. Venom is certainly the one that has attracted the most interest due to the complexity of its chemical composition. Several types of research have been conducted utilizing biological (cellular) systems to figure out the properties of bee venom in vitro. Primarily, cell lines of various sorts and origins are used for this purpose. Afterward, experiments on murine models paved the way for clinical trials on humans. Therefore, there are numerous reviews summarising the uses of venom for human medicine, but none have focused on its use in veterinary medicine. This review aims to gather the relevant publications on the use of bee venom in veterinary medicine.

Abstract: Apitherapy is a branch of alternative medicine that consists of the treatment of diseases through products collected, processed, and secreted by bees, specifically pollen, propolis, honey, royal jelly, and bee venom. In traditional medicine, the virtues of honey and propolis have been well-known for centuries. The same, however, cannot be said for venom. The use of bee venom is particularly relevant for many therapeutic aspects. In recent decades, scientific studies have confirmed and enabled us to understand its properties. Bee venom has anti-inflammatory, antioxidant, central nervous system inhibiting, radioprotective, antibacterial, antiviral, and antifungal properties, among others. Numerous studies have often been summarised in reviews of the scientific literature that have focused on the results obtained with mouse models and their subsequent transposition to the human patient. In contrast, few reviews of scientific work on the use of bee venom in veterinary medicine exist. This review aims to take stock of the research achievements in this particular discipline, with a view to a recapitulation and stabilisation in the different research fields.

Keywords: apitherapy; alternative medicine; bee venom; antioxidant activity; antimicrobial and antiviral activity; anti-inflammatory activity; anti-cancer effects

1. Introduction

A third of our food is produced directly or indirectly by honeybees, one of the most abundant and effective pollinator species. Additionally, these insects are bred, creating worthwhile products and job prospects in rural regions [1–3]. Various bee products are used in alternative medicine, as they possess interesting healing and disease-preventive properties. The term "Apitherapy" is used to describe a group of therapeutic and preventative procedures used in both human and animal medicine to improve health [4,5].

The use of honey, pollen, and royal jelly spans the fields of nutrition and food sciences as well as pharmacology (desensitization, anti-inflammatory therapies, and treatments for autoimmune diseases).

The medicinal and nutritional benefits of hive products have recently been thoroughly studied. Numerous studies have been conducted, not least due to the rising problem of drug resistance, which has necessitated the search for novel pharmacologically active substances [6,7]. Additionally, in some parts of the world, drug expenses are prohibitive, whereas apitherapy cost is typically reasonable. Consequently, apitherapy has been used as a "supplemental medication" in many different nations (Brazil, China, Japan) [5]. However, there is no shared consensus on the medical application of apitherapy [5]. The methods of administration and use of hive products vary widely. Use must be based on an understanding of the unique physiological reactions of humans and animals, in addition to age and weight [8]. Because bee products are multi-substance mixes with several unknown components, they provide a challenge [9]. It is important to bear in mind that, in the absence of products with standardized chemical composition, the therapeutic effects of bee products may fluctuate according to the source. Soil, climate, harvesting and storage practices, botanical sources, etc., all affect the quality and effectiveness of the products used in apitherapy. To maximize outcomes and protect the patient from hazards, it is crucial to understand the conditions under which the products are generated. In any case, researching potential and standardizing products seem promising alternatives for the near future.

Honey, propolis, pollen, bee bread, royal jelly, apilarnil, beeswax, and venom are some of the bee products utilized in apitherapy [10]. Bee venom and its clinical veterinary medicinal uses are the main topics of this review. Bee venom's medicinal benefits have a very long history. Since 3000 BC, bee venom has been utilized in traditional Eastern medicine to treat inflammatory illnesses [11]. In this context, ancient civilizations such as Nibia, Babylon, and Assyria would also have been familiar with bee venom. The Greek Hippocrates, who is considered the "father of medicine," employed it to treat arthritis and other inflammatory conditions [10]. The Roman Pliny the Elder (23–79 AD) describes it in his *Naturalis Historia* [8,12]. Charlemagne is said to have used bee venom to cure his gout [13]. The first collecting attempts occurred in the 19th century. Between 1897 and 1899, J. Langer of the University of Prague made the first attempt to harvest the venom without killing the bee, collecting the poison in droplets inside capillary tubes. His first technique involved pressing a bee's lower abdomen so that she would protrude a sting with a drop of poison at the end. In the early 1900s, apitherapy began to be used to treat rheumatic disorders. This practice quickly expanded throughout Europe. Demand for the product has become stronger. The poison was first made available for purchase in 1930 by the Mack company in southern Germany [14]. The first methods of manual extraction of the poison were followed by more articulate ones [15]. Using a light electric shock to induce the bees to inject the venom was a time-saving method. The drawback was that the bees lost their stinger and, in part, their abdominal guts, resulting in death. This method was perfected in Czechoslovakia in 1960 when the mean used for collection allowed the bees to stay alive and maintain their stinger [14]. Bee venom therapy was pioneered by Dr. Bodog Beck, a naturalized Hungarian-American who published the influential book, *Bee Venom Therapy*, in 1930. Dr. Joseph Broadman of New York began using bee therapy to treat arthritis in the early 1950s and wrote about his experiences in the 1962 book, *Bee Venom, the Natural Curative for Arthritis and Rheumatism* [11]. Since 1971, at least 12 nations in Europe, three in Asia, and three in America have used bee venom [14].

Bee venom has traditionally been used to treat inflammatory diseases such as rheumatism [16,17]. However, bee venom has also been known to be used as an adjunct in the treatment of neurological disorders, asthma, and infectious diseases such as malaria. There are limited research evaluations on the use of bee venom in veterinary medicine. In contrast, many published studies have addressed its potential application in human medicine. In light of the latter consideration, this study aims to summarise published research on the potential application of bee venom in animal therapies.

2. Venom Source

Bee venom is produced by the venom gland located in the abdominal cavity of female honeybees [4]. The gland is connected to a containment sac. The veliniferous apparatus of social insects belonging to the genus *Apis* is an essential defence mechanism. Bees sting in the vicinity of the apiary in an attitude of colony defence [18]. The queen, on the other hand, stings to kill rivals [19]. Each hive can only have one queen, and when several queens are born at once, either some of them escape along with a specific number of bees, a born queen kills the unborn queens who are still within their cell, or two queens engage in a death battle [20]. The protein concentration of queen bee venom is highest in the first (0–3) days of life and diminishes after 7 days (a necessary condition shortly after emergence to kill the eldest queen and twin queens in competition for hive domination). As the gland degenerates, the protein content of the venom in honeybees diminishes during the following days. In contrast, the venom is not detectable at the time of emergence in the female honeybees. Instead, it increases quickly over the following two days, remains constant for the first 14 days, and then drops. Therefore, older honeybees produce less poison than younger ones [18]. The venom's composition changes throughout time with age. For instance, melittin is released in an inactive precursor form, which transforms into an active form with growth and the passage into the guardian stage, which happens about day 20 of age [18].

Honeybees have a pointed stinger that is extracted from the abdomen during stinging along with the venom sac. Unlike wasps and hornets, they can only sting once before dying [21]. When a bee stings a person or a mammal in general, the stinger remains embedded in the skin, and the bee dies as a result of ripping out its intestines, muscles, and nerve center in an effort to detach. The bee dies because such a large amount of its body is lost. The stinger's pointed end features tiny hooks that keep it from being removed without damage. Once embedded, it uses a separate piston mechanism to push the venom into the wound [22]. The stinger self-incorporates into the tissue and there is a simultaneous release of the contents of the venom sac, which is usually expelled completely within a few minutes [21]. Additionally, the alarm pheromone message conveyed by bee venom activates other bees to defend the hive. The alarm pheromone is made up of the mandibular gland's 2-heptanone molecule and other substances, such as isopentyl acetate, released by the gland connected to the stinging apparatus [21,23]. Bee venom cause localized inflammation with symptoms like pain, heat, and itching to systemic allergic reactions that can end in anaphylactic shock and, in extreme cases of hypersensitivity, can be fatal [24,25]. In popular culture, bee venom is frequently connected to these phenomena. However, it is one of the most priceless gifts the beehive has given us. It can be helpful in the treatment of a wide range of illnesses when used in tiny dosages. Its use in the treatment of many illnesses states is intriguing due to its complex composition of chemicals with significant pharmacological and biochemical activity.

Freshly secreted bee venom is a clear, colourless liquid that forms a light yellow powder when it dries [26]. It has the pungent aromatic odour of honey and is acidic (between 4.5 and 5.5). The water content in bee venom varies between 55 and 70 percent [27]. The active components of the venom of various hymenoptera are peptides, proteins, enzymes, low molecular weight substances, and aliphatic constituents in varying quantities [18,28]. No exemption applies to bee venom. It is a very complicated composition that is largely (80%) made up of proteins. These latter compounds have high (proteins) or low (peptide) molecular weights. Biogenic amines are the most important low-molecular-weight substances. The peptides in bee venom adolapine, melittin, apamin, and peptide 401 have undergone extensive research [29] Table 1 summarises the composition of bee venom.

Table 1. Composition of bee venom: dry matter data according to Dotimas and Hider (1987) [27].

Substance	%	Substance	%
Enzymes		**Biogenic amines**	
Phospholipase A2	10–12	Histamine	0.5–2
Hyaluronidase	1.5–2	Dopamine	0.2–1
Phosphatase, glucosidase	1-2	Noradrenaline	0.1–0.5
Proteins		**Carbohydrates**	
Mast cell degranulating Peptide	1–2	Sugar (glucose, fructose)	2
Melittin	40–50	**Phospholipids**	5
		Amino acids	
Secapine	0.5	Aminobutyric acid and α-amino acids	0.4
Tertiapine, apamin, procamine	2–5	**Volatile substances** (pheromones)	4–8
Other small peptides	13–15	**Mineral substances**	3–4

The right collection is the crucial element in obtaining the best quality bee venom. Pollen, honey, and other colony products must be free of impurities. As pointed out by Krell [15], there are no official quality standards, as bee venom is not recognised as an official drug or foodstuff. A quantitative study of its more stable or readily quantifiable components, such as melittin, dopamine, histamine, noradrenaline, or those for which contamination is suspected, can be used to determine a substance's degree of purity. Standardization and quality control techniques for the efficacy and purity of hymenoptera venom, particularly those of bees, were discussed by Guralnick et al. in 1986 [30].

3. Venom Constituents and Their Biological Activities
3.1. Melittin

The more abundant element is melittin. It makes up roughly 50% of the peptides in the venom and consequently 50% of the dry BV [31]. The sequencing of the peptide by Habermann and Jentsch (1967) revealed that it included 26 amino acid residues [32].

The carboxy-terminal region (residues 21–26) is hydrophilic due to the presence of a positively charged amino acid stretch, whereas the amino-terminal region (residues 1–20) is hydrophobic [33,34]. Melittin is soluble in water as a monomer or tetramer due to its amphoteric nature. The polypeptide spontaneously integrates into the phospholipid bilayer of cell membranes, damaging them [35–37]. Thus, the molecule's primary structure resembles the fundamental form of a detergent-type molecule. By changing the phospholipid composition of the cell membrane, melittin accumulation leads to cell lysis. Neumann and Habermann (1953) discovered that it was a haemolytic factor for the first time [38]. Melittin is a member of the class of compounds known as amphiphilic due to its distinctive structure. Each melittin chain has two α-helical segments and resembles a bent rod overall. Melittin is monomeric at the lowest concentrations necessary for cell lysis and tetrameric at the amounts found in the bee venom sac [39]. To describe the precise steps involved in membrane permeation by amphipathic α-helical lytic peptides, two different pathways were put forth. They are theoretically quite different from one another.

The first one, known as the "barrel-stave" model, is characterized by the insertion of amphipathic α-helices into the membrane's hydrophobic core to create transmembrane holes. In the second, known as the "carpet" model, the peptides are in touch with the lipid head group during the whole process of membrane permeation and do not integrate into the hydrophobic core of the membrane, even if they are not required to acquire an amphipathic α-helical structure [40]. The cytotoxic and anti-inflammatory actions of melittin on tumor cells may be significantly influenced by these structural characteristics. By facilitating an enhanced Ca^{2+} ion influx, melittin also activates phospholipase A2 and adenylate cyclase [41]. All of the above characteristics make melittin interesting due to its currently known anti-cancer, anti-inflammatory, antiviral, antibacterial, and neuroprotective properties [42–45].

3.2. Apamin

Eighteen amino acids make up the polypeptide apamin, which also has two disulfide bridges in it. It is the smallest neurotoxin in bee venom and makes up less than 2% of the weight of dry venom [46]. Apamin functions as an allosteric inhibitor since it has long been recognized as a highly selective blocker of small-conductance Ca^{2+}-activated K^+ (SK) channels [47]. These channels help control the ionic balance in the cell membrane, which regulates the resting and action potentials in vital cells as well as signal transmission through neurons and muscle contraction. Through this route, apamin produces a neurotoxic impact by mediating long-term after-hyperpolarization in neurons and muscle cells. This polypeptide can also pass the blood–brain barrier and affect how the central nervous system functions through a variety of mechanisms. For instance, it has been shown in rats to have neurotoxic effects that result in hyperactivity and convulsions [48]. Apamin also affects the permeability of the cell membrane to potassium (K+) ions by inhibiting calcium-activated K+ channels. Through the Akt and Erk signaling pathways, the toxin can prevent vascular smooth muscle cells from proliferating and migrating [49]. This finding emphasizes apamin's potential for use in atherosclerosis treatment plans. Generally speaking, pathophysiological responses, including atherosclerosis and Parkinson's disease involve a significant function for apamin target channels.

3.3. Mast Cell Degranulation Peptide

It also is known as "peptide 401". It is a polypeptide with 22 amino acid residues and a molecular structure that resembles an apamin with two disulfide bridges [50]. It only makes up a small portion of the venom, roughly 2–3% of the dry matter volume. The name MCD refers to the physiologic process by which mast cells release histamine; the peptide promotes mast cell degranulation and sets off inflammatory responses. In animal trials, MCD has been proven to significantly lower blood pressure [51]. In this context, it is the component considered responsible for the hypotension observed in BV intoxication [52].

3.4. Adolapin

It is a polypeptide of 103 amino acids and makes up around 1% of dry BV. By inhibiting prostaglandin synthesis and cyclooxygenase activity, adolapin exerts anti-inflammatory, analgesic, antinociceptive, and antipyretic effects [53,54]. Because naloxone has been shown to partially suppress the analgesic effect of adolapin, a central mechanism may be involved in the drug's action [55]. According to Koburova (1985), adolapin, like aspirin and other comparable substances, has antipyretic actions, most likely via inhibiting the synthesis of cerebral prostaglandins [56].

3.5. Phospholipase A2

The enzyme that is most prevalent in bee venom is phospholipase A2. It is an alkaline component that makes up 12–15% of the dry BV. It has four disulfide bridges and 128 amino acid residues [57]. It is highly aggressive against the cell membrane, resulting in cytolysis, together with melittin and lysolecithin, which are produced when phospholipase acts. Furthermore, phospholipase is the most significant allergen and hence the most toxic element of bee venom. Phospholipases A2 (PLA2) are enzymes capable of hydrolysing the ester linkage of glycerophospholipids leading to the liberation of free fatty acids and lysophospolipids, including arachidonic acid, a precursor necessary for the biosynthesis of eicosanoids through the intervention of cyclooxygenase, molecules involved in the inflammatory cascade. Phospholipase A2 is therefore involved in the synthesis of prostaglandins and leukotrienes. Pure phospholipase A2 is not poisonous, but when it is near melittin, it becomes a haemolytic factor [21]. It works in concert with melittin to lyse erythrocytes by causing breaches in the cell membrane that let melittin flow through. Melittin does this by dissolving the phospholipid layers that make up the majority of the cell membranes. This haemolytic effect of bee venom is inhibited by heparin [58]. Additionally, it has been demonstrated that phospholipase A2 has anti-inflammatory, anti-tumor, and anti-parasitic properties [59,60].

3.6. Hyaluronidase

Hyaluronidase is a 350 amino acid residue polypeptide that makes up 1% to 2% of the BV. Human hyaluronidase, which is involved in the turnover of hyaluronic acid, and bee venom hyaluronidase share a 30% sequence identity [61]. Hyaluronidase acts as an adjuvant to venom diffusion. Certain acidic mucopolysaccharides in connective tissues have intrinsic glycolide linkages that the enzyme hyaluronidase breaks down, decreasing the viscosity of the tissue and allowing the venom to enter the tissues [62]. Additionally, because hydrolyzed hyaluronic acid particles have pro-inflammatory, pro-angiogenic, and immune-stimulating capabilities, they accelerate systemic poisoning [21]. It is known to promote blood vessel dilatation, increasing permeability and hence, blood circulation, which in turn enhances BV circulation [60].

The Table 2 below summarizes the key characteristics of the bee venom's constituent parts and the associated biological effects.

Table 2. Biological effects of bee venom and its components.

Components	Effect
Melittin	Peptide with biological activity. Melittin prevents blood from clotting, works well against germs, shields against radiation. Melittin works as an anti-inflammatory in small dosages. It has a haemolytic action and is clearly cytotoxic.
Phospholipase A2	Phospholipase is the most important allergen and therefore the most harmful component of bee venom.
Hyaluronidase	It is an enzyme that allows venom to enter tissues and causes blood vessels to widen and tissues to become more permeable, increasing blood flow.
Acid phosphatase	Allergen.
Apamin	Biologically active peptide; a neurotoxin.
Mast cell degranulating peptide	Peptide that degranulates mast cells by releasing biogenic amines.
Protease inhibitor	It has anti-inflammatory and hemorrhagic properties and inhibits the action of various proteases, including trypsin, chymotrypsin, plasmin, and thrombin.
Adolapin	Anti-inflammatory, anti-rheumatic, and analgesic.
Histamine	It dilates blood vessels and increases capillary permeability. It is an allergen.
Dopamine, noradrenaline	Neurotransmitters that affect the behaviour and physiology of the senses.
Alarm pheromone	It puts the colony on high alert.

4. Collection of Bee Venom

The final product has varying properties depending on the extraction process used. The most effective venom appears to be that which is collected under water to prevent the evaporation of the highly volatile components. Venom from venom sacs that had been surgically excised had a different protein composition than venom obtained using the electric shock technique [15].

The venom gland was traditionally removed surgically from bees, or bees were individually squeezed until a drop of venom was extracted from the stinger tip. Electroshock extraction has gradually gained popularity since the early 1960s and is now considered the norm. The bees are induced to release venom by touching wires covered in a fine wire mesh through which low-voltage electric current discharges (20–30 volts) pass; the venom is then periodically collected from a glass plate beneath the wires, such as every ten minutes. Ten thousand stings produce one gram of venom in an hour or two [27].

The method of using electrical shocks with bees to extract their venom was first described by Markovic and Mollnar (1954) [63]. There are different models and installations [64–66]. Depending on the author describing the technique, different parameters are sought to collect bee venom. Typically, the voltage is between 24 and 30 volts, the pulse lasts between 2 and 3 s, there is a 3 to 6 s gap, and the pulse frequency is between 50 and 1000 hertz. The bees are not harmed throughout the operation, making it safe for them. One hundred fifty milligrams of honeybee venom can be collected after 3 h of harvesting. Twenty hives may yield one gram of venom over the course of two hours [67]. Four grams of dried bee venom can be acquired if venom is collected three to four times each month for three hours between April and October [68]. However, the price to pay is a 10% to 15% decrease in brood activity and honey production. Bee productivity is unaffected by less frequent harvesting (3 to 4 times each season).

Individual bee venom active ingredients can be extracted for specialized medical and biological purposes using chromatographic separation techniques or molecular genetic techniques [27,69].

Electric shock extraction techniques momentarily disturb hive life because the bees become hostile and produce the alarm pheromone [18,70]. The venom obtained in this manner, known as "apitoxin," becomes more unstable and loses some of its volatile components when compared to the venom preserved pure in the bee's sac (the esters, whose therapeutic value is antispasmodic, calming, tonic, anti-arhythmic). When the venom is ready, it can be administered using acupuncture needles that inject the poison right into the affected area. A conventional and affordable method of delivering the active ingredients in their most complete and fresh form involves the bee directly stinging the patient.

5. Effects and Applications in Veterinary Medicine

One of the products that has undergone the most extensive investigation in the fields of biology and medicine is bee venom. It is also a traditional medicinal product that is most well-known around the world [71]. Many research investigations have been conducted during the past 20 years employing animal models, particularly murine models. Bee venom or its components are used in apitherapy, allergology, as well as in experimental biology [72,73]. Bee venom has a variety of diverse and perhaps contradictory biological effects. It is necessary to employ certain bee venom components to produce particular biological effects. Like many medications, bee venom has adverse effects that must be taken into account in addition to the intended therapeutic effects. Crude bee venom has substantially lesser toxicity when compared to the combined action of its constituent parts. Bee venom has toxic effects if the dose provided is 200–500 times more than the therapeutic dose, whereas individual bee venom components have toxic effects if the dose used is 20–50 times greater than recommended [74]. Bee venom therapies are currently accessible throughout the world, although they are most popular in Asia, Eastern Europe, and South America. In addition to treating "traditional" musculoskeletal illnesses like arthritis and rheumatism, diverse therapeutic uses also extend into grey areas, as in the case of a new study that suggests bee venom as a supplemental treatment for COVID-19 [75–77]. In the next section, the antioxidant, anti-inflammatory, anti-pathogenic, and anti-carcinogenic activities aimed at resolving neurological disorders of bee venom will be analysed (Figure 1).

5.1. Antioxidant Activity

Bee venom contains substances with strong antioxidant activity (AOA) [78]. Phospholipase A2, apamin, and melittin are responsible for this reaction. A variety of methods, including free-radical scavenging, hydrogen donation, metal ion chelation, single oxygen quenching, and acting as a substrate for superoxide and hydroxyl radicals, underpin the antioxidant activity. The antioxidant effect may result from the compounds' ability to inhibit lipid peroxidation (a process involving those chemical species with an independent existence and one or more unpaired electrons or an odd number of electrons, the so-called free radicals) and boost superoxide dismutase activity (an important enzyme that reduces radical damage by removing the superoxide radical in almost all cells exposed to oxygen). However, bee venom also contains additional substances that function as antioxidants in addition to these. For instance, vitellogenin demonstrates antioxidant action in mammalian cells by directly protecting the cell from oxidative stress, providing the cells with a defense against reactive oxygen molecules.

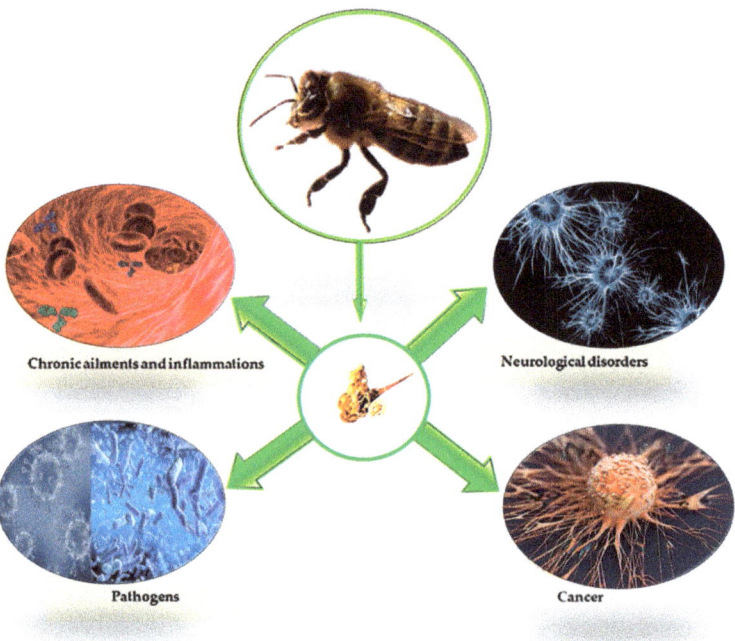

Figure 1. Schematic illustration of bee venom properties.

Only three recent investigations have used conventional tests to measure the AOA of bee venom [79–81]. Antioxidant qualities were present in all samples, which appeared to be unrelated to any of the specific components that were discovered and measured in the same samples. According to certain evidence, melittin alone exerts very low AOA compared to bee venom extracts, and this may be because other venom components also play a role [82]. Therefore, some other small compounds may be implicated in the observed bioactivities, along with synergistic or antagonistic actions at certain dosages, leading to various outcomes across bee venom samples.

Among the first studies conducted, we have that of Rekka et al. (1990) [83]. Rekka et al. demonstrated that honeybee venom had a considerable inhibitory effect on nonenzymatic lipid peroxidation. Additionally, it has strong hydroxyl radical scavenging abilities, as demonstrated by its competition with dimethyl sulfoxide for HO (hydroxyl radicals). These findings may further support the idea that antioxidant activity plays a role in the anti-inflammatory properties of honey bee venom, which is mostly known for its ability to decrease interleukin-1 production in vitro [83].

Other studies have investigated antioxidant activity in conjunction with other parameters. For example, El-Hanoun et al. (2020) [84] administered 0.1, 0.2, and 0.3 mg per rabbit subcutaneously twice a week for a total of 20 weeks. The total antioxidant capacity (TAC), glutathione S-transferase (GST), glutathione content (GSH), glutathione peroxidase (GPx), superoxide dismutase (SOD), malondialdehyde (MDA), and TBARS were all tested during the experiment to determine any potential changes in the antioxidant activity. The GST and GSH levels in the treated rabbits increased, according to the findings. MDA and TBARS values were also lower. These findings supported BV's antioxidant properties. Additionally, BV resulted in an enhancement in reproductive performance that was directly associated with the semen's increased antioxidant activity. Similar evidence of improvement of several parameters was obtained by subcutaneous administration of bee venom in rabbits by Elkomy et al. (2021) [85]. Particularly, compared to the control group, milk yield, litter size at birth, litter weight, and survival rate at weaning age were all considerably higher in the BV groups. When compared to the control group, serum estradiol 17- (E2) levels in the rabbit treated with BV were 15% higher, which was statistically significant. In comparison to the control, the does who were given any study dosages of BV saw a gradual and significant drop (12%) in serum progesterone levels (P4). Additionally, compared to the control group, they demonstrated a statistically significant rise in conception (17%) and fertility rates (10%). When BV was administered to the rabbit, the activity of the liver enzymes aspartate aminotransferase (AST) (16%) and alanine aminotransferase (37%) gradually decreased and became significantly lower. Results also showed that BV caused a significant decrease in malondialdehyde (MDA) and thiobarbituric acid reactive substances (TBARS) in BV groups compared to the control group, as well as a gradual and significant increase in total antioxidant capacity (TAC), antioxidative enzymes like glutathione S-transferase (GST) and glutathione peroxidase (GPx), serum IgG, IgM, and Ig [85].

Instead, the study by El-Speiy et al. (2022) investigated the possibilities of supplementing bee venom (BV) to the drinking water of rabbits [86]. The association of BV with oxytetracycline (OXY) was proposed in an experimental group of investigation. Subsequently, it was looked at how weaned rabbits' immunological status, bacterial count, antioxidant activity, and haemato-biochemical profile had changed. The findings showed that, except for the rise in ALT in the OXY group compared to the control group, weaned rabbits treated with OXY and BV had significantly higher levels of total plasma protein (TP) and globulin (Glo) while having lower levels of AST and ALT. Triglycerides (TG), total cholesterol (TC), and very low-density lipoprotein (VLDL) were dramatically reduced in rabbits treated with OXY or BV (VLDL-c). IgG, total antioxidant capacity (TAC), superoxide dismutase (SOD), catalase (CAT), and glutathione peroxidase all increased in the BV-treated groups (GPX).

The broiler has also been used to assess the antioxidant capabilities of bee venom. In particular, in the research of Kim et al. (2019) [87], increasing concentrations from 10 to 500 micrograms per kilogram have been added to the basic diet. Numerous serum markers and antioxidant activity were assessed after 21 days. Additionally, the liver was removed to analyze the fatty acid content and quantify the malondialdehyde levels. Except for triglycerides and non-esterified fatty acids, the blood parameters did not change by adding dietary bee venom. Bee venom consumption quadratically enhanced the content of stearic acid in the diet but also lowered the concentrations of palmitoleic, oleic, and linoleic acids as well as monounsaturated and polyunsaturated fatty acids. Finally, eating bee venom tended to quadratically reduce hepatic malondialdehyde levels. The authors concluded that eating bee venom enhanced antioxidant capacity and changed the metabolism of fatty acids in broilers [87].

5.2. Antimicrobial and Antiviral Activity

Antimicrobial resistance is a global public health challenge, accelerated by antibiotic misuse [88]. Infections caused by multi-drug resistance bacteria have resulted in an increase in fatalities in recent years, and the issue seems to be getting worse [89]. These resistant bacteria are also a concern in the food chain, as the bacteria can resist common biocides used in the food industry and reach consumers [90]. In such a scenario, bee venom proves to be a promising ally. The peptide melittin is primarily responsible for the antibacterial properties of bee venom [91]. Melittin's capacity to disrupt cellular membranes serves as the primary mechanism of its antibacterial effect. Due to the structure of the cell membrane, Gram-positive bacteria are more sensitive to melittin than Gram-negative bacteria. Melittin can more readily pass through the peptidoglycan layer of Gram-positive cells' membrane than it can through the lipopolysaccharide layer that protects Gram-negative cells' membrane. According to Fennell et al. (1968) [45], melittin and bee venom were effective at killing 86% of Gram-positive bacteria and 46% of Gram-negative bacteria. One milligram of melittin has the same antibacterial action as 0.1 to 93 units of penicillin on Gram-positive microorganisms. It has been demonstrated that the proline residue at position 14 is crucial to melittin's antimicrobial action. Its absence in a melittin analogue significantly reduced the anti-microbial activity compared to the native peptide.

Melittin's effectiveness as an antibacterial agent has been investigated against several bacteria, including *Escherichia coli*, *S. aureus*, and *B. burgdorferi* [92–95]. At MICs of 0.5–4, 0.5–4, and 1–8 g/mL, respectively, melittin shows antibacterial activity against methicillin-sensitive *S. aureus* (MSSA), MRSA, and *Enterococcus spp.* bacteria [96]. *B. burgdorferi*, the cause of Lyme disease, has been found to be affected by both BV and melittin alone in terms of the form and size of its biofilms [93]. BV's antibacterial and antibiofilm properties against 16 *Salmonella* strains obtained from chickens were also investigated. The MIC for BV was between 256 and 1024 g/mL. In 14 of the 16 *Salmonella* strains that were examined, sub-inhibitory doses of BV considerably decreased biofilm production while significantly increasing motility. The motility of *Salmonella isangi I G1* and *S. infantis Lhica I17* was unaffected by BV [97]. The therapeutic efficacy of bee venom (BV) was also investigated against clinical and subclinical mastitis in dairy cows. In the study by Han et al. (2009), mastitic cows selected on the basis of a somatic cell count above 200,000 cells/mL milk were used [98]. Fifteen lactating mastitic cows were subcutaneously injected with four different BV dosages (3, 6, 12, and 24 mg per treatment) to examine the effects of the BV dose. It was shown that the action of BV enhanced the number of clinically cured quarters with less than 0.2 million/mL somatic cell count (SCC) during the duration of the treatment period. Within two weeks of receiving BV therapy, a considerable decrease in the detection of *Staphylococcus aureus* and other Gram-positive bacteria was seen. The authors concluded that the mammary defense systems of dairy cows with mastitis may have been compromised by BV therapy [98]. The findings demonstrated that bee venom significantly inhibits seven main bacterial mastitis pathogens. In comparison to normal pharmaceuticals, the minimal inhibitory concentrations (MIC) against methicillin-resistant *Staphylococcus aureus* (MRSA), *Staphylococcus aureus*, and *Escherichia coli* exhibited a greater effect. Therefore, apitoxin may have antibacterial properties, which justifies testing it as an alternative to antibiotics for the treatment of bovine mastitis.

Bee venom has proven to be equally effective in the treatment of canine bacterial otitis. In particular, it was observed that dogs treated with apitoxin injection three times a week for a fortnight had a similar bacterial count to the experimental control group treated with conventional antibiotics [99].

Along with other similarly active components, the enzyme phospholipase A2 also possesses antibacterial characteristics [100]. In addition, vitellogenin acts as an antimicrobial peptide, causing damage to the cell membranes of bacteria [71]. The enzyme phospholipase A2 also has antifungal properties against some species of the *Candida* genus and can also be employed as an anti-parasitic drug in the treatment of specific organisms like *Trypanosoma* and *Plasmodium falciparum* [101–103]. Studies on the use of bee venom against *Toxoplasma gondii* should also be highlighted. Bee venom exerts damaging effects on live tachyzoites, as shown by Hegazi et al. (2014) [104].

It is important to concentrate our attention on viruses, which are likewise deserving of discussion. Studies on animal and plant viruses have already shown mellitin's capacity to damage cell membranes and interact with cell surface molecules; the latter is a key component in antiviral therapy [43]. Mellitin has proven to be effective against Papillomaviruses and the vesicular stomatitis virus [105,106]. Mellitin has also shown antiviral properties against viruses without a viral membrane. Through a significant up-regulation of Th1 cytokines (IFN- and IL-12) and several immune cell types, including CD3+ CD8+

T-cells, CD4+CD8+, BV and its component melittin, can induce immunity against porcine reproductive and respiratory syndrome viruses (PRRSV), resulting in a decrease in viral load and a milder form of interstitial pneumonia in pigs infected with PRRSV [107].

A final consideration can be made about the use of antibiotics for auxinic purposes, aimed at preventing diseases and promoting weight gain in animals with low dosage administrations. This use of antibiotics was banned in the European Union in 2006, but was used in the past [108]. The study conducted by Kim et al. (2018) was designed to evaluate purified bee venom (BV) as an alternative to antibiotics in broilers [109]. To obtain 0, 10, 50, 100, and 500 g of BV per kg of food, BV was added to a diet of soybean meal and corn meal. Dietary BV enhanced body weight gain to 1–21 days as the amount in the diet improved the feed conversion ratio quadratically. Secretory immunoglobulin A (sIgA) content on the ileal mucosa rose linearly with the addition of BV to the diet at 21 days and 1.5 months. With increasing toxicity in the meals at 21 days, the total amount of short-chain fatty acids (SCFA) in the cecal digesta decreased. Except for creatinine, none of the serum values were impacted by the BV diet [109]. Similarly, Han et al. (2010), who added bee venom to water acquired comparable proof of weight growth in broilers [110]. Finally, positive effects on growth performance and immunocompetence blood parameters were also recorded in young pigs [111]. Bee venom could also be interesting in this capacity as a growth promoter.

5.3. Anti-Inflammatory Activity

Bee venom contains at least four substances that have anti-inflammatory effects. Among the most important, we have melittin, apamin, adolapin, and phospholipase A2. Mellitin has been extensively studied for its anti-inflammatory properties against liver inflammation, amyotrophic lateral sclerosis, atherosclerosis, and neuroinflammation [112–115].

Inflammation can largely be seen as the manifestation of a genetic transcriptional programme activated by tissue danger signals. Nuclear factor-kappa B (NF-κB) is a protein complex functioning as a transcription factor. NF-kB plays a significant role in the regulation of inflammatory genes (cyclooxygenase-2 (COX-2), cytosolic phosphatase A2 (cPLA2), and tumor necrotic factor-a) [116]. It is located in the cytosol, bound to an inhibitory protein called inhibitor of κB (IκB). A variety of extracellular signals reaching the membrane receptors of the Toll family can activate the enzyme IκB kinase (IKK). IκB kinase (IKK) phosphorylates IκB, which detaches. NF-κB is then free to migrate to the nucleus, where it binds to NF-κB consensus sites located upstream of several inflammatory genes. The inhibition of nuclear factor kappa B (NF-B) by the enzyme kinase IkB (IKK) may be how the possible anti-inflammatory mechanism function works. IKK activity is inhibited by melittin's interaction with the enzyme. These protein–protein interactions were linked to the inhibition of IKKa and IKKb activity as well as the prevention of IkB release in response to an inflammatory stimulation [116]. Inhibition of IKK reduces the production of phospho-p38, the cytokines interleukin-1 (IL-1), and interleukin-6 (IL-6), as well as reducing the release of tumour necrosis factor (TNF) [113,117,118].

Melittin significantly inhibits MAPKs (Mitogen-activated protein kinases), including ERK and p38 MAPK [119]. MAPKs (Mitogen-activated protein kinases) are enzymes widely present in the body and involved in numerous physiological and pathological processes. In particular, p38 represents a very interesting pharmacological target, being a protein involved in various cellular responses. Its enzymatic activity occurs both in the cytoplasm and in the nucleus. It is involved in various cellular processes, such as the regulation of mRNA, apoptosis, protein degradation, and the organisation of the cytoskeleton and chromatin. The activation of p38, in particular p38α, has been correlated with inflammation by in vivo and in vitro studies, which have demonstrated its ability to intervene at transcriptional and post-transcriptional levels. It induces COX-2 activity and regulates the biosynthesis of numerous proinflammatory cytokines (IL-1β, IL-6, TNF-α, INF-gamma) that are fundamental in the pathogenesis of autoimmune diseases (such as rheumatoid arthritis, multiple sclerosis, Crohn's disease), asthma and COPD (chronic obstructive pulmonary disease), but also of cardiovascular disorders such as atherosclerosis [120–122].

Therefore, treatments with melittin modulate TLR pathway activation and prevent inflammatory cytokine expression [123]. Melittin has the ability to block nuclear NF-kB p65 activation and MAPK serine p38 inhibition in vitro [124]. As a result, this function has anti-inflammatory effects. By modifying the transcription factors NF-kB and AP-1 in vivo, melittin also showed anti-inflammatory capabilities [125]. Recent research has revealed that using BV topically for atopic dermatitis has anti-inflammatory effects. IgE concentrations, cytokine release, and the activity of NF-kB and MAP kinases are all decreased, which has an anti-inflammatory impact. Both the TNF-/IFN-dependent inflammatory response and the lipopolysaccharide (LPS)-induced inflammatory responses are inhibited by the lowering of NF-kB and MAPK activity. A decrease in MAPK activity also affects the expression of the inflammatory genes COX-2 and iNOS, as well as the control of NF-kB signals that affect cytokine release [126,127]. Studies on the anti-inflammatory properties are among the most numerous. A large portion of the controlled clinical research on how bee venom affects arthritis has been carried out on arthritic animals (mice, rats, and guinea pigs). One of the most popular test models in scientific research to create new substances that can be utilized to treat arthritis and other inflammatory disorders is adjuvant-induced arthritic rats.

Bee venom was used in investigations on the prevention and treatment of adjuvant-induced arthritis in rats by Lorenzetti et al. (1972) [128]. The authors demonstrated that administering bee venom subcutaneously to arthritic rats three times a week has a significant impact on both avoiding the onset of arthritis and reducing the severity of an already present case. The anti-inflammatory impact of bee venom, according to these investigators, was far more prominent when it was applied as a preventative measure.

Similar findings have emerged in subsequent studies. According to Zurier et al. (1973) [129], daily injections of three distinct bee venom components—melittin, apamin, and phospholipase A 2—along with daily injections of entire bee venom, delayed the onset of adjuvant arthritis in rats.

Chang and Bliven (1979) [130] investigated the mechanism of action of bee venom on adjuvant-induced arthritis and came to the conclusion that at least two processes were involved. They discovered that a single bee venom injection given the day before or the day of the adjuvant injection significantly prevented the development of arthritis in rats. According to their findings, this suppression was caused by an altered immune response in addition to the bee venom's anti-inflammatory effects [130]. In the following years, numerous independent studies on the anti-inflammatory benefits of entire bee venom have been conducted using rat models. In the rat adjuvant-induced arthritis and carrageenan footpad edema tests, these investigations showed that entire bee venom has an anti-inflammatory effect. Chang and Bliven (1979) [130] discovered that using these in vivo assays that bee venom (0.5 mg/rat subcutaneously) and cyclophosphamide (60 mg/kg orally) behaved similarly in suppressing adjuvant-induced arthritis in rats and showed a distinctly different temporal pattern of activity from steroid therapy, even when considering the theory that the effects were caused by stress-induced steroid production. Additionally, their findings indicated that this suppression may have been caused by changes in the immune system, in addition to the bee venom's anti-inflammatory effects.

Eiseman et al. (1982) [131] investigated how bee venom affected the progression of adjuvant-induced arthritis and drug metabolism depression in rats. The main and secondary inflammatory responses to the adjuvant hind paws were shown to be reduced by bee venom, according to the investigators. Additionally, they noticed variations in heme metabolism brought on by the venom, which is strongly suggestive of immune system disturbances leading to modifications in the hepatic microsomal enzymes.

Studies in mouse models were followed by clinical trials in animals. Melittin contains anti-inflammatory effects that activate the pituitary-adrenal system and causes it to release cortisol, as Vick et al. showed in monkeys as early as 1972 [132]. Based on findings from animal models, it is estimated to be 100 times more effective than hydrocortisone [132].

Another study by Vick et al. (1976) describes an application of bee venom in the treatment of canine arthritis [133]. In particular, a group of 24 dogs was enlisted, of whom 8 were verified to have arthritis by radiographic examination and a thorough physical examination, and 16 were randomly chosen as normal dogs. On days 30, 37, 50, and 60, 1 mg of whole bee venom was given subcutaneously to the arthritic dogs. Weekly assessments of motor activity in the cage were made using a pedometer, and plasma cortisol levels was registered. Plasma cortisol levels rose 15 days following bee venom injection treatment. Prior to therapy, the arthritic dogs travelled, on average, about four miles per day compared to the normal canines, who covered roughly twelve miles per day. The average activity of the arthritic dogs resembled that of the healthy dog population after just three doses of bee venom. Additionally, this increase in activity persisted for sixty to ninety days after the final injection, suggesting that the venom had a long-lasting impact [133].

Results of the treatment of 17 arthritic dogs were reported by Short et al. in 1979 [134]. Fourteen out of seventeen dogs considerably recovered after receiving bee venom treatment, recovering to normal or almost normal mobility. All dogs with disc complications recovered to normal or nearly normal conditions after a series of bee venom injections were given at the sites of pain and stiffness. Four of five dogs treated for joint complications (hip dysplasia and arthritic joints) showed improved movement. Four of six dogs treated for poor surgical recovery responded well. The authors of this study came to the conclusion that some canine arthritic disorders may be greatly improved by bee venom treatment.

Anti-inflammatory effects have also been studied in large animals. In the study of Jeong (2017), apitoxin was employed in mastitis treatment [135]. The idea was that BV would lessen inflammation in the cells of the cow mammary epithelium (MAC-T). Cells were treated with LPS (1 g/mL) to cause an inflammatory response, and the anti-inflammatory effects of BV (2.5 and 5 g/mL) were investigated to test the theory. The cellular defenses of BV against LPS-induced inflammation were also investigated. The findings demonstrated that BV can reduce the production of COX2, a protein associated with inflammation, as well as pro-inflammatory cytokines, including IL-6 and TNF-. In LPS-treated cells, BV dramatically reduced the activation of NF-B, an inflammatory transcription factor, via dephosphorylating ERK1/2. Additionally, pretreatment with BV reduced the amount of intracellular reactive oxygen species that were LPS-induced (e.g., superoxide anion). These results support the idea that BV may suppress oxidative stress, NF-B, ERK1/2, and COX-2 signaling to diminish LPS-induced inflammatory responses in bovine mammary epithelial cells [135].

In research by Von Bredow et al. (1978) [136], the authors evaluated the effects of bee venom injections on eight arthritic horses with ages ranging from 8 to 17. Three of the six horses who showed a significant improvement—out of the eight, six—showed full recovery. Finally, bee venom has also been investigated against important horse diseases. Kim et al. (2006) [137] describe a case of a 13-year-old male Arabian horse suffering from laminitis. The subject was injected with bee venom at several sites. After the third session, the patient showed almost normal walking.

Between 12 and 25% of the racing population of horses were estimated to have chronic obstructive pulmonary disease (COPD). However, since the fibrobronchoscope was developed, it is now conservatively believed that 50% of horses at racetracks have COPD. This ailment needs to be taken into account if a horse performs below standard. Since drugs are prohibited in racing, COPD poses a significant concern for racehorses. The effectiveness of bee venom in treating COPD in racehorses was the subject of a randomised controlled trial. From among the horses competing on the Ontario Jockey Club circuit, some were chosen at random. In total, 3.0 milliliters of bee venom were subcutaneously injected, 0.5 milliliters per site, into three bilateral acupuncture points. The performance of 76% of the horses improved as their COPD decreased [138]. Therefore, bee venom has also demonstrated valuable properties in this direction.

5.4. Neurodegenerative Disorders

The neuroinflammation caused by persistent glial cell and microglial activation is associated with neurodegenerative diseases. Pla2 and apamin, two components of BV, have been investigated as anti-neuroinflammatory medicines, and as an adjuvant to increase the effectiveness of some medications against neurodegenerative illnesses and/or to lessen adverse effects [139]. The use of BV was investigated in neurodegenerative diseases by Tsai et al. in 2015 [140]. To treat dogs with intervertebral disc disease, the authors used bee venom. Intervertebral disc disease is a disorder characterized by algia that calls for the use of analgesics and anti-inflammatory medications to lessen pain and nociceptive signals. The study's authors found that BVA efficiently reduces pain symptoms. Forty dogs with neurological conditions brought on by intervertebral disc disease were enlisted and split into experimental groups to get this information. The myelopathy scoring system and the functional number scale scores of the dogs receiving BV treatment dramatically improved and were comparable to those of the group receiving traditional therapy [140].

Other research has focused on non-immune mediated nerve palsy. For example, Jun et al. (2007) [141] studied the effects of bee venom on facial nerve paralysis (FNP) [141]. Twelve dogs were enlisted for this study and split into three experimental groups: a control group with four dogs, a dexamethasone group with four dogs, and a bee venom group with four dogs. In the control group, saline solution (1 mL) was intramuscularly injected into the head muscle following FNP induction. Clinical ratings, drawn up in the form of treatment points, were used to track changes in the clinical symptoms of FNP after the injection of 100 g apitoxin. Bee venom was successful in resolving the condition. Comparisons were also made between the groups treated with apitoxin and dexamethasone. However, there was no discernible difference between the groups treated with apitoxin and dexamethasone [141]. The same outcome was attained in an apitoxin-treated 6-year-old male Shih Tzu dog that had the left side of his face paralyzed and tilted. Following bee venom acupuncture therapy, the clinical symptoms gradually became better. Eight weeks after beginning bee venom acupuncture, the patient's face sensory and neurological indicators improved [142]. This case study demonstrates the potential benefit of using bee venom in acupuncture for canine idiopathic facial paralysis.

It has also been demonstrated that BV is effective in treating peripheral neuropathy that develops in association with vincristine therapy. Due to damage to the sensory and motor neurons in the peripheral nervous system, several chemotherapy drugs do cause peripheral neuropathy. The effects and mechanism of bee venom injection (BVA) were examined in the study by Li et al. (2020) to treat peripheral neuropathic pain brought on by repeated intraperitoneal vincristine (1 mg/kg/day, days 1–5 and 8–12) infusions in rats [143]. Bee venom (BV, 1.0 mg/kg) administered subcutaneously at therapeutic site ST36 reduced mechanical and cold sensitivities. Extracellular vivo recording demonstrated that bee venom acupuncture (BVA) prevented vincristine-treated rats' abnormal spinal wide-range dynamic (WDR) neuron hyperexcitation brought on by cold cutaneous (acetone) and mechanical (brush, push, and pinch) stimuli. Additionally, BVA's effects on mechanical and cold hypersensitivity were reversed by lidocaine microinjection into the ipsilateral locus coeruleus or by antagonists of spinal 2-adrenergic receptors, demonstrating the critical role of descending noradrenergic regulation in analgesia [143]. These results suggest that BVA could be a potential therapeutic option for vincristine-induced peripheral neuropathy.

5.5. Anti-Cancer Activity

In recent years, there has been a great deal of interest in finding natural compounds having anti-cancer potential. Mellitin and phospholipase A2 are the components of bee venom that have antitumor action [144–146]. The interactions between them also lead to other antitumor effects, such as the production of apoptosis and necrosis, as well as the suppression of the proliferation of different tumor cells.

The most appealing action for slowing the proliferation of cancer cells is apoptosis. The part of BV with the highest level of cytotoxic action against cancer cells is melittin.

The first study establishing the antitumor impact of melittin revealed that leukemic cells' inhibition of calmodulin caused cancer cells to undergo apoptosis. This Ca^{2+} channel pump blockage led to a massive increase in Ca^{2+} concentration, which ultimately caused cell death. [147]. Since that time, several investigations on the antitumor effects of melittin and their mechanisms of action have been carried out using various types of tumor cell lines.

Nowadays, it is known that different bee venom components stimulate various and distinct cell signaling pathways in different ways. At the cell surface, many growth factor receptors (epidermal growth factor receptor, TNF receptor, etc.) are activated during carcinogenesis. These receptors' activation triggers multiple downstream signaling cascades. The Ras-MAPK (including ERK and JNK) pathways, the PI3K-AKT pathways, PLC-γ-CaM, and the NF-kB are significant and are the targets of bee venom components among these pathways. Some components of bee venom inhibit surface receptors either by dephosphorylating them or by causing their degradation, which in turn modifies the signaling pathways downstream that are crucial for proliferation, metastasis, angiogenesis, and apoptosis (for example, the synergistic effect of BV sPLA2 and PtdIns(3,4)P2); PtdIns(3,4)P2 and bv-sPLA2 are responsible for the cytotoxic action because they cause cell death as a result of membrane integrity loss, absence of signal transmission, and production of cytotoxic lyso-PtdIns(3,4)P2. Bee venom components frequently inhibit AKT and ERK signaling, albeit frequently, this inhibition is the consequence of growth factor inhibition. Another typical target of bee venom components is the inhibition of the NF-kB signaling pathway by interfering with several signaling targets. Certain bee venom components produce reactive oxygen species (ROS), which activate members of the p53 family and cause cell cycle arrest and death [148]. The anti-cancer activity of bee venom is also expressed in its ability to modulate cell apoptosis.

The growth of multicellular organisms and the maintenance of good tissue homeostasis both depend on apoptosis. Two molecular programs that ultimately result in the activation of particular members of the caspase family are in charge of controlling the execution of this route in mammals. This subsequently results in the cleavage of key cell substrates, leading to cell death. The intrinsic pathway, which is triggered by a wide variety of stress signals, and the extrinsic pathway, which functions downstream of death receptors like Fas and the tumour necrosis factor receptor family, are the two molecular programs. The identification of cytochrome c as an apoptogenic factor released by mitochondria marked a crucial breakthrough in the discovery of the importance of these organelles in the intrinsic pathway of apoptosis. The 'point of no return' in this pathway is defined by mitochondrial outer membrane permeabilisation (MOMP), which leads to the release of cytochrome c.

The intrinsic (mitochondrial) pathway of apoptosis is controlled by the BCL-2 family of proteins, which operate within a complex network of protein-protein and protein-membrane interactions. The BCL-2 family includes both pro- and anti-apoptotic regulators of the intrinsic apoptosis pathway. The BCL-2 family of proteins regulates MOMP and thus determines the cellular commitment to apoptosis. Indeed, BCL-2 proteins play a key role in mediating the delicate balance between cell survival and death.

Several cytotoxic stimuli, including oncogenic stress and chemotherapeutic agents, as well as developmental signals, involve the mitochondrial pathway, which is regulated by members of the BCL-2 family. These stimuli activate BH3-only (initiator) proteins, which inhibit pro-apoptotic BCL-2 proteins (guardians), thus allowing the activation of the pro-apoptotic effectors BAX and BAK, which subsequently disrupt the outer mitochondrial membrane. Cytochrome c released from the mitochondria promotes caspase-9 activation on the scaffold protein Apaf-1, while the released protein SMAC (second mitochondria-derived activator of caspases) blocks the caspase inhibitor XIAP (X-linked inhibitor of apoptosis protein). BH3-only proteins, which are transcriptionally or post-translationally induced by cytotoxic stress signals, exert their pro-apoptotic function by two mechanisms: the neutralisation of pro-apoptotic BCL-2 proteins and the direct activation of the pro-apoptotic effectors BAX and BAK. Bee venom and melittin have been shown to increase the expression and levels of a number of pro- and apoptotic mediators, including cytochrome C (Cyt C), protein 53 (p53), Bcl-2-associated X protein (Bax), Bcl-2 homologues antagonist/killer (Bak), caspase-3, caspase-9, and various death receptors, while decreasing the anti-apoptotic mediator Bcl-2 [17,148,149]. Other mechanisms are involved in the apoptotic activity of bee venom. The expression of metalloproteinases, enzymes involved in the breakdown of collagen and thus in pathological invasion processes (tumour metastasis), is suppressed by bee venom. Matrix metalloproteinase-9 (MMP-9) expression and activity can be suppressed by inhibiting extracellular/mitogen-activated protein kinase p38 (ERK/p38 MAP) regulated protein kinases and NF-B pathways [150,151].

Furthermore, in relation to tumour progression, by suppressing vascular endothelial growth factor (VEGF), VEGFR-2, and preventing the latter's signaling pathways, bee venom significantly reduced angiogenesis and metastasis [152]. Melittin has been shown to increase $[Ca^{2+}]$ and activate phospholipase A2 (PLA2) in numerous cancer cell types. Melittin's membrane-disrupting activity causes cell membranes to become more permeable, which appears to open specific kinds of Ca^{2+} channels and raise intracellular Ca^{2+} concentration. Apoptosis or necrosis of mammalian cells is then brought on by changes in the cytosolic free Ca^{2+} level [148]. In prostate cancer, BV and melittin demonstrated tumor cell growth inhibition. The down-regulation of anti-apoptotic gene products such as Bcl-2, XIAP, iNOS, and COX-2 was the source of this impact [17,153]. As a result, this down-regulation inhibited NF-kB transcriptional activity, which is correlated with apoptosis, the process through which cells die. By preventing the translocation of p50 and p65, IkB phosphorylation was impaired, which in turn led to the deactivation of NF-kB signalling [17]. In ovarian cancer cells, a different mechanism of BV and melittin-induced apoptosis was investigated. Melittin had an antitumor impact in this study by activating death receptors and inhibiting the JAK2/STAT3 pathway [154]. Inactivation of STAT3 and increased expression of the death receptors DR3, DR4, and DR6 were the major strategies used to slow the proliferation of ovarian cancer cells. When these DRs were expressed, apoptosis was activated in a caspase-8-dependent manner [155].

Alternately, melittin employs additional cancer-fighting pathways in addition to apoptosis. Melittin reduced tumor cell growth without apoptosis in murine animal models of Lewis lung carcinoma. The amount of tumor-associated macrophages (TAMs), particularly CD206+ M2-like TAMs in the tumor stroma, was decreased by melittin therapy. Because there were less CD206 + M2-like TAMs, there were fewer VEGF+ and CD31+ cells in the tumor tissue. This fact reveals melittin's anti-angiogenic properties [155]. The capacity of melittin to interact with phospholipid membranes is linked to further processes that result in the death of cancer cells. This interaction results in holes that have the potential to cause cell lysis by collapsing the cell membrane [144,156]. This capability was investigated in relation to colorectal and stomach cancer. Melittin produced granulation, blebbing, and cell swelling in cancer cells in vitro in about one minute at a dosage of 20 g/mL, which was very quick. Additionally, full death happened 15 min after the commencement of the therapy [157].

This lytic action, meanwhile, is not limited to cancer cells and can also result in the lysis of healthy cells. In this regard, using vectors like nanoparticles to restrict melittin's activity in target cells is one possible answer. In a recent study, melittin and nanographene oxide, as well as melittin and nanodiamonds were combined to combat breast cancer [158]. Compared to melittin alone, this combination increased the harmful impact on cancer cells. Furthermore, melittin with nanodiamonds was able to shield healthy cells from melittin's lytic action. Additionally, it was seen that the degree of necrosis had diminished.

5.6. Activities on Other Diseases

Bee venom and melittin have anti-inflammatory effects on digestive disorders linked to inflammation, such as gastric ulceration, nonalcoholic steatohepatitis, ulcerative colitis, acute liver failure, etc.

When acetylsalicylic acid caused gastric ulcers in rats, BV demonstrated gastroprotective properties. In acetylsalicylic acid-treated rats, it attenuated the haematological, haemostatic, and histopathological changes, decreased tissue eosinophil levels, as well as the ulcer index, fluid volumes, and pepsin concentrations. This was attributed to its anti-inflammatory and antioxidant effects by lowering TNF-, MPO levels, and MDA concentration, and increasing SOD activity and glutathione (GSH) concentration, as well as its anti-apoptotic property by downregulating Bax and Caspase-3 level [159].

In streptozotocin-induced diabetic rats, beeswax-coated water-soluble fraction of BV (BWCBVA) reduced blood glucose levels, restored serum biochemical markers, and raised body weight. Additionally, BWCBVA treatment raised the number of islet cells and decreased the damage to cells in the pancreas while decreasing the expression of PI3K-p85 and glucokinase in the liver. Additionally, by boosting calcium ion influx and blocking the potassium ion channel, co-administering BWCBVA with nifedipine and nicorandil caused insulin secretion [160].

The kidney has also been shown to benefit from the effects of bee venom. Acute kidney injury and renal fibrosis have been demonstrated to be protected by BV and its key ingredients, such as MEL and apamin. LPS endotoxin causes systemic inflammatory reactions in sepsis. By reducing oxidative stress, inflammation, and cell death in mice, BV, MEL, and apamin reduced the acute kidney injury brought on by LPS. Consider MEL as an example. It reduced structural and functional damage to the kidneys while attenuating the levels of direct tubular injury indicators in LPS-treated mice. MEL reduced the buildup of immune cells in the kidney and inhibited the NF-B pathway in addition to lowering TNF- and IL-6 levels in the body and the kidney. Following LPS treatment, MEL decreased MDA levels, suppressed the production of nicotinamide adenine dinucleotide phosphate oxidase 4 (NOX4), supported Nrf2-mediated antioxidant defenses, and avoided apoptosis and necrosis [161–163].

6. Current Limits in Use

Despite its potential for therapeutic benefit, potential side effects and allergic responses connected to its composition must always be taken into account. The development of safe practices depends on this factor. The investigations on the usage of bee venom and its harmful effects were summarized by Park et al. (2015) in a comprehensive literature review [164]. The study's analysis of 145 articles revealed that 28.87% of patients receiving bee venom had negative side effects. The same evaluation highlighted the subpar nature of research conducted in this field and the subsequent difficulties in result analysis. Additionally, due to the allergenicity of the ingredients, both allergic and anaphylactic reactions happened. Noble and Armstrong (1999) [165] observed clinical signs such as lethargy, haematuria, ataxia, and convulsions in two dogs that had been poisoned by bee stings. One of the two dogs succumbed to death. Nair et al. (2019) [166] observed acute and delayed onset of haemolytic anaemia, echinocytosis, spherocytosis, thrombocytopenia, haemoglobinaemia, and haemoglobinuria following poisoning. Kaplinsky et al. (1977) [167] observed in dogs and cats that high doses of bee venom (above 1 mg per kg) cause an immediate drop in blood pressure to irreversible shock levels. Several types of changes in the electrocardiogram (ECG) were noted: marked shifts of the ST-T segments, the occurrence of varying degrees of atrioventricular block, and severe ventricular arrhythmias. Therefore, a possible contraindication is not knowing whether the patient is allergic to bee venom or not.

In light of the comprehensiveness of the overview provided, the following are some recommended solutions and holes in the area to be filled. First of all, the purification of bee venom is a crucial step. For various applications, it is vital to produce purified bee venom, which is free of histamine and phospholipase A2, to reduce allergic responses and other negative consequences while keeping significant anti-inflammatory efficacy. Secondarily, some components such as melittin have no specific action. In addition to lysing red blood cells, melittin has shown cytotoxicity against both normal and malignant cells. More specialized analogues for therapeutic use can be created by researching melittin's effects in model systems. The utilization of model systems and live cells can give information to stimulate the invention of novel melittin analogues or hybrid peptides for therapeutic reasons, despite the apparent differences between the actions of melittin in model systems and living cells.

Moreover, it is important to accurately identify and measure the components of bee venom; it is necessary to use processes that allow one to be certain of the substance one is working with. Regarding the latter consideration, standardizing bee venom is necessary to ensure the reproducibility of the outcome. Another aspect to consider is the relatively short plasma half-life of bee venom and the problem of determining the final dose. These critical issues can be overcome with the combination of polymers or nanoparticles [168]. Finally, to increase the effectiveness and safety of the carried substance and lower the likelihood of negative consequences, it is important to understand the precise paths followed by the bee venom or its components follow in the body.

7. Conclusions

Bee venom proves to be a promising remedy and/or adjunct for the treatment of numerous ailments. Its antibacterial, antiviral, and anti-parasitic capacities make it extremely attractive for reducing the use of conventional drugs and associated drug-resistance phenomena. Moreover, its use for one condition can also have positive implications for other concomitant diseases, as shown in this in-depth dissertation on its anti-inflammatory, anti-tumour, etc., properties. Certainly, its use in the clinical setting must follow careful efficacy studies aimed at determining the best doses to achieve the pharmacological response while avoiding the side effects associated with its use. As in human medicine, therefore, the already numerous in vitro studies must be followed by clinical trials to determine a conscious and effective use of bee venom in veterinary clinical practice.

Author Contributions: Conceptualization, R.B. and F.C.; methodology, R.B., F.C., E.P. and D.B.; writing—original draft preparation, R.B., F.C., V.M., C.L., E.P. and D.B.; writing—review and editing, R.B., F.C., V.M., C.L., E.P. and D.B.; supervision E.P. and D.B. All authors have read and agreed to the published version of the manuscript.

Funding: This research received no external funding.

Institutional Review Board Statement: Not applicable.

Informed Consent Statement: Not applicable.

Conflicts of Interest: The authors declare no conflict of interest.

References

1. Bava, R.; Castagna, F.; Piras, C.; Palma, E.; Cringoli, G.; Musolino, V.; Lupia, C.; Perri, M.R.; Statti, G.; Britti, D.; et al. In vitro evaluation of acute toxicity of five *citrus* spp. Essential oils towards the parasitic mite *varroa destructor*. *Pathogens* **2021**, *10*, 1182. [CrossRef] [PubMed]
2. Castagna, F.; Bava, R.; Piras, C.; Carresi, C.; Musolino, V.; Lupia, C.; Marrelli, M.; Conforti, F.; Palma, E.; Britti, D. Green Veterinary Pharmacology for Honey Bee Welfare and Health: *Origanum heracleoticum* L.(Lamiaceae) Essential Oil for the Control of the *Apis mellifera* Varroatosis. *Vet. Sci.* **2022**, *9*, 124. [CrossRef] [PubMed]
3. Morse, R.A.; Calderone, N.W. The Value of Honey Bees As Pollinators of U.S. Crops in 2000. *Bee Cult.* **2000**, *128*, 1–15.
4. Abdela, N.; Jilo, K. Bee venom and its therapeutic values: A review. *Adv. Life Sci. Technol.* **2016**, *44*, 18–22.
5. Weis, W.A.; Ripari, N.; Conte, F.L.; da Silva Honorio, M.; Sartori, A.A.; Matucci, R.H.; Sforcin, J.M. An overview about apitherapy and its clinical applications. *Phytomed. Plus* **2022**, *2*, 100239. [CrossRef]
6. Boukraâ, L. Bee products: The rediscovered antibiotics. *Anti-Infect. Agents* **2015**, *13*, 36–41. [CrossRef]
7. Szweda, P.; Kot, B. Bee products and essential oils as alternative agents for treatment of infections caused by *S. aureus*. *Front. Staphylococcus Aureus* **2017**, 203–223.
8. Hellner, M.; Winter, D.; von Georgi, R.; Münstedt, K. Apitherapy: Usage and experience in German beekeepers. *Evid. Based Complement. Altern. Med.* **2008**, *5*, 475–479. [CrossRef]
9. Münstedt, K. Bee products—An overview of their pharmacological properties and medicinal applications. *Bee Prod. Their Appl. Food Pharm. Ind.* **2022**, 1–23.
10. Gokulakrishnaa, R.; Thirunavukkarasu, S. Apitherapy: A valuable gift from honey bee. *J. Entomol. Zool. Stud.* **2020**, *8*, 2317–2323.
11. Zhang, S.; Liu, Y.; Ye, Y.; Wang, X.-R.; Lin, L.-T.; Xiao, L.-Y.; Zhou, P.; Shi, G.-X.; Liu, C.-Z. Bee venom therapy: Potential mechanisms and therapeutic applications. *Toxicon* **2018**, *148*, 64–73. [CrossRef]
12. Bogdanov, S. Biological and therapeutic properties of bee venom. *Bee Prod. Sci.* **2016**, 1–23.

13. Clark, C.C. *Encyclopedia of Complementary Health Practice P*; Springer: Berlin/Heidelberg, Germany, 1999; ISBN 0826117228.
14. Crane, E. The past and present importance of bee products to man. In *Bee Products*; Springer: Berlin/Heidelberg, Germany, 1997; pp. 1–13.
15. Krell, R. *Value-Added Products from Beekeeping*; Food and Agriculture Organization: Rome, Italy, 1996; ISBN 9251038198.
16. Kwon, Y.; Lee, J.; Lee, H.; Han, H.; Mar, W.; Kang, S.; Beitz, A.J.; Lee, J. Bee venom injection into an acupuncture point reduces arthritis associated edema and nociceptive responses. *Pain* 2001, *90*, 271–280. [CrossRef]
17. Park, M.H.; Choi, M.S.; Kwak, D.H.; Oh, K.; Yoon, D.Y.; Han, S.B.; Song, H.S.; Song, M.J.; Hong, J.T. Anti-cancer effect of bee venom in prostate cancer cells through activation of caspase pathway via inactivation of NF-κB. *Prostate* 2011, *71*, 801–812. [CrossRef]
18. Piek, T. *Venoms of the Hymenoptera: Biochemical, Pharmacological and Behavioural Aspects*; Elsevier: Amsterdam, The Netherlands, 2013; ISBN 1483263703.
19. Schmidt, J.O. Toxinology of venoms from the honeybee genus Apis. *Toxicon* 1995, *33*, 917–927. [CrossRef] [PubMed]
20. Tarpy, D.R.; Gilley, D.C.; Seeley, T.D. Levels of selection in a social insect: A review of conflict and cooperation during honey bee (*Apis mellifera*) queen replacement. *Behav. Ecol. Sociobiol.* 2004, *55*, 513–523. [CrossRef]
21. Elieh Ali Komi, D.; Shafaghat, F.; Zwiener, R.D. Immunology of bee venom. *Clin. Rev. Allergy Immunol.* 2018, *54*, 386–396. [CrossRef] [PubMed]
22. Lee, J.A.; Singletary, E.; Charlton, N. Methods of honey bee stinger removal: A systematic review of the literature. *Cureus* 2020, *12*, e8078. [CrossRef]
23. Lensky, Y.; Cassier, P. The alarm pheromones of queen and worker honey bees. *Bee World* 1995, *76*, 119–129. [CrossRef]
24. Annila, I.T.; Karjalainen, E.S.; Annila, P.A.; Kuusisto, P.A. Bee and wasp sting reactions in current beekeepers. *Ann. Allergy Asthma Immunol.* 1996, *77*, 423–427. [CrossRef] [PubMed]
25. Fitzgerald, K.T.; Flood, A.A. Hymenoptera stings. *Clin. Technol. Small Anim. Pract.* 2006, *21*, 194–204. [CrossRef] [PubMed]
26. Hider, R.C. Honeybee venom: A rich source of pharmacologically active peptides. *Endeavour* 1988, *12*, 60–65. [CrossRef] [PubMed]
27. Dotimas, E.M.; Hider, R.C. Honeybee venom. *Bee world* 1987, *68*, 51–70. [CrossRef]
28. Silva, J.; Monge-Fuentes, V.; Gomes, F.; Lopes, K.; dos Anjos, L.; Campos, G.; Arenas, C.; Biolchi, A.; Gonçalves, J.; Galante, P. Pharmacological alternatives for the treatment of neurodegenerative disorders: Wasp and bee venoms and their components as new neuroactive tools. *Toxins* 2015, *7*, 3179–3209. [CrossRef]
29. Hoffman, D.R. Hymenoptera venom proteins. *Nat. Toxins 2* 1996, 169–186.
30. Guralnick, M.W.; Mulfinger, L.M.; Benton, A.W. Collection and standardization of *Hymenoptera venoms*. *Folia Allergol. Immunol. Clin* 1986, *33*, 9–18.
31. White, J.; Meier, J. *Handbook of Clinical Toxicology of Animal Venoms and Poisons*; CRC Press: Boca Raton, FL, USA, 2017; ISBN 1351443143.
32. Habermann, E.; Jentsch, J. Sequenzanalyse des Melittins aus den tryptischen und peptischen Spaltstücken. *Physiol. Chem.* 1967, *348*, 37–50. [CrossRef]
33. Raghuraman, H.; Chattopadhyay, A. Melittin: A membrane-active peptide with diverse functions. *Biosci. Rep.* 2007, *27*, 189–223. [CrossRef]
34. Terwilliger, T.C.; Eisenberg, D. The structure of melittin. I. Structure determination and partial refinement. *J. Biol. Chem.* 1982, *257*, 6010–6015. [CrossRef]
35. Bernheimer, A.W.; Rudy, B. Interactions between membranes and cytolytic peptides. *Biochim. Biophys. Acta (BBA)-Rev. Biomembr.* 1986, *864*, 123–141. [CrossRef]
36. Dempsey, C.E. The actions of melittin on membranes. *Biochim. Biophys. Acta (BBA)-Rev. Biomembr.* 1990, *1031*, 143–161. [CrossRef]
37. Sansom, M.S. The biophysics of peptide models of ion channels. *Prog. Biophys. Mol. Biol.* 1991, *55*, 139–235. [CrossRef] [PubMed]
38. Neumann, W.; Habermann, E.; Hansen, H. Differentiation of two hemolytic factors in the bee's venom. *Naunyn. Schmiedebergs. Arch. Exp. Pathol. Pharmakol.* 1953, *217*, 130–143. [PubMed]
39. Terwilliger, T.C.; Eisenberg, D. The structure of melittin. II. Interpret. *J. Biol. Chem.* 1982, *257*, 6016–6022. [CrossRef]
40. Shai, Y. Mechanism of the binding, insertion and destabilization of phospholipid bilayer membranes by α-helical antimicrobial and cell non-selective membrane-lytic peptides. *Biochim. Biophys. Acta (BBA)-Biomembr.* 1999, *1462*, 55–70. [CrossRef]
41. Kajita, S.; Iizuka, H. Melittin-induced alteration of epidermal adenylate cyclase responses. *Acta Derm. Venereol.* 1987, *67*, 295–300. [CrossRef]
42. Zhang, S.; Chen, Z. Melittin exerts an antitumor effect on non-small cell lung cancer cells. *Mol. Med. Rep.* 2017, *16*, 3581–3586. [CrossRef]
43. Memariani, H.; Memariani, M.; Moravvej, H.; Shahidi-Dadras, M. Melittin: A venom-derived peptide with promising anti-viral properties. *Eur. J. Clin. Microbiol. Infect. Dis.* 2020, *39*, 5–17. [CrossRef] [PubMed]
44. Nguyen, C.D.; Lee, G. Neuroprotective Activity of Melittin—The Main Component of Bee Venom—Against Oxidative Stress Induced by Aβ25–35 in In Vitro and In Vivo Models. *Antioxidants* 2021, *10*, 1654. [CrossRef]
45. Fennell, J.F.; Shipman, W.H.; Cole, L.J. Antibacterial action of melittin, a polypeptide from bee venom. *Proc. Soc. Exp. Biol. Med.* 1968, *127*, 707–710. [CrossRef]
46. Azam, M.N.K.; Ahmed, M.N.; Biswas, S.; Ara, N.; Rahman, M.M.; Hirashima, A.; Hasan, M.N. A review on bioactivities of honey bee venom. *Annu. Res. Rev. Biol.* 2018, 1–13. [CrossRef]

47. Gu, H.; Han, S.M.; Park, K.-K. Therapeutic effects of apamin as a bee venom component for non-neoplastic disease. *Toxins* **2020**, *12*, 195. [CrossRef] [PubMed]
48. Mourre, C.; Nehlig, A.; Lazdunski, M. Cerebral glucose utilization after administration of apamin, a toxin active on Ca^{2+}-dependent K^+ channels. *Brain Res.* **1988**, *451*, 261–273. [CrossRef] [PubMed]
49. Kim, J.-Y.; Kim, K.-H.; Lee, W.-R.; An, H.-J.; Lee, S.-J.; Han, S.-M.; Lee, K.-G.; Park, Y.-Y.; Kim, K.-S.; Lee, Y.-S. Apamin inhibits PDGF-BB-induced vascular smooth muscle cell proliferation and migration through suppressions of activated Akt and Erk signaling pathway. *Vascul. Pharmacol.* **2015**, *70*, 8–14. [CrossRef]
50. Walde, P.; Jäckle, H.; Luisi, P.L.; Dempsey, C.J.; Banks, B.E.C. Spectroscopic investigations of peptide 401 from bee venom. *Biopolym. Orig. Res. Biomol.* **1981**, *20*, 373–385. [CrossRef]
51. Hanson, J.M.; Morley, J.; Soria-Herrera, C. Anti-inflammatory property of 401 (MCD-peptide), a peptide from the venom of the bee *Apis mellifera* (L.). *Br. J. Pharmacol.* **1974**, *50*, 383. [CrossRef] [PubMed]
52. Wehbe, R.; Frangieh, J.; Rima, M.; El Obeid, D.; Sabatier, J.-M.; Fajloun, Z. Bee venom: Overview of main compounds and bioactivities for therapeutic interests. *Molecules* **2019**, *24*, 2997. [CrossRef]
53. Bellik, Y. Bee venom: Its potential use in alternative medicine. *Anti-Infect. Agents* **2015**, *13*, 3–16. [CrossRef]
54. Cherniack, E.P.; Govorushko, S. To bee or not to bee: The potential efficacy and safety of bee venom acupuncture in humans. *Toxicon* **2018**, *154*, 74–78. [CrossRef]
55. Son, D.J.; Lee, J.W.; Lee, Y.H.; Song, H.S.; Lee, C.K.; Hong, J.T. Therapeutic application of anti-arthritis, pain-releasing, and anti-cancer effects of bee venom and its constituent compounds. *Pharmacol. Ther.* **2007**, *115*, 246–270. [CrossRef]
56. Koburova, K.L.; Michailova, S.G.; Shkenderov, S.V. Further investigation on the antiinflammatory properties of adolapin—Bee venom polypeptide. *Acta Physiol. Pharmacol. Bulg.* **1985**, *11*, 50–55. [PubMed]
57. Shipolini, R.A.; Callewaert, G.L.; Cottrell, R.C.; Vernon, C.A. The amino-acid sequence and carbohydrate content of phospholipase A_2 from bee venom. *Eur. J. Biochem.* **1974**, *48*, 465–476. [CrossRef] [PubMed]
58. Sergeeva, L.I. Heparin-induced inhibition of the hemolytic activity of bee venom. *Uch. Gor'k. Gos. Univ* **1974**, *175*, 130.
59. Dudler, T.; Chen, W.-Q.; Wang, S.; Schneider, T.; Annand, R.R.; Dempcy, R.O.; Crameri, R.; Gmachl, M.; Suter, M.; Gelb, M.H. High-level expression in *Escherichia coli* and rapid purification of enzymatically active honey bee venom phospholipase A_2. *Biochim. Biophys. Acta (BBA)-Lipids Lipid Metab.* **1992**, *1165*, 201–210. [CrossRef]
60. Hossen, M.; Gan, S.H.; Khalil, M. Melittin, a potential natural toxin of crude bee venom: Probable future arsenal in the treatment of diabetes mellitus. *J. Chem.* **2017**, *2017*, 4035626. [CrossRef]
61. Marković-Housley, Z.; Miglierini, G.; Soldatova, L.; Rizkallah, P.J.; Müller, U.; Schirmer, T. Crystal structure of hyaluronidase, a major allergen of bee venom. *Structure* **2000**, *8*, 1025–1035. [CrossRef] [PubMed]
62. Bala, E.; Hazarika, R.; Singh, P.; Yasir, M.; Shrivastava, R. A biological overview of Hyaluronidase: A venom enzyme and its inhibition with plants materials. *Mater. Today Proc.* **2018**, *5*, 6406–6412. [CrossRef]
63. Markovic, O.; Mollnar, L. Isolation of and determination of bee venom. *Chem. Zvesti* **1954**, *8*, 80–90.
64. Benton, A.W.; Morse, R.A.; Stewart, J.D. Venom collection from honey bees. *Science* **1963**, *142*, 228–230. [CrossRef]
65. Fakhim-Zadeh, K. Improved device for venom extraction. *Bee World* **1998**, *79*, 52–56. [CrossRef]
66. Simics, M. Commercial bee venom collection. *Bee Biz* **1998**, *7*, 19–20.
67. Ali, M. Studies on bee venom and its medical uses. *Int. J. Adv. Res. Technol.* **2012**, *1*, 69–83.
68. Krivtzov, N.; Lebedev, V. *Bienenprodukte*; Editing House: Niwa Niwa, Russia, 1995.
69. Müller, U.; Fricker, M.; Wymann, D.; Blaser, K.; Crameri, R. Increased specificity of diagnostic tests with recombinant major bee venom allergen phospholipase A_2. *Clin. Exp. Allergy* **1997**, *27*, 915–920. [CrossRef] [PubMed]
70. Nawaz, A.; Khan, M.A.; Naz, R.; Zeb, S. Extraction of venom from honey bee in district swat, Khyber Pakhtunkhwa, Pakistan. *Extraction* **2019**, *4*.
71. Carpena, M.; Nuñez-Estevez, B.; Soria-Lopez, A.; Simal-Gandara, J. Bee venom: An updating review of its bioactive molecules and its health applications. *Nutrients* **2020**, *12*, 3360. [CrossRef]
72. Müller, U.; Akdis, C.A.; Fricker, M.; Akdis, M.; Blesken, T.; Bettens, F.; Blaser, K. Successful immunotherapy with T-cell epitope peptides of bee venom phospholipase A_2 induces specific T-cell anergy in patients allergic to bee venom. *J. Allergy Clin. Immunol.* **1998**, *101*, 747–754. [CrossRef]
73. Gu, H.; Kim, W.; An, H.; Kim, J.; Gwon, M.; Han, S.M.; Leem, J.; Park, K. Therapeutic effects of bee venom on experimental atopic dermatitis. *Mol. Med. Rep.* **2018**, *18*, 3711–3718. [CrossRef]
74. Skenderov, S.; Und Ivanov, T. Bienenprodukte Zemizdat Verlag, Sofia (Bulg.). 1983.
75. Lima, W.G.; Brito, J.C.M.; da Cruz Nizer, W.S. Bee products as a source of promising therapeutic and chemoprophylaxis strategies against COVID-19 (SARS-CoV-2). *Phyther. Res.* **2021**, *35*, 743–750. [CrossRef]
76. Kasozi, K.I.; Niedbała, G.; Alqarni, M.; Zirintunda, G.; Ssempijja, F.; Musinguzi, S.P.; Usman, I.M.; Matama, K.; Hetta, H.F.; Mbiydzenyuy, N.E. Bee venom—A potential complementary medicine candidate for SARS-CoV-2 infections. *Front. Public Health* **2020**, *8*, 594458. [CrossRef] [PubMed]
77. Lee, J.-D.; Park, H.-J.; Chae, Y.; Lim, S. An overview of bee venom acupuncture in the treatment of arthritis. *Evid. Based Complement. Altern. Med.* **2005**, *2*, 79–84. [CrossRef]
78. Martinello, M.; Mutinelli, F. Antioxidant activity in bee products: A review. *Antioxidants* **2021**, *10*, 71. [CrossRef]

79. Frangieh, J.; Salma, Y.; Haddad, K.; Mattei, C.; Legros, C.; Fajloun, Z.; El Obeid, D. First characterization of the venom from *apis mellifera* syriaca, a honeybee from the middle east region. *Toxins* **2019**, *11*, 191. [CrossRef]
80. Sobral, F.; Sampaio, A.; Falcão, S.; Queiroz, M.J.R.P.; Calhelha, R.C.; Vilas-Boas, M.; Ferreira, I.C.F.R. Chemical characterization, antioxidant, anti-inflammatory and cytotoxic properties of bee venom collected in Northeast Portugal. *Food Chem. Toxicol.* **2016**, *94*, 172–177. [CrossRef]
81. Somwongin, S.; Chantawannakul, P.; Chaiyana, W. Antioxidant activity and irritation property of venoms from Apis species. *Toxicon* **2018**, *145*, 32–39. [CrossRef] [PubMed]
82. Pavel, C.I.; Mărghitaş, L.A.; Dezmirean, D.S.; Tomoş, L.I.; Bonta, V.; Şapcaliu, A.; Buttstedt, A. Comparison between local and commercial royal jelly—Use of antioxidant activity and 10-hydroxy-2-decenoic acid as quality parameter. *J. Apic. Res.* **2014**, *53*, 116–123. [CrossRef]
83. Rekka, E.; Kourounakis, L.; Kourounakis, P. Antioxidant activity of and interleukin production affected by honey bee venom. *Arzneimittelforschung* **1990**, *40*, 912–913. [PubMed]
84. El-Hanoun, A.; El-Komy, A.; El-Sabrout, K.; Abdella, M. Effect of bee venom on reproductive performance and immune response of male rabbits. *Physiol. Behav.* **2020**, *223*, 112987. [CrossRef] [PubMed]
85. Elkomy, A.; El-Hanoun, A.; Abdella, M.; El-Sabrout, K. Improving the reproductive, immunity and health status of rabbit does using honey bee venom. *J. Anim. Physiol. Anim. Nutr.* **2021**, *105*, 975–983. [CrossRef] [PubMed]
86. El-Speiy, M.; Elsawy, M.; Sadaka, T.; Elkomy, A.; Hassan, S. Impact of bee venom and oxytetracycline on blood parameters, antioxidant, immunity status and bacterial count of weaning rabbits. *Egypt. J. Rabbit Sci.* **2022**, *32*, 181–199. [CrossRef]
87. Kim, D.; Han, S.; Choi, Y.-S.; Kang, H.-K.; Lee, H.-G.; Lee, K. Effects of dietary bee venom on serum characteristic, antioxidant activity and liver fatty acid composition in broiler chickens. *Korean J. Poult. Sci.* **2019**, *46*, 39–46. [CrossRef]
88. Llor, C.; Bjerrum, L. Antimicrobial resistance: Risk associated with antibiotic overuse and initiatives to reduce the problem. *Ther. Adv. Drug Saf.* **2014**, *5*, 229–241. [CrossRef] [PubMed]
89. Jasovský, D.; Littmann, J.; Zorzet, A.; Cars, O. Antimicrobial resistance—A threat to the world's sustainable development. *Ups. J. Med. Sci.* **2016**, *121*, 159–164. [CrossRef]
90. Bennani, H.; Mateus, A.; Mays, N.; Eastmure, E.; Stärk, K.D.C.; Häsler, B. Overview of evidence of antimicrobial use and antimicrobial resistance in the food chain. *Antibiotics* **2020**, *9*, 49. [CrossRef] [PubMed]
91. Terwilliger, T.C.; Weissman, L.; Eisenberg, D. The structure of melittin in the form I crystals and its implication for melittin's lytic and surface activities. *Biophys. J.* **1982**, *37*, 353–361. [CrossRef] [PubMed]
92. Han, S.; Yeo, J.; Baek, H.; Lin, S.-M.; Meyer, S.; Molan, P. Postantibiotic effect of purified melittin from honeybee (*Apis mellifera*) venom against *Escherichia coli* and *Staphylococcus aureus*. *J. Asian Nat. Prod. Res.* **2009**, *11*, 796–804. [CrossRef]
93. Socarras, K.M.; Theophilus, P.A.S.; Torres, J.P.; Gupta, K.; Sapi, E. Antimicrobial activity of bee venom and melittin against *Borrelia burgdorferi*. *Antibiotics* **2017**, *6*, 31. [CrossRef]
94. Lubke, L.L.; Garon, C.F. The antimicrobial agent melittin exhibits powerful in vitro inhibitory effects on the Lyme disease spirochete. *Clin. Infect. Dis.* **1997**, *25*, S48–S51. [CrossRef]
95. Choi, J.H.; Jang, A.Y.; Lin, S.; Lim, S.; Kim, D.; Park, K.; Han, S.; Yeo, J.; Seo, H.S. Melittin, a honeybee venom-derived antimicrobial peptide, may target methicillin-resistant *Staphylococcus aureus*. *Mol. Med. Rep.* **2015**, *12*, 6483–6490. [CrossRef]
96. Issam, A.-A.; Zimmermann, S.; Reichling, J.; Wink, M. Pharmacological synergism of bee venom and melittin with antibiotics and plant secondary metabolites against multi-drug resistant microbial pathogens. *Phytomedicine* **2015**, *22*, 245–255.
97. El-Seedi, H.; Abd El-Wahed, A.; Yosri, N.; Musharraf, S.G.; Chen, L.; Moustafa, M.; Zou, X.; Al-Mousawi, S.; Guo, Z.; Khatib, A. Antimicrobial properties of *Apis mellifera*'s bee venom. *Toxins* **2020**, *12*, 451. [CrossRef]
98. Han, S.M.; Lee, K.G.; Yeo, J.H.; Hwang, S.J.; Chenoweth, P.J.; Pak, S.C. Somatic cell count in milk of bee venom treated dairy cows with mastitis. *J. ApiProduct ApiMed Sci.* **2009**, *1*, 104–109. [CrossRef]
99. Kim, S.-H.; Jun, H.-K.; Kim, S.; You, M.-J.; Jun, M.-H.; Kim, D.-H. Therapeutic effect of injection-acupuncture with bee-venom (apitoxin) in cases of canine otitis externa. *J. Vet. Clin.* **2008**, *25*, 159–164.
100. Perumal Samy, R.; Gopalakrishnakone, P.; Thwin, M.M.; Chow, T.K.V.; Bow, H.; Yap, E.H.; Thong, T.W.J. Antibacterial activity of snake, scorpion and bee venoms: A comparison with purified venom phospholipase A_2 enzymes. *J. Appl. Microbiol.* **2007**, *102*, 650–659. [CrossRef] [PubMed]
101. Boutrin, M.-C.; Foster, H.A.; Pentreath, V.W. The effects of bee (*Apis mellifera*) venom phospholipase A_2 on *Trypanosoma brucei brucei* and enterobacteria. *Exp. Parasitol.* **2008**, *119*, 246–251. [CrossRef] [PubMed]
102. Guillaume, C.; Calzada, C.; Lagarde, M.; Schreével, J.; Deregnaucourt, C. Interplay between lipoproteins and bee venom phospholipase A_2 in relation to their anti-plasmodium toxicity. *J. Lipid Res.* **2006**, *47*, 1493–1506. [CrossRef] [PubMed]
103. Lee, S.-B. Antifungal activity of bee venom and sweet bee venom against clinically isolated *Candida albicans*. *J. Pharmacopunct.* **2016**, *19*, 45. [CrossRef]
104. Hegazi, A.G.; El-Fadaly, H.A.; Barakat, A.M.; Abou-El-Doubal, S.K.A. In vitro effects of some bee products on T. gondii Tachyzoites. *Glob. Vet.* **2014**, *13*, 1043–1050.
105. Uddin, M.B.; Lee, B.-H.; Nikapitiya, C.; Kim, J.-H.; Kim, T.-H.; Lee, H.-C.; Kim, C.G.; Lee, J.-S.; Kim, C.-J. Inhibitory effects of bee venom and its components against viruses in vitro and in vivo. *J. Microbiol.* **2016**, *54*, 853–866. [CrossRef]
106. Kim, Y.-W.; Chaturvedi, P.K.; Chun, S.N.; Lee, Y.G.; Ahn, W.S. Honeybee venom possesses anticancer and antiviral effects by differential inhibition of HPV E6 and E7 expression on cervical cancer cell line. *Oncology Reports* **2015**, *33.4*, 1675–1682. [CrossRef]

107. Lee, J.; Kim, Y.-M.; Kim, J.-H.; Cho, C.-W.; Jeon, J.-W.; Park, J.-K.; Lee, S.-H.; Jung, B.-G.; Lee, B.-J. Nasal delivery of chitosan/alginate nanoparticle encapsulated bee (*Apis mellifera*) venom promotes antibody production and viral clearance during porcine reproductive and respiratory syndrome virus infection by modulating T cell related responses. *Vet. Immunol. Immunopathol.* **2018**, *200*, 40–51. [CrossRef]
108. Scicutella, F.; Mannelli, F.; Daghio, M.; Viti, C.; Buccioni, A. Polyphenols and Organic Acids as Alternatives to Antimicrobials in Poultry Rearing: A Review. *Antibiotics* **2021**, *10*, 1010. [CrossRef]
109. Kim, D.-H.; Han, S.-M.; Keum, M.C.; Lee, S.; An, B.-K.; Lee, S.-R.; Lee, K.-W. Evaluation of bee venom as a novel feed additive in fast-growing broilers. *Br. Poult. Sci.* **2018**, *59*, 435–442. [CrossRef] [PubMed]
110. Han, S.M.; Lee, K.G.; Yeo, J.H.; Oh, B.Y.; Kim, B.S.; Lee, W.; Baek, H.J.; Kim, S.T.; Hwang, S.J.; Pak, S.C. Effects of honeybee venom supplementation in drinking water on growth performance of broiler chickens. *Poult. Sci.* **2010**, *89*, 2396–2400. [CrossRef] [PubMed]
111. Han, S.M.; Lee, K.G.; Yeo, J.H.; Hwang, S.J.; Jang, C.H.; Chenoweth, P.J.; Pak, S.C. Effects of bee venom treatment on growth performance of young pigs. *Am. J. Chin. Med.* **2009**, *37*, 253–260. [CrossRef] [PubMed]
112. Kim, J.-I.; Yang, E.J.; Lee, M.S.; Kim, Y.-S.; Huh, Y.; Cho, I.-H.; Kang, S.; Koh, H.-K. Bee venom reduces neuroinflammation in the MPTP-induced model of Parkinson's disease. *Int. J. Neurosci.* **2011**, *121*, 209–217. [CrossRef]
113. Yang, E.J.; Jiang, J.H.; Lee, S.M.; Yang, S.C.; Hwang, H.S.; Lee, M.S.; Choi, S.-M. Bee venom attenuates neuroinflammatory events and extends survival in amyotrophic lateral sclerosis models. *J. Neuroinflamm.* **2010**, *7*, 69. [CrossRef]
114. Cai, M.; Lee, J.H.; Yang, E.J. Bee venom ameliorates cognitive dysfunction caused by neuroinflammation in an animal model of vascular dementia. *Mol. Neurobiol.* **2017**, *54*, 5952–5960. [CrossRef]
115. Chung, E.S.; Lee, G.; Lee, C.; Ye, M.; Chung, H.; Kim, H.; Bae, S.S.; Hwang, D.-S.; Bae, H. Bee venom phospholipase A_2, a novel Foxp3+ regulatory T cell inducer, protects dopaminergic neurons by modulating neuroinflammatory responses in a mouse model of Parkinson's disease. *J. Immunol.* **2015**, *195*, 4853–4860. [CrossRef]
116. Park, H.J.; Son, D.J.; Lee, C.W.; Choi, M.S.; Lee, U.S.; Song, H.S.; Lee, J.M.; Hong, J.T. Melittin inhibits inflammatory target gene expression and mediator generation via interaction with IκB kinase. *Biochem. Pharmacol.* **2007**, *73*, 237–247. [CrossRef]
117. Lee, G.; Bae, H. Anti-inflammatory applications of melittin, a major component of bee venom: Detailed mechanism of action and adverse effects. *Molecules* **2016**, *21*, 616. [CrossRef]
118. Kim, E.-J.; Kim, G.-Y. Regulation of inflammatory cytokine production by bee venom in rat chondrocytes. *J. Physiol. Pathol. Korean Med.* **2011**, *25*, 132–137. [CrossRef]
119. Moon, D.-O.; Park, S.-Y.; Lee, K.-J.; Heo, M.-S.; Kim, K.-C.; Kim, M.-O.; Lee, J.-D.; Choi, Y.H.; Kim, G.-Y. Bee venom and melittin reduce proinflammatory mediators in lipopolysaccharide-stimulated BV2 microglia. *Int. Immunopharmacol.* **2007**, *7*, 1092–1101. [CrossRef]
120. Cuenda, A.; Rousseau, S. p38 MAP-kinases pathway regulation, function and role in human diseases. *Biochim. Biophys. Acta (BBA)-Mol. Cell Res.* **2007**, *1773*, 1358–1375. [CrossRef] [PubMed]
121. Schindler, J.F.; Monahan, J.B.; Smith, W.G. p38 pathway kinases as anti-inflammatory drug targets. *J. Dent. Res.* **2007**, *86*, 800–811. [CrossRef] [PubMed]
122. Gupta, J.; Nebreda, A.R. Roles of p38α mitogen-activated protein kinase in mouse models of inflammatory diseases and cancer. *FEBS J.* **2015**, *282*, 1841–1857. [CrossRef] [PubMed]
123. Kim, J.-Y.; Lee, W.-R.; Kim, K.-H.; An, H.-J.; Chang, Y.-C.; Han, S.-M.; Park, Y.-Y.; Pak, S.C.; Park, K.-K. Effects of bee venom against *Propionibacterium acnes*-induced inflammation in human keratinocytes and monocytes. *Int. J. Mol. Med.* **2015**, *35*, 1651–1656. [CrossRef]
124. Lee, W.-R.; Kim, K.-H.; An, H.-J.; Kim, J.; Chang, Y.-C.; Chung, H.; Park, Y.-Y.; Lee, M.-L.; Park, K. The protective effects of Melittin on *Propionibacterium acnes*–induced inflammatory responses in vitro and in vivo. *J. Investig. Dermatol.* **2014**, *134*, 1922–1930. [CrossRef]
125. Jeong, Y.-J.; Shin, J.-M.; Bae, Y.-S.; Cho, H.-J.; Park, K.-K.; Choe, J.-Y.; Han, S.-M.; Moon, S.-K.; Kim, W.-J.; Choi, Y.H. Melittin has a chondroprotective effect by inhibiting MMP-1 and MMP-8 expressions via blocking NF-κB and AP-1 signaling pathway in chondrocytes. *Int. Immunopharmacol.* **2015**, *25*, 400–405. [CrossRef] [PubMed]
126. Lee, Y.J.; Oh, M.J.; Lee, D.H.; Lee, Y.S.; Lee, J.; Kim, D.-H.; Choi, C.-H.; Song, M.J.; Song, H.S.; Hong, J.T. Anti-inflammatory effect of bee venom in phthalic anhydride-induced atopic dermatitis animal model. *Inflammopharmacology* **2020**, *28*, 253–263. [CrossRef]
127. Ozturk, A.B.; Bayraktar, R.; Gogebakan, B.; Mumbuc, S.; Bayram, H. Comparison of inflammatory cytokine release from nasal epithelial cells of non-atopic non-rhinitic, allergic rhinitic and polyp subjects and effects of diesel exhaust particles in vitro. *Allergol. Immunopathol.* **2017**, *45*, 473–481. [CrossRef]
128. Lorenzetti, O.J. Influence of bee venom in the adjuvant-induced arthritic rat model. *Res. Commun. Chem. Pathol. Pharmacol.* **1972**, *4*, 339–352.
129. Zurier, R.B.; Mitnick, H.; Bloomgarden, D.; Weissmann, G. Effect of bee venom on experimental arthritis. *Ann. Rheum. Dis.* **1973**, *32*, 466. [CrossRef] [PubMed]
130. Chang, Y.-H.; Bliven, M.L. Anti-arthritic effect of bee venom. *Agents Actions* **1979**, *9*, 205–211. [CrossRef]
131. Eiseman, J.L.; Von Bredow, J.; Alvares, A.P. Effect of honeybee (*Apis mellifera*) venom on the course of adjuvant-induced arthritis and depression of drug metabolism in the rat. *Biochem. Pharmacol.* **1982**, *31*, 1139–1146. [CrossRef]

132. Vick, J.A.; Mehlman, B.; Brooks, R.; Phillips, S.J.; Shipman, W. Effect of bee venom and melittin on plasma cortisol in the unanesthetized monkey. *Toxicon* **1972**, *10*, 581–586. [CrossRef] [PubMed]
133. Vick, J.A.; Warren, G.B.; Brooks, R.B. The effect of treatment with whole bee venom on cage activity and plasma cortisol levels in the arthritic dog. *Inflammation* **1976**, *1*, 167–174. [CrossRef] [PubMed]
134. Short, T.; Jackson, R.; Beard, G. Usefulness of bee venom therapy in canine arthritis. *NAAS Proc.* **1979**, *2*, 13–17.
135. Jeong, C.H.; Cheng, W.N.; Bae, H.; Lee, K.W.; Han, S.M.; Petriello, M.C.; Lee, H.G.; Seo, H.G.; Han, S.G. Bee venom decreases LPS-induced inflammatory responses in bovine mammary epithelial cells. *J. Microbiol. Biotechnol.* **2017**, *27*, 1827–1836. [CrossRef]
136. Von Bredow, J.; Bradford, C.; Froehlich, H.; Vick, J. Treatment of Equine Arthritis with Bee Venom. *Proc. Apiotherapy Conf.* **1978**, 76–79.
137. Kim, D.-H.; Liu, J.-Z.; Choi, S.-H.; MacManus, P.; Jennings, P.; Darcy, K.; Burke, F.; Leorald, N.; Rogers, P.A.M. Acupuncture treatment in a case with equine laminitis. *J. Vet. Clin.* **2006**, *23*, 6–8.
138. Mizrahi, A.; Fulder, S.; Sheinman, N.; Sheinman, N. *Potentiating Health and the Crisis of the Immune System*; Springer Science & Business Media: Berlin/Heidelberg, Germany, 1997; ISBN 0306456028.
139. Mohammadi-Rad, M.; Ghasemi, N.; Aliomrani, M. Evaluation of apamin effects on myelination process in C57BL/6 mice model of multiple sclerosis. *Res. Pharm. Sci.* **2019**, *14*, 424.
140. Tsai, L.-C.; Lin, Y.-W.; Hsieh, C.-L. Effects of bee venom injections at acupoints on neurologic dysfunction induced by thoracolumbar intervertebral disc disorders in canines: A Randomized, Controlled Prospective Study. *Biomed Res. Int.* **2015**, *2015*, 363801. [CrossRef] [PubMed]
141. Jun, H.; Oh, H.; Han, J.; Lee, H.; Jeong, S.-M.; Choi, S.-H.; Kim, C.M.-H.; Kim, D.-H. Therapeutic effect of bee-venom and dexamethasone in dogs with facial nerve paralysis. *J. Vet. Clin.* **2007**, *24*, 503–508.
142. Sung, H.-J.; Park, H.-M. Therapeutic Trial of Bee Venom Acupuncture for Idiopathic Facial Paralysis in a Dog. *J. Vet. Clin.* **2013**, *30*, 107–110.
143. Li, D.; Chung, G.; Kim, S.K. The involvement of central noradrenergic pathway in the analgesic effect of bee venom acupuncture on vincristine-induced peripheral neuropathy in rats. *Toxins* **2020**, *12*, 775. [CrossRef]
144. Gajski, G.; Garaj-Vrhovac, V. Melittin: A lytic peptide with anticancer properties. *Environ. Toxicol. Pharmacol.* **2013**, *36*, 697–705. [CrossRef] [PubMed]
145. Rady, I.; Siddiqui, I.A.; Rady, M.; Mukhtar, H. Melittin, a major peptide component of bee venom, and its conjugates in cancer therapy. *Cancer Lett.* **2017**, *402*, 16–31. [CrossRef] [PubMed]
146. Kim, Y.-M.; Lee, J.-D.; Park, D.-S. The Anti-Cancer Effect of Apamin in Bee-Venom on Melanoma cell line SK-MEL-2 and Inhibitory Effect on the MAP-Kinase Signal Pathway. *J. Acupunct. Res.* **2001**, *18*, 101–115.
147. Hait, W.N.; Grais, L.; Benz, C.; Cadman, E.C. Inhibition of growth of leukemic cells by inhibitors of calmodulin: Phenothiazines and melittin. *Cancer Chemother. Pharmacol.* **1985**, *14*, 202–205. [CrossRef]
148. Oršolić, N. Bee venom in cancer therapy. *Cancer Metastasis Rev.* **2012**, *31*, 173–194. [CrossRef]
149. Ip, S.; Chu, Y.; Yu, C.; Chen, P.; Ho, H.; Yang, J.; Huang, H.; Chueh, F.; Lai, T.; Chung, J. Bee venom induces apoptosis through intracellular Ca^{2+}-modulated intrinsic death pathway in human bladder cancer cells. *Int. J. Urol.* **2012**, *19*, 61–70. [CrossRef] [PubMed]
150. Lin, T.-Y.; Hsieh, C.-L. Clinical applications of bee venom acupoint injection. *Toxins* **2020**, *12*, 618. [CrossRef] [PubMed]
151. Cho, H.-J.; Jeong, Y.-J.; Park, K.-K.; Park, Y.-Y.; Chung, I.-K.; Lee, K.-G.; Yeo, J.-H.; Han, S.-M.; Bae, Y.-S.; Chang, Y.-C. Bee venom suppresses PMA-mediated MMP-9 gene activation via JNK/p38 and NF-κB-dependent mechanisms. *J. Ethnopharmacol.* **2010**, *127*, 662–668. [CrossRef] [PubMed]
152. Huh, J.-E.; Baek, Y.-H.; Lee, M.-H.; Choi, D.-Y.; Park, D.-S.; Lee, J.-D. Bee venom inhibits tumor angiogenesis and metastasis by inhibiting tyrosine phosphorylation of VEGFR-2 in LLC-tumor-bearing mice. *Cancer Lett.* **2010**, *292*, 98–110. [CrossRef]
153. Pahl, H.L. Activators and target genes of Rel/NF-κB transcription factors. *Oncogene* **1999**, *18*, 6853–6866. [CrossRef]
154. Jo, M.; Park, M.H.; Kollipara, P.S.; An, B.J.; Song, H.S.; Han, S.B.; Kim, J.H.; Song, M.J.; Hong, J.T. Anti-cancer effect of bee venom toxin and melittin in ovarian cancer cells through induction of death receptors and inhibition of JAK2/STAT3 pathway. *Toxicol. Appl. Pharmacol.* **2012**, *258*, 72–81. [CrossRef]
155. Lee, C.; Bae, S.-J.S.; Joo, H.; Bae, H. Melittin suppresses tumor progression by regulating tumor-associated macrophages in a Lewis lung carcinoma mouse model. *Oncotarget* **2017**, *8*, 54951. [CrossRef]
156. Liu, J.; Xiao, S.; Li, J.; Yuan, B.; Yang, K.; Ma, Y. Molecular details on the intermediate states of melittin action on a cell membrane. *Biochim. Biophys. Acta (BBA)-Biomembr.* **2018**, *1860*, 2234–2241. [CrossRef]
157. Soliman, C.; Eastwood, S.; Truong, V.K.; Ramsland, P.A.; Elbourne, A. The membrane effects of melittin on gastric and colorectal cancer. *PLoS ONE* **2019**, *14*, e0224028. [CrossRef]
158. Daniluk, K.; Kutwin, M.; Grodzik, M.; Wierzbicki, M.; Strojny, B.; Szczepaniak, J.; Bałaban, J.; Sosnowska, M.; Chwalibog, A.; Sawosz, E. Use of selected carbon nanoparticles as melittin carriers for MCF-7 and MDA-MB-231 human breast cancer cells. *Materials* **2019**, *13*, 90. [CrossRef]
159. Mohamed, W.A.; Abd-Elhakim, Y.M.; Ismail, S.A.A. Involvement of the anti-inflammatory, anti-apoptotic, and anti-secretory activity of bee venom in its therapeutic effects on acetylsalicylic acid-induced gastric ulceration in rats. *Toxicology* **2019**, *419*, 11–23. [CrossRef] [PubMed]

160. Balamurugan, R.; Kim, J.H.; Jo, M.; Xue, C.; kyu Park, J.; Lee, J.K. Bee wax coated water-soluble fraction of bee venom improved altered glucose homeostasis in streptozotocin-induced diabetic rats. *J. Tradit. Chin. Med.* **2019**, *39*, 842.
161. Kim, J.-Y.; Leem, J.; Hong, H.-L. Melittin ameliorates endotoxin-induced acute kidney injury by inhibiting inflammation, oxidative stress, and cell death in mice. *Oxid. Med. Cell. Longev.* **2021**, *2021*, 8843051. [CrossRef]
162. Kim, J.-Y.; Lee, S.-J.; Maeng, Y.-I.; Leem, J.; Park, K.-K. Protective effects of bee venom against endotoxemia-related acute kidney injury in mice. *Biology* **2020**, *9*, 154. [CrossRef] [PubMed]
163. Kim, J.-Y.; Leem, J.; Park, K.-K. Antioxidative, antiapoptotic, and anti-inflammatory effects of apamin in a murine model of lipopolysaccharide-induced acute kidney injury. *Molecules* **2020**, *25*, 5717. [CrossRef] [PubMed]
164. Park, J.H.; Yim, B.K.; Lee, J.-H.; Lee, S.; Kim, T.-H. Risk associated with bee venom therapy: A systematic review and meta-analysis. *PLoS ONE* **2015**, *10*, e0126971. [CrossRef] [PubMed]
165. Noble, S.J.; Armstrong, P.J. Bee sting envenomation resulting in secondary immune-mediated hemolytic anemia in two dogs. *J. Am. Vet. Med. Assoc.* **1999**, *214*, 1026–1027.
166. Nair, R.; Riddle, E.A.; Thrall, M.A. Hemolytic anemia, spherocytosis, and thrombocytopenia associated with honey bee envenomation in a dog. *Vet. Clin. Pathol.* **2019**, *48*, 620–623. [CrossRef]
167. Kaplinsky, E.; Ishay, J.; Ben-Shachar, D.; Gitter, S. Effects of bee (*Apis mellifera*) venom on the electrocardiogram and blood pressure. *Toxicon* **1977**, *15*, 251–256. [CrossRef]
168. Khalil, A.; Elesawy, B.H.; Ali, T.M.; Ahmed, O.M. Bee Venom: From Venom to Drug. *Molecules* **2021**, *26*, 4941. [CrossRef]

Disclaimer/Publisher's Note: The statements, opinions and data contained in all publications are solely those of the individual author(s) and contributor(s) and not of MDPI and/or the editor(s). MDPI and/or the editor(s) disclaim responsibility for any injury to people or property resulting from any ideas, methods, instructions or products referred to in the content.

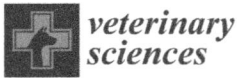

Article

Perceptions of Veterinarians and Veterinary Students on What Risk Factors Constitute Medical Disputes and Comparisons between 2014 and 2022

Zih-Fang Chen [1], Yi-Hsin Elsa Hsu [2,3,*], Jih-Jong Lee [4] and Chung-Hsi Chou [1,*]

[1] Zoonoses Research Center, School of Veterinary Medicine, National Taiwan University, Taipei 10617, Taiwan
[2] Executive Master Program of Business Administration in Biotechnology, Taipei Medical University, Taipei 11031, Taiwan
[3] School of Healthcare Administration, Taipei Medical University, Taipei 11031, Taiwan
[4] Institute of Veterinary Clinical Science, School of Veterinary Medicine, National Taiwan University, Taipei 10617, Taiwan
* Correspondence: elsahsu@tmu.edu.tw (Y.-H.E.H.); cchou@ntu.edu.tw (C.-H.C.)

Simple Summary: This study investigated the risk factors for medical disputes in the veterinary profession in Taiwan. The research aimed to compare the perceptions of veterinarians and veterinary students and to examine any differences between two surveys conducted in 2014 and 2022. Online validity-tested questionnaires were used to collect data, with 106 (73 veterinarians and 33 students) and 157 (126 veterinarians and 31 students) surveys collected in 2014 and 2022, respectively. The study found that the main causes of medical disputes were poor communication and complaints management, rather than the quality of veterinary care provided. The study also revealed a difference in perceptions between experienced veterinarians and veterinary students, with the latter considering medical skills and clients' perspectives to be the primary risk factors. However, both groups identified attitudes during interactions and complaint management as key issues. The authors suggest that veterinary education should provide students with more practical experience in medical disputes and complaint management to help bridge the gap in perception between experienced veterinarians and veterinary students. Results from this study have important implications for improving the quality of veterinary care, reducing the risk of medical disputes, and promoting the continuing education of veterinary professionals.

Abstract: This study compared the risk perceptions of medical disputes among veterinarians and veterinary students in Taiwan between 2014 and 2022. Online validity-tested questionnaires were used to collect data, with 106 (73 veterinarians and 33 students) and 157 (126 veterinarians and 31 students) surveys collected in 2014 and 2022, respectively. Respondents would be asked to rate their perceptions on how likely each risk factor constitutes a medical dispute according to their past experiences on a five-point Likert scale from 1 to 5: "Very unlikely, unlikely, neutral, likely, very likely." The results showed that overall risk perceptions increased significantly in 2022 compared to 2014, with the top risk factors being attitudes during interactions and complaint management among experienced veterinarians. In contrast, students considered medical skills and clients' perspectives as the top two risk factors, with complaints management ranking as the least significant factor. The findings suggest that effective communication and complaint management are crucial in preventing medical disputes, highlighting the importance of developing these skills in young veterinarians and veterinary students to reduce medical disputes. The study also recommends increasing practical experiences of medical disputes and complaint management in veterinary education to bridge the gap between the perceptions of experienced veterinarians and students.

Keywords: Taiwan; questionnaire; veterinarians; veterinary students; cross-section study; medical disputes; factors; complaints; communication education; risk perceptions; Likert scale

Citation: Chen, Z.-F.; Hsu, Y.-H.E.; Lee, J.-J.; Chou, C.-H. Perceptions of Veterinarians and Veterinary Students on What Risk Factors Constitute Medical Disputes and Comparisons between 2014 and 2022. *Vet. Sci.* **2023**, *10*, 200. https://doi.org/10.3390/vetsci10030200

Academic Editors: Simona Sacchini and Ayoze Castro-Alonso

Received: 7 January 2023
Revised: 16 February 2023
Accepted: 26 February 2023
Published: 6 March 2023

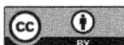

Copyright: © 2023 by the authors. Licensee MDPI, Basel, Switzerland. This article is an open access article distributed under the terms and conditions of the Creative Commons Attribution (CC BY) license (https://creativecommons.org/licenses/by/4.0/).

1. Introduction

The number of medical disputes among veterinarians has increased dramatically over the past several decades. As a result, the clients have become increasingly litigious, especially those with companion animals. Compared to economic animals, companion animals are "their families", [1] not "pets or functional animals" [2] to clients, so the small animal medical disputes pressures are as enormous as human medicine. These medical disputes might cause veterinarians many negative impacts, including mental stress and physical problems [3–7].

Medical disputes include malpractices, such as medical errors, and inadequate communication, such as insufficiently informed and emotional conflicts. Previous research revealed evidence that 80% of claims contained an element of communication breakdown [8] caused by client dissatisfaction [9,10], indicating that communication issues might cause client complaints. The quality of care is not the primary determinant in a client's decision to initiate a malpractice claim. Instead, most complaints and medical disputes are related to poor communication [8,9,11,12]. Past research outcomes also revealed that emotional conflicts might be caused by disappointing experiences [13,14], dissatisfaction [10–12,15], lack of communication [8], and feeling uncared for [4,8,16,17]. These medical disputes may have severe effects on veterinarians. Veterinarians who experienced medical disputes will be more concerned about client complaints and fear litigation, which might cause veterinarians to have intense relationships with future clients, heavier work stress, and even career burnout.

In the past, it was generally believed that communication skills were common sense, but it gradually transformed into one of the core competencies of veterinary professionals [18–21]. Therefore, the world organization for animal health (WOAH, founded as OIE) announced the core veterinary education curriculum in May 2012, which included "clinical communication courses" to improve communication effectiveness, reduce work pressure and prevent clients' complaints [16,17,22–26].

Students' successful transition into clinical practice depends on communication competence by improving client satisfaction and reducing the risk of medical disputes [27]. However, recent veterinary graduates may need more communication skills or abilities from veterinary education or training to manage the inevitable distress in daily work [18]. For example, they try to deliver bad news, talk about euthanasia or terminal disease, show empathetic attitudes, deal with complaints, and even medical expense arguments [28]. Nevertheless, they might learn with "real clients" with colossal stress and gradually become aware of the medical dispute risk and causes [29]. In contrast to the curriculum at school, they have to develop the perceptions of medical disputes via clinical practice and learn the experiences of senior veterinarians as a hidden curriculum [19,30]. Thus, it is essential to understand the differences in perceptions among veterinarians and students to improve communication education and decrease the stress from learning in reality.

Furthermore, this study investigates the perceptions of risk factors that constitute medical disputes and the differences between veterinarians and veterinarians-to-be, the veterinary students. Also, the differences in time are investigated with a comparison of perceptions surveyed in different years. This study primarily focuses on the medical dispute risk factors of companion animals.

2. Materials and Methods

2.1. Study Design and Questionnaire

The cross-sectional web-based surveys were used to separately investigate the perceptions of risk factors constituting medical disputes among veterinarians and veterinary students in Taiwan in 2014 and 2022. The 2014 survey was financially supported by a project granted by the National Science and Technology Council in Taiwan (NSC 102-2633-S-038-001), and the 2022 survey was completed without government-supporting funds. The questionnaire (which may be found in Supplementary Material) adopted in this study was developed by Hsu (2014) [31]. The questionnaire was developed by literature review and research team discussion and then revised and finalized by focus groups of experts, professors, and veterinarians. The final version questionnaire was valid and reliability tested. The questionnaire included two parts: the first part was the demographic characteristics, including the age, gender, veterinarian or veterinary student, the experience of medical disputes, and the outcomes of medical disputes. The second part was the measures of the perceptions on risk factors constituting medical disputes, including twenty-three risk factors questions belonging to six dimensions: (1) medical skills, (2) modes of communication, (3) the attitude of stakeholders during interactions, (4) medical expenses, (5) complaints management, and 6) clients' perceptions (see Table 1).

Table 1. Six dimensions of the questionnaire for measures of perceptions towards medical disputes.

	Dimensions	Content
1.	Medical skills	Misdiagnosis leading to worsening of patient condition. Inappropriate/improper hospital care or treatment procedures.
2.	Modes of communication	Explanations from the veterinarians to the clients are too simple. Use of too many medical terms during explanation with no clear supplementary explanation. The clients have doubts about the treatment but fail to enquire or get an unsatisfactory answer from the veterinarians before the treatment. A gap between clients' expected and actual treatment outcomes due to a lack of information for decision-making before the treatment. No precise decision being made by the clients' families during the discussion of subsequent treatment procedures with the veterinarian. The veterinarians do not provide supplementary paper documents to the clients to raise their knowledge level about the treatment.
3.	The attitude of stakeholders during interactions	The veterinarians try to make the clients reluctantly accept the recommended diagnosis and treatments. The veterinarians do not respond appropriately or take appropriate steps to solve the clients' concerns. The veterinarians do not give feelings of support and encouragement during interactions, resulting in the clients' thinking that the veterinarian may not be concerned about the health of sick animals. When the clients' and veterinarians' views on the animals' condition differ, the client tends to stick with their subjective perception.
4.	Medical expenses	The veterinarians do not explain to the clients in advance the possible total medical expenses. The veterinarians do not clearly explain the possible medical costs for each treatment procedure. The disparity between clients' expected and actual medical costs.
5.	Complaints management	The veterinarians did nothing to respond to the complaints in time. Absence of senior staff to attend to the complaints. The complaint resolution process was done with inappropriate attitudes and improper ways. Staff members do not have relevant professional training to handle the complaints.
6.	Clients' perceptions	The clients depend on self-gathered information. The clients have many questions about treatment and lack trust in the interaction. The clients' misconception of pets being taken care of by the veterinarian. The clients may have the motives of extortion.

Respondents would be asked to answer their perceptions on how likely each risk factor constitutes medical disputes according to their past experiences on a five-point Likert scale from 1 to 5: "Very unlikely, unlikely, neutral, likely, very likely". The Likert scale is commonly used to measure the phenomenon in medical science [32]. Past studies have different analyzing approaches to the Likert scale [33–35]. The measurement of Likert scales could be analyzed as ordinal or interval data [33–35]; some researchers suggested the central tendency could be measured better by using the mean than the median [35–38] while some suggest vice versa [33,34]. The study was approved by the Research Ethics Committee of National Taiwan University (NTU-REC No.: 202209HS024).

2.2. Respondents

This study has surveyed two stakeholders: veterinarians and veterinary students. The questionnaire is an anonymous, self-administered online google form survey. The questionnaire was distributed through the following channels: universities, associations, and social media, such as Facebook and LINE, distributed to the survey participants. The veterinarians who participated were invited by email or social networks, such as clubs of veterinary medical associations and animal hospitals. The participants, veterinary students from five veterinary medicine departments in Taiwan, were invited by email. All participants were asked to answer the online Google questionnaire. The informed consent was shown before replying to the questionnaire, including the survey details, such as the time to complete and confidentiality. They would answer the questionnaire when they accepted the informed consent. The response rate was not reported due to the questionnaire being an anonymous online google form.

2.3. Analysis

Demographic characteristics such as age, gender, experiences of medical disputes, and the outcomes of medical disputes in 2014 and 2022 were summarized as numbers, means, and percentages using descriptive statistics. Participants' perceptions of risk factors in six dimensions were assessed using a five-point Likert scale, and results were analyzed using descriptive statistics (mean and standard deviation) and inferential statistics. The *t*-test was used to compare risk factor perceptions among stakeholders, genders, and experiences of medical disputes in 2014 and 2022. Furthermore, *t*-tests were conducted to compare risk factor perception differences between the two periods for each subgroup (e.g., veterinarians, students, genders, and experiences) separately. All statistical analyses were conducted using SPSS statistical software with a significance level of $p < 0.05$.

3. Results

A total of 263 participants completed the survey, with 108 respondents in 2014 and 158 in 2022. However, three participants were excluded from the analysis due to various reasons, such as being less than 20 years old, completing the study in an unrealistic short time (within 1 min), or having too many missing responses. Therefore, the analysis was conducted on 106 respondents in 2014 and 157 in 2022.

3.1. Demographic Characteristics

A total of 263 cases responded to the questionnaire, with 106 in 2014 and 157 in 2022. In 2022, there were 126 veterinarians and 31 senior veterinary students, while in 2014, there were 106 veterinarians and 33 senior veterinary students, as shown in Table 2. In 2014, the 20–29 age group and 30–39 age group accounted for 84% of all respondents. In contrast, there were 35 respondents (22%) in the 40–49 age group in 2022, which was five times the percentage in 2014. In 2022, 121 respondents (77%) reported experiencing medical disputes, twice the number in 2014. Simple communication and monetary compensation resolved 75% of medical disputes in 2022, which is about twice the percentage in 2014 (16% and 18%). However, the number of cases resolved by third-party mediation decreased dramatically to one, while the number of cases filed in court increased from one in 2014 to eight in 2022 (5%), a five-fold increase from 2014.

3.2. Ranking of the Perceptions of Risk Factors in Six Dimensions

Participants' perceptions of risk factors in six dimensions were evaluated using a five-point Likert scale, and the results were analyzed using mean and standard deviation. The higher scores indicated that the risk factor was more likely to lead to medical disputes. The six dimensions of risk factors were ranked by the mean score from highest to lowest (see Table 3). When comparing the top risk factors identified by veterinarians in different years, a noteworthy observation emerged. In 2014, respondents identified medical expenses, clients' perspectives, and attitudes during interactions as the top three risk factors most likely to lead to medical disputes.

Table 2. Demographic characteristics distribution of participants in 2014 and 2022.

Characteristics	2014 (n = 106)		2022 (n = 157)	
	n	%	n	%
Stakeholder's position				
Veterinarian	73	68.90%	126	80.30%
Veterinary student	33	31.10%	31	19.70%
Age				
20–29 years old	53	50.00%	58	36.90%
30–39 years old	36	34.00%	56	35.70%
40–49 years old	5	4.70%	35	22.30%
50+ years old	12	11.30%	8	5.10%
Gender				
Male	51	48.10%	66	42.00%
Female	55	51.90%	91	58.00%
Experiences of medical disputes				
Experienced	53	50.00%	121	77.10%
Inexperienced	53	50.00%	36	22.90%
Outcomes of medical disputes				
No idea	54	50.90%	12	7.60%
Resolved by simple communication	17	16.00%	56	35.70%
Resolved by communication and reconciliation via money compensation or medical fee reduction	19	17.90%	63	40.10%
Resolved by simple third-party involvement/mediation	7	6.60%	1	0.60%
Resolved by third party involvement and reconciliation via money compensation or medical fee reduction	8	7.50%	17	10.80%
Unresolved even with third party involvement and the complaint was filed in the court	1	0.90%	8	5.10%

Table 3. Ranking of the perceptions of risk factors in six dimensions for veterinarians and students in 2014 and 2022.

Risk Factors Dimensions	Veterinarians				Students			
	2014 (n = 73)		2022 (n = 126)		2014 (n = 33)		2022 (n = 31)	
	Mean	Rank [1]	Mean	Rank	Mean	Rank	Mean	Rank
Clients' perspectives	3.70	1	4.07	5	3.53	1	4.17	2
Medical expenses	3.65	2	4.17	3	3.07	5	4.14	3
Attitudes during interactions	3.45	3	4.26	1	3.22	4	4.14	3
Modes of communication	3.20	4	3.98	6	2.99	6	3.84	6
Medical skills	3.12	5	4.14	4	3.50	2	4.61	1
Complaints management	3.09	6	4.20	2	3.31	3	4.07	5

[1] Rank by the mean from highest to lowest.

In contrast, the top three risk factors in 2022 were attitudes during interactions, complaint management, and medical expenses. Furthermore, the least significant risk factors, or those considered least likely to contribute to medical disputes, were medical skills in 2014 and modes of communication in 2022.

Inexperienced veterinarians and students in 2014 shared similar perceptions of the risk factors most likely to lead to medical disputes. However, in 2022, medical skills were identified as the top risk factor for both groups. When comparing inexperienced veterinarians and students in 2014 and 2022, the top two risk factors identified by students without experience of medical disputes were medical skills and clients' perspectives, while modes of communication were the least significant risk factor (see Table 4). Interestingly, students ranked complaint management as the fifth risk factor instead of the top first risk ranking among veterinarians with dispute experiences.

Table 4. Ranking of the perceptions of risk factors in six dimensions for inexperienced Veterinarians and students in 2014 and 2022.

Risk Factors Dimensions	Students without Experience				Veterinarians without Experience			
	2014 $n = 32$		2022 $n = 24$		2014 $n = 21$		2022 $n = 12$	
	Mean	Rank [1]	Mean	Rank	Mean	Rank	Mean	Rank
Clients' perspectives	3.48	1	4.18	3	3.58	1	4.17	5
Medical skills	3.45	2	4.60	1	3.45	2	4.29	1
Complaints management	3.27	3	4.02	5	3.20	5	4.25	3
Attitudes during interactions	3.16	4	4.23	2	3.33	3	4.23	4
Medical expenses	3.01	5	4.14	4	3.25	4	4.28	2
Modes of communication	2.96	6	3.80	6	3.17	6	4.01	6

[1] Rank by the mean from highest to lowest.

3.3. Differences in Risk Factor Perception by Demographic Variables in 2014 and 2022

In 2014, 73 veterinarians and 33 students out of the 106 interviewees had significantly different perceptions of the risk of medical disputes caused by medical expenses ($p < 0.022$). For instance, veterinarians gave a risk score of 3.65 ± 1.10 points, ranking it the second-highest level of risk, whereas veterinary students gave 3.07 ± 1.35 points, ranking it fifth. This indicates that veterinarians considered medical expenses to be more likely to lead to medical disputes than the students in 2014.

In 2022, the risk factor with a significant difference in the risk scores given by 126 veterinarians and 31 students was medical skill ($p < 0.001$), with veterinary students giving a score of 4.06 ± 0.53 points, ranking it first, while veterinarians gave 4.14 ± 0.84 points, ranking it fourth. Conversely, regarding the risk of medical skill in 2014, veterinarians ranked it fifth (3.12 ± 1.35), while students ranked it second (3.50 ± 1.36), showing no significant change in the ranking. Nevertheless, there was a difference in risk perception in 2014 that became significantly different in 2022 (see Table 5).

Table 5. The risk factor perception differences between veterinarians and students in 2014 and 2022.

Risk Factors Dimensions	2014 Stakeholder's Position					2022 Stakeholder's Position				
	Veterinarians $n = 73$		Students $n = 33$			Veterinarians $n = 126$		Students $n = 31$		
	Mean	SD	Mean	SD	p	Mean	SD	Mean	SD	p
Risk_all [1]	3.37	0.80	3.27	0.97	0.599	4.14	0.40	4.16	0.56	0.769
client_p	3.70	1.05	3.53	1.38	0.492	4.07	0.65	4.17	0.59	0.417
inter_att	3.45	1.00	3.22	1.25	0.324	4.26	0.57	4.14	0.78	0.324
med_exp	3.65	1.10	3.07	1.35	0.022 *	4.17	0.67	4.14	0.89	0.823
med_sk	3.12	1.35	3.50	1.36	0.179	4.14	0.84	4.61	0.53	<0.001 ***
complaint	3.09	1.10	3.31	1.33	0.364	4.20	0.60	4.07	0.75	0.309
commu	3.20	0.92	2.99	0.91	0.279	3.98	0.56	3.84	0.73	0.251

[1] Risk_all: Average scores of all the risk factors including medical skills (med_sk), modes of communication (commu), attitudes of stakeholders during the interaction (inter_att), medical expenses (med_exp), complaints management (complaint), and clients' perceptions (client_p). p value < 0.05 *; p value < 0.001 ***.

In 2014, there was no difference in risk factor perceptions among males and females across the six dimensions. However, in 2022, women (4.22 ± 0.37) had a significantly higher degree of risk perception for overall risk factors ($p = 0.005$) compared to men (4.04 ± 0.50). Additionally, they had a significantly higher score for the risk of disputes arising from clients' perspectives ($p = 0.01$) than men (see Table 6). In 2014, respondents with experience

(3.83 ± 0.97) believed that the degree of risk caused by medical expenses was significantly higher than that of inexperienced respondents (3.11 ± 1.32) ($p < 0.002$). Consequently, the medical expenses factor ranked first in the group with experience and fifth in the group without experience. Conversely, in 2022, experienced respondents (4.15 ± 0.84) believed that the degree of risk of medical skill factors ($p = 0.023$) was significantly lower than that of inexperienced respondents (4.50 ± 0.64), and the factor ranked fourth, while the no-experience group ranked it first (see Table 7).

Table 6. The risk factor perception differences by gender in 2014 and 2022.

Risk Factors Dimensions	2014 Gender					2022 Gender				
	Male $n = 51$		Female $n = 55$			Male $n = 66$		Female $n = 91$		
	Mean	SD	Mean	SD	p	Mean	SD	Mean	SD	p
Risk_all [1]	3.43	0.76	3.25	0.93	0.302	4.04	0.50	4.22	0.37	0.017 *
client_p	3.71	0.87	3.59	1.38	0.607	3.93	0.71	4.20	0.56	0.01 **
inter_att	3.49	0.99	3.27	1.16	0.295	4.14	0.72	4.30	0.53	0.133
med_exp	3.62	1.01	3.33	1.36	0.212	4.06	0.79	4.25	0.65	0.101
med_sk	3.29	1.19	3.18	1.50	0.67	4.13	0.88	4.31	0.75	0.173
complaint	3.24	1.11	3.08	1.24	0.478	4.11	0.63	4.22	0.64	0.289
commu	3.21	0.94	3.08	0.89	0.466	3.86	0.62	4.01	0.57	0.105

[1] Risk_all: Average scores of all the risk factors including medical skills (med_sk), modes of communication (commu), attitudes of stakeholders during the interaction (inter_att), medical expenses (med_exp), complaints management (complaint), and clients' perceptions (client_p). p value < 0.05 *; p value < 0.01 **.

Table 7. The risk factor perception differences in experiences of medical disputes in 2014 and 2022.

Risk Factors Dimensions	2014 Experiences of Medical Disputes					2022 Experiences of Medical Disputes				
	Experienced $n = 53$		Inexperienced $n = 53$			Experienced $n = 121$		Inexperienced $n = 36$		
	Mean	SD	Mean	SD	p	Mean	SD	Mean	SD	p
Risk_all [1]	3.41	0.79	3.27	0.92	0.411	4.13	0.40	4.18	0.55	0.587
client_p	3.77	1.04	3.52	1.27	0.279	4.06	0.62	4.17	0.69	0.348
inter_att	3.52	0.94	3.23	1.20	0.173	4.24	0.59	4.23	0.72	0.943
med_exp	3.83	0.97	3.11	1.32	0.002 **	4.16	0.68	4.19	0.82	0.852
med_sk	3.02	1.37	3.45	1.32	0.1	4.15	0.84	4.50	0.64	0.023 *
complaint	3.07	1.09	3.25	1.26	0.435	4.20	0.59	4.10	0.77	0.393
commu	3.23	0.95	3.05	0.88	0.306	3.97	0.55	3.87	0.73	0.368

[1] Risk_all: Average scores of all the risk factors including medical skills (med_sk), modes of communication (commu), attitudes of stakeholders during the interaction (inter_att), medical expenses (med_exp), complaints management (complaint), and clients' perceptions (client_p). p value < 0.05 *; p value < 0.01 **.

3.4. Compare Risk Factor Perception Differences between the Two Periods for Each Subgroup

To investigate differences in risk factor perception between the two periods (2014 and 2022) for each subgroup (e.g., males, females, veterinarians, students, experienced and inexperienced in medical disputes), a separate analysis was conducted. All subgroups in 2022 showed significantly higher risk scores than those in 2014 (see Tables 8–10). Males in 2014 ($n = 51$) perceived clients' perspectives and medical expenses as the top two risk factors, while in 2022 ($n = 66$), they considered attitudes during interactions and medical skills as the top two risks. Interestingly, there was no significant difference in risk perception regarding the "clients' perspective" dimension between the two periods, but the order changed from the first in 2014 to the fifth in 2022. Females had a similar perception of the top two risk factors as males.

Table 8. Comparisons of the risk factor perceptions differences between 2014 and 2022 for gender subgroups.

Risk Factors Dimensions	Gender									
	Male n = 117					Female n = 146				
	2014 n = 51		2022 n = 66		p	2014 n = 55		2022 n = 91		p
	Mean	SD	Mean	SD		Mean	SD	Mean	SD	
Risk_all [1]	3.43	0.76	4.04	0.50	<0.001 ***	3.25	0.93	4.22	0.37	<0.001 ***
client_p	3.71	0.87	3.93	0.71	0.131	3.59	1.38	4.20	0.56	0.003 **
inter_att	3.49	0.99	4.14	0.72	<0.001 ***	3.27	1.16	4.30	0.53	<0.001 ***
med_exp	3.62	1.01	4.06	0.79	0.013 **	3.33	1.36	4.25	0.65	<0.001 ***
med_sk	3.29	1.19	4.13	0.88	<0.001 ***	3.18	1.50	4.31	0.75	<0.001 ***
complaint	3.24	1.11	4.11	0.63	<0.001 ***	3.08	1.24	4.22	0.64	<0.001 ***
commu	3.21	0.94	3.86	0.62	<0.001 ***	3.08	0.89	4.01	0.57	<0.001 ***

[1] Risk_all: Average scores of all the risk factors including medical skills (med_sk), modes of communication (commu), attitudes of stakeholders during the interaction (inter_att), medical expenses (med_exp), complaints management (complaint), and clients' perceptions (client_p). p value < 0.01 **; p value < 0.001 ***.

Table 9. Comparisons of the risk factor perceptions differences between 2014 and 2022 for veterinarians and students subgroup.

Risk Factors Dimensions	Stakeholder's Position									
	Veterinarians					Students				
	2014 n = 73		2022 n = 126		p	2014 n = 33		2022 n = 31		p
	Mean	SD	Mean	SD		Mean	SD	Mean	SD	
Risk_all [1]	3.37	0.80	4.14	0.40	<0.001 ***	3.27	0.97	4.16	0.56	<0.001 ***
client_p	3.70	1.05	4.07	0.65	0.008 **	3.53	1.38	4.17	0.59	0.019 *
inter_att	3.45	1.00	4.26	0.57	<0.001 ***	3.22	1.25	4.14	0.78	<0.001 ***
med_exp	3.65	1.10	4.17	0.67	<0.001 ***	3.07	1.35	4.14	0.89	<0.001 ***
med_sk	3.12	1.35	4.14	0.84	<0.001 ***	3.50	1.36	4.61	0.53	<0.001 ***
complaint	3.09	1.10	4.20	0.60	<0.001 ***	3.31	1.33	4.07	0.75	0.006 **
commu	3.20	0.92	3.98	0.56	<0.001 ***	2.99	0.91	3.84	0.73	<0.001 ***

[1] Risk_all: Average scores of all the risk factors including medical skills (med_sk), modes of communication (commu), attitudes of stakeholders during the interaction (inter_att), medical expenses (med_exp), complaints management (complaint), and clients' perceptions (client_p). p value < 0.05 *; p value < 0.01 **; p value < 0.001 ***.

Table 10. Comparisons of the risk factor perceptions differences between 2014 and 2022 for medical disputes experience subgroup.

Risk Factors Dimensions	Experiences of Medical Disputes									
	Experienced					Inexperienced				
	2014 n = 53		2022 n = 121		p	2014 n = 53		2022 n = 36		p
	Mean	SD	Mean	SD		Mean	SD	Mean	SD	
Risk_all [1]	3.41	0.79	4.13	0.40	<0.001 ***	3.27	0.92	4.18	0.55	<0.001 ***
client_p	3.77	1.04	4.06	0.62	0.061	3.52	1.27	4.17	0.69	0.003 **
inter_att	3.52	0.94	4.24	0.59	<0.001 ***	3.23	1.20	4.23	0.72	<0.001 ***
med_exp	3.83	0.97	4.16	0.68	0.028 *	3.11	1.32	4.19	0.82	<0.001 ***
med_sk	3.02	1.37	4.15	0.84	<0.001 ***	3.45	1.32	4.50	0.64	<0.001 ***
complaint	3.07	1.09	4.20	0.59	<0.001 ***	3.25	1.26	4.10	0.77	<0.001 ***
commu	3.23	0.95	3.97	0.55	<0.001 ***	3.05	0.88	3.87	0.73	<0.001 ***

[1] Risk_all: Average scores of all the risk factors including medical skills (med_sk), modes of communication (commu), attitudes of stakeholders during the interaction (inter_att), medical expenses (med_exp), complaints management (complaint), and clients' perceptions (client_p). p value < 0.05 *; p value < 0.01 **; p value < 0.001 ***.

In the mean ranking of experienced respondents' risk perception (see Table 10), those with experience in 2014 (n = 53) and inexperienced respondents in 2014 (n = 53) both believed that the top two risk factors were medical expenses and clients' perspectives. In contrast, experienced respondents in 2022 (n = 121) perceived attitudes during interactions and complaints management as the top two risks. However, inexperienced respondents (n = 36) ranked medical skills as their top risk factor.

In the mean ranking of experienced veterinarians' risk perception (see Table 11), those with experience in 2014 ($n = 52$) perceived medical expenses and clients' perspectives as the top two risk factors. In 2022, experienced veterinarians ($n = 114$) perceived attitudes during interactions and complaints management as the top two risks. Inexperienced veterinarians in 2014 ($n = 21$) and students perceived clients' perspectives and medical skills as the top two risks. In 2022, the top two risk factors perceived by inexperienced veterinarians ($n = 12$) were medical skills and medical expenses, which were similar to students' perceptions.

Table 11. Comparisons of the risk factor perceptions differences between 2014 and 2022 for veterinarians with/without experiences subgroup.

Risk Factors Dimensions	Veterinarians with Experiences					Veterinarians without Experiences				
	2014 $n = 52$		2022 $n = 114$			2014 $n = 21$		2022 $n = 12$		
	Mean	SD	Mean	SD	p	Mean	SD	Mean	SD	p
Risk_all [1]	3.38	0.77	4.13	0.41	<0.001 ***	3.33	0.90	4.20	0.37	0.003 **
client_p	3.75	1.03	4.05	0.64	0.05 *	3.58	1.12	4.17	0.76	0.12
inter_att	3.49	0.93	4.26	0.59	<0.001 ***	3.33	1.18	4.23	0.36	0.003 **
med_exp	3.81	0.96	4.16	0.68	0.02 *	3.25	1.32	4.28	0.62	0.005 **
med_sk	2.98	1.36	4.12	0.85	<0.001 ***	3.45	1.30	4.29	0.75	0.05
complaint	3.04	1.08	4.20	0.60	<0.001 ***	3.20	1.18	4.25	0.68	0.003 **
commu	3.21	0.95	3.97	0.56	<0.001 ***	3.17	0.85	4.01	0.60	0.005 **

[1] Risk_all: Average scores of all the risk factors including medical skills (med_sk), modes of communication (commu), attitudes of stakeholders during the interaction (inter_att), medical expenses (med_exp), complaints management (complaint), and clients' perceptions (client_p). p value < 0.05 *; p value < 0.01 **; p value < 0.001 ***.

4. Discussion

This study explores the perceptions of veterinarians and veterinary students in Taiwan on the factors that lead to medical disputes. The study is unique as it compares the perceptions of these two groups using online questionnaires from two different periods. The study's objectives were to recognize the most significant risk factors, distinguish between the perceptions of veterinarians and veterinary students, and compare the findings of two surveys conducted in 2014 and 2022.

The study's results revealed that the most significant risk factors for medical disputes among veterinarians and veterinary students were attitudes during interactions, complaint management, and medical expenses. These results differ from the previous survey conducted in 2014, which identified medical expenses, clients' perspectives, and attitudes during interactions as the top three risk factors for medical disputes. The results suggest that the perception of risk factors has changed over time, and veterinarians and veterinary students have become more aware of the importance of effective communication and complaints management in preventing medical disputes.

Compared to the results obtained from veterinarians in 2014 and 2022; there was a significant increase in overall risk perceptions. This increase in risk perceptions may have been influenced by the continuous veterinary education program implemented since 2016. The Taiwan Veterinarian Act may be one of the reasons for this increase. It requires veterinarians to engage in continuing education and renew their practice license every six years by presenting certificates of completed continuing education to remain eligible to practice last year (2016–2022). In addition, the continuous veterinary education program provides veterinarians with 120 h of training, including 24 h of courses on medical quality improvement, ethics, and laws. Therefore, veterinarians may have been influenced to change their perception of the top two risk factors during interactions with stakeholders and customer complaints management. The increased risk perception may result from the greater emphasis placed on improving the quality of veterinary care and ensuring compliance with ethical and legal standards.

The study found that medical skills and modes of communication were the least significant risk factors that constituted medical disputes. These results suggest that the quality of care provided by veterinarians and veterinary students is not the primary determinant of medical disputes. Instead, poor communication and complaints management were the leading causes of medical disputes, similar to previous studies [11,39]. The findings highlight the importance of improving the communication skills of veterinarians and veterinary students, developing effective complaint management strategies, and reducing the risk of medical disputes. On the other hand, the modes of communication mean the process of informed consent, such as explanations and information. Effective modes of communication might have become the standard operation procedure (SOP) and online-friendly tools to help clients get information during these years, as previously reported [26,40].

The study's results also revealed significant differences in the perception of risk factors between veterinarians and veterinary students. For instance, in 2014, veterinarians considered medical expenses ($p = 0.022$) more likely to lead to medical disputes than veterinary students [28]. However, in 2022, veterinary students ranked medical skills ($p < 0.001$) as the top risk factor, while veterinarians ranked it fourth. Moreover, the study found that experienced veterinarians had a different perception of risk factors than inexperienced veterinarians and veterinary students. Experienced veterinarians perceived attitudes during interactions and complaint management as the top risk factors for medical disputes. In contrast, inexperienced veterinarians and veterinary students ranked clients' perspectives and medical skills as the top risk factors. These results suggest that the perception of risk factors may change as veterinarians gain more experience and become more aware of the importance of effective communication and complaint management. Although veterinary students' successful transition into clinical practice depends on communication competence, their perceptions seem significantly different from senior veterinarians; it was similar to previous studies [27,41]. Thus, increased employer cooperation in regard to continued education and research into best practices for tertiary institution–employer collaboration needs to be developed.

The study is not without limitations. One limitation is that it was conducted in Taiwan, and the population of veterinarians and veterinary students is relatively small compared to other countries. Therefore, the results may not be generalizable to other countries with different healthcare systems and cultural backgrounds. Another limitation is that the study used a cross-sectional survey design, which cannot establish causality. As a result, the causal relationships between the variables cannot be determined. A third limitation is that the study relied on self-reported data, which may be subject to social desirability bias. Participants may have provided answers that they believed were socially desirable rather than reflecting their true perceptions. Fourth, the study did not investigate the factors contributing to the change in perception of risk factors over time. Understanding these factors could provide valuable insights into the reasons for the changes in perception. Lastly, the Likert scale is commonly used as interval data in the medical area, although it is considered ordinal data. Therefore, the data were analyzed as a median rather than a mean.

Despite these limitations, the study provides valuable insights into the perception of risk factors that cause medical disputes among veterinarians and veterinary students. Future research can explore the factors contributing to changes in risk perception over time, compare the perception of risk factors in different countries, and examine the effectiveness of communication strategies and complaint management skills in reducing the risk of medical disputes. Additionally, further research could investigate the efficacy of different educational programs in developing effective communication and complaint management skills in young veterinarians and veterinary students. Understanding these factors can help improve the quality of care for companion animals, reduce the risk of medical disputes, and enhance the competency of veterinary professionals.

In conclusion, the study provides valuable insights into the perception of risk factors that cause medical disputes among veterinarians and veterinary students. The results suggest effective communication and complaint management are crucial in preventing medical disputes. The study highlights the importance of developing effective communication strategies and complaint management skills for young veterinarians and veterinary students, reducing the risk of medical disputes, and improving the quality of care for companion animals. Veterinary education might be suggested to increase the practical experience of medical disputes and complaint management to help students overcome the gaps and gain the competency to transition into clinical practice successfully.

Supplementary Materials: The following are available online at https://www.mdpi.com/xxx/s1, Supplementary Material: Questionnaire.

Author Contributions: Conceptualization, Z.-F.C., Y.-H.E.H., J.-J.L. and C.-H.C.; Methodology, Z.-F.C., Y.-H.E.H., J.-J.L. and C.-H.C.; Validation, Y.-H.E.H. and C.-H.C.; Resources, Y.-H.E.H. and C.-H.C.; Data curation, Z.-F.C.; Writing—original draft, Z.-F.C.; Writing—review & editing, Y.-H.E.H., J.-J.L. and C.-H.C.; Supervision, Y.-H.E.H., J.-J.L. and C.-H.C.; All authors have read and agreed to the published version of the manuscript.

Funding: This research received no external funding.

Institutional Review Board Statement: The protocol had been approved by Research Ethics Committee of National Taiwan University. The committee is organized under, and operates in accordance with, Social and Behavioral Research Ethical Principles and Regulations of National Taiwan University and government laws and regulations. [NTU-REC No.: 202209HS024 and date of approval: 11 October 2022, to 31 July 2023].

Informed Consent Statement: Participants indicated their informed consent by partaking in the survey.

Data Availability Statement: Data sharing not applicable.

Conflicts of Interest: The authors declare no conflict of interest.

References

1. Park, R.M.; Gruen, M.E.; Royal, K. Association between Dog Owner Demographics and Decision to Seek Veterinary Care. *Vet. Sci.* **2021**, *8*, 7. [CrossRef]
2. Ritter, C.; Jansen, J.; Roche, S.; Kelton, D.F.; Adams, C.L.; Orsel, K.; Barkema, H.W. Invited review: Determinants of farmers' adoption of management-based strategies for infectious disease prevention and control. *J. Dairy Sci* **2017**, *100*, 3329–3347. [PubMed]
3. Irwin, A. Managing client complaints: Identifying and mitigating their detrimental impacts on veterinary practitioners. *Vet. Rec* **2022**, *191*, 157–159. [CrossRef]
4. Bryce, A.R.; Rossi, T.A.; Tansey, C.; Murphy, R.A.; Murphy, L.A.; Nakamura, R.K. Effect of client complaints on small animal veterinary internists. *J. Small Anim. Pract.* **2019**, *60*, 167–172. [CrossRef] [PubMed]
5. Moses, L.; Malowney, M.J.; Wesley Boyd, J. Ethical conflict and moral distress in veterinary practice: A survey of North American veterinarians. *J. Vet. Intern.* **2018**, *32*, 2115–2122. [CrossRef]
6. Kipperman, B.S.; Kass, P.H.; Rishniw, M. Factors that influence small animal veterinarians' opinions and actions regarding cost of care and effects of economic limitations on patient care and outcome and professional career satisfaction and burnout. *J. Am. Vet. Med. Assoc.* **2017**, *250*, 785–794. [CrossRef]
7. Kogan, L.R.; Wallace, J.E.; Hellyer, P.W.; Richards, M. Veterinary Technicians and Occupational Burnout. *Front. Vet. Sci.* **2020**, *7*, 328. [CrossRef]
8. Shaw, J.R.; Adams, C.L.; Bonnett, B.N. What can veterinarians learn from studies of physician-patient communication about veterinarian-client-patient communication? *J. Am. Vet. Med. Assoc.* **2004**, *224*, 676–684. [CrossRef]
9. Levinson, W.; Roter, D.L.; Mullooly, J.P.; Dull, V.T.; Frankel, R.M. Physician-patient communication: The relationship with malpractice claims among primary care physicians and surgeons. *JAMA* **1997**, *277*, 553–559. [CrossRef]
10. Shaw, J.R.; Barley, G.E.; Hill, A.E.; Larson, S.; Roter, D.L. Communication skills education onsite in a veterinary practice. *Patient Educ. Couns.* **2010**, *80*, 337–344. [CrossRef]
11. Gibson, J.; White, K.; Mossop, L.; Oxtoby, C.; Brennan, M. 'We're gonna end up scared to do anything': A qualitative exploration of how client complaints are experienced by UK veterinary practitioners. *Vet. Rec.* **2022**, *191*, e1737. [CrossRef]
12. Andela, M. Burnout, somatic complaints, and suicidal ideations among veterinarians: Development and validation of the Veterinarians Stressors Inventory. *J. Vet. Behav.* **2020**, *37*, 48–55. [CrossRef]
13. Sahu, P.K.; Phillips Savage, A.C.N.; Sa, B. Exploring students' perceptions of the educational environment in a caribbean veterinary school: A cross-sectional study. *J. Vet. Med. Educ.* **2020**, *47*, 668–677. [CrossRef] [PubMed]
14. O'Connell, D.; Bonvicini, K.A. Addressing disappointment in veterinary practice. *Vet. Clin. N. Am. Small Anim.* **2007**, *37*, 135–149. [CrossRef]
15. Lyu, S.Y.; Liao, C.K.; Chang, K.P.; Tsai, S.T.; Lee, M.B.; Tsai, F.C. Analysis of medical litigation among patients with medical disputes in cosmetic surgery in Taiwan. *Aesthetic Plast. Surg.* **2011**, *35*, 764–772. [CrossRef] [PubMed]

16. Stackhouse, N.; Chamberlain, J.; Bouwer, A.; Mexas, A.M. Development and validation of a novel measure for the direct assessment of empathy in veterinary students. *J. Vet. Med. Educ.* **2020**, *47*, 452–464. [CrossRef]
17. Matthew, S.M.; Bok, H.G.; Chaney, K.P.; Read, E.K.; Hodgson, J.L.; Rush, B.R.; Molgaard, L.K. Collaborative development of a shared framework for competency-based veterinary education. *J. Vet. Med. Educ.* **2020**, *47*, 578–593. [CrossRef]
18. Stevens, B.J.; Kedrowicz, A.A. Evaluation of fourth-year veterinary students' client communication skills: Recommendations for scaffolded instruction and practice. *J. Vet. Med. Educ.* **2018**, *45*, 85–90. [CrossRef]
19. World Organisation for Animal Health (OIE). OIE Recommendations on the Competencies of Graduating Veterinarians ("Day 1 Graduates") to Assure National Veterinary Services of Quality. 2012. Available online: https://www.woah.org/app/uploads/2021/03/dayone-b-ang-vc.pdf (accessed on 12 January 2022).
20. Caple, I.W. Continuing professional development for veterinarians. *Aust. Vet. J.* **2005**, *83*, 200–202. [CrossRef]
21. Torres, C.G.; Laytte, M.J.; Tadich, T.A. Perceptions of small animal practitioners and pet owners on professional competencies in veterinary practice: An essential component for curricula design. *Vet. Mex.* **2020**, *6*, 14. [CrossRef]
22. Kates, F.R.; Samuels, S.K.; Case, J.B.; Dujowich, M. Lessons Learned from a pilot study implementing a team-based messaging application (Slack) to improve communication and teamwork in Veterinary Medical Education. *J. Vet. Med. Educ.* **2020**, *47*, 18–26. [CrossRef] [PubMed]
23. Englar, R.E. Tracking veterinary students' acquisition of communication skills and clinical communication confidence by comparing student performance in the first and twenty-seventh standardized client encounters. *J. Vet. Med. Educ.* **2019**, *46*, 235–257. [CrossRef] [PubMed]
24. Russell, E.; Mossop, L.; Forbes, E.; Oxtoby, C. Uncovering the 'messy details' of veterinary communication: An analysis of communication problems in cases of alleged professional negligence. *Vet. Rec.* **2022**, *190*, e1068. [CrossRef] [PubMed]
25. Coe, J.B.; Adams, C.L.; Bonnett, B.N. A focus group study of veterinarians' and pet owners' perceptions of the monetary aspects of veterinary care. *J. Am. Vet. Med. Assoc.* **2007**, *231*, 1510–1518. [CrossRef] [PubMed]
26. Routh, J.; Paramasivam, S.J.; Cockcroft, P.; Nadarajah, V.D.; Jeevaratnam, K. Stakeholder perceptions on veterinary student preparedness for workplace clinical training–a qualitative study. *BMC Vet. Res.* **2022**, *18*, 1–18. [CrossRef]
27. Adams, C.L.; Kurtz, S.M. *Skills for Communicating in Veterinary Medicine*; Otmoor: Oxford, UK, 2017; pp. 1–3.
28. Alec Martin, E. Managing client communication for effective practice: What skills should veterinary graduates have acquired for success? *J. Vet. Med. Educ.* **2006**, *33*, 45–49. [CrossRef]
29. Fogelberg, K.; Farnsworth, C.C. Faculty and students' self-assessment of client communication skills and professional ethics in three veterinary medical schools. *J. Vet. Med. Educ.* **2009**, *36*, 423–428. [CrossRef]
30. Whitcomb, T.L. Raising awareness of the hidden curriculum in veterinary medical education: A review and call for research. *J. Vet. Med. Educ.* **2014**, *41*, 344–349. [CrossRef]
31. Hsu, Y.-H.E. Innovation communication education in veterinary medicine: A client-centered model. In *NSTC Medical Education Conference*, 1st ed.; Government Research Bulletin; National Science and Technology Council: Tainan, Taiwan, 2014; pp. 125–130. Available online: https://www.grb.gov.tw/search/planDetail?id=3170065&docId=426656 (accessed on 13 July 2022).
32. May, T.W.; Pfäfflin, M.; Bien, C.G.; Hamer, H.M.; Holtkamp, M.; Rating, D.; Schulze-Bonhage, A.; Straub, H.B.; Strzelczyk, A.; Thorbecke, R. Attitudes toward epilepsy assessed by the SAPE questionnaire in Germany—Comparison of its psychometric properties and results in a web-based vs. face-to-face survey. *Epilepsy Behav.* **2022**, *130*, 108665. [CrossRef]
33. Jakobsson, U. Statistical presentation and analysis of ordinal data in nursing research. *Scand. J. Caring Sci.* **2004**, *18*, 437–440. [CrossRef]
34. South, L.; Saffo, D.; Vitek, O.; Dunne, C.; Borkin, M.A. Effective use of Likert scales in visualization evaluations: A systematic review. *Comput Graph Forum.* **2022**, *41*, 43–55. [CrossRef]
35. Lewis, J.R. Multipoint scales: Mean and median differences and observed significance levels. *Int. J. Hum. Comput. Int.* **1993**, *5*, 383–392. [CrossRef]
36. Bentley, H.; Lee, J.; Supersad, A.; Yu, H.; Dobson, J.L.; Wong, S.A.; Stewart, M.; Vatturi, S.S.; Lebel, K.; Crivellaro, P.; et al. Preparedness of residents and medical students for the transition to competence by design in diagnostic radiology post-graduate medical education. *Can. Assoc. Radiol. J.* **2022**, 08465371221119139. [CrossRef] [PubMed]
37. Senos, R.; Leite, C.A.R.; dos Santos Tolezano, F.; Roberto-Rodrigues, M.; Pérez, W. Using videos in active learning: An experience in veterinary anatomy. *Anat. Histol. Embryol.* **2022**, *52*, 50–54. [CrossRef]
38. Schoenfeld-Tacher, R.M.; Dorman, D.C. Effect of Delivery Format on Student Outcomes and Perceptions of a Veterinary Medicine Course: Synchronous Versus Asynchronous Learning. *Vet. Sci.* **2021**, *8*, 13. [CrossRef] [PubMed]
39. Gordon, S.; Gardner, D.; Weston, J.; Bolwell, C.; Benschop, J.; Parkinson, T. Fostering the Development of Professionalism in Veterinary Students: Challenges and Implications for Veterinary Professionalism Curricula. *Educ. Sci.* **2021**, *11*, 720. [CrossRef]

40. Rogers, C.W.; Murphy, L.A.; Murphy, R.A.; Malouf, K.A.; Natsume, R.E.; Ward, B.D.; Tansey, C.; Nakamura, R.K. An analysis of client complaints and their effects on veterinary support staff. *Vet. Med. Sci.* **2022**, *8*, 925–934. [CrossRef]
41. Springer, S.; Sandøe, P.; Bøker Lund, T.; Grimm, H. "Patients' interests first, but . . . "–Austrian Veterinarians' Attitudes to Moral Challenges in Modern Small Animal Practice. *Animals* **2019**, *9*, 241. [CrossRef]

Disclaimer/Publisher's Note: The statements, opinions and data contained in all publications are solely those of the individual author(s) and contributor(s) and not of MDPI and/or the editor(s). MDPI and/or the editor(s) disclaim responsibility for any injury to people or property resulting from any ideas, methods, instructions or products referred to in the content.

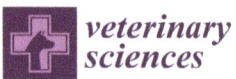

Article

Are They Thinking Differently? The Perceptions and Differences in Medical Disputes between Veterinarians and Clients

Zih-Fang Chen [1], Yi-Hsin Elsa Hsu [2,3,*], Jih-Jong Lee [4] and Chung-Hsi Chou [1,*]

[1] Zoonoses Research Center, School of Veterinary Medicine, National Taiwan University, Taipei 10617, Taiwan
[2] Executive Master Program of Business Administration in Biotechnology, Taipei Medical University, Taipei 11031, Taiwan
[3] School of Healthcare Administration, Taipei Medical University, Taipei 11031, Taiwan
[4] Institute of Veterinary Clinical Science, School of Veterinary Medicine, National Taiwan University, Taipei 10617, Taiwan
* Correspondence: elsahsu@tmu.edu.tw (Y.-H.E.H.); cchou@ntu.edu.tw (C.-H.C.)

Simple Summary: This study explored the perceptions of veterinarians and clients regarding risk factors and potential solutions for medical disputes in veterinary practices. A total of 245 respondents in Taiwan, including 125 veterinarians and 120 clients, completed an electronic questionnaire in 2022. The questionnaire covered six dimensions: medical skills, complaint management, the attitudes of stakeholders during interactions, medical expenses, clients' perspectives, and communication modes. The results showed significant differences in the perceptions of inducing medical dispute risk factors between clients and veterinarians in veterinary practice. Both young veterinarians and clients perceived medical skills as the highest risk factor for inducing medical disputes, while experienced veterinarians disagreed. Veterinarians with medical dispute experience identified stakeholders' attitudes during interactions as the top contributing factor. The possible solutions for veterinarians included providing clients with cost estimates and fostering empathy and compassion for clients. In contrast, clients emphasized being informed consent of treatment and expenses. They suggested that their veterinarians should provide detailed written information. The study emphasizes the importance of understanding stakeholders' perceptions to reduce medical disputes and highlights the need for enhanced communication by young veterinarians. The findings provide valuable insights for veterinarians and clients into preventing and managing medical disputes in veterinary practices.

Abstract: Medical disputes in veterinary practices are widespread; yet, a limited amount of research has been conducted to investigate the factors contributing to medical disputes. This study examined veterinarians' and clients' perceptions regarding risk factors and possible solutions to medical disputes. A total of 245 respondents from Taiwan, including 125 veterinarians and 120 clients, completed an electronic self-administered, semi-structured questionnaire in 2022. The questionnaire covered six dimensions: medical skills, complaint management, the attitudes of stakeholders during interactions, medical expenses, clients' perspectives, and communication modes. The results highlighted significant differences in the perceptions of risk factors for inducing medical disputes and possible solutions between clients and veterinarians in veterinary practice. First, young veterinarians and clients perceived medical skills as the highest risk factor for inducing medical disputes, while experienced veterinarians disagreed ($p < 0.001$). In addition, veterinarians with medical dispute experience identified stakeholders' attitudes during interactions as the top contributing factor. Second, regarding possible solutions, all veterinarians preferred offering clients cost estimates and cultivating empathy and compassion towards them. On the other hand, clients underscored the importance of obtaining informed consent for treatments and expenses and suggested that veterinarians should supply comprehensive written information to facilitate this process. This study underlies the importance of understanding stakeholders' perceptions to mitigate medical disputes and advocates for improved communication education and training for young veterinarians. These findings provide valuable

Citation: Chen, Z.-F.; Hsu, Y.-H.E.; Lee, J.-J.; Chou, C.-H. Are They Thinking Differently? The Perceptions and Differences in Medical Disputes between Veterinarians and Clients. *Vet. Sci.* **2023**, *10*, 367. https://doi.org/10.3390/vetsci10050367

Academic Editors: Simona Sacchini and Ayoze Castro-Alonso

Received: 11 April 2023
Revised: 15 May 2023
Accepted: 22 May 2023
Published: 22 May 2023

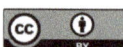

Copyright: © 2023 by the authors. Licensee MDPI, Basel, Switzerland. This article is an open access article distributed under the terms and conditions of the Creative Commons Attribution (CC BY) license (https://creativecommons.org/licenses/by/4.0/).

insights for veterinarians and clients, contributing to preventing and managing medical disputes in veterinary practices.

Keywords: medical dispute; risk factor for medical disputes; questionnaire; veterinarians; clients; pet owner; veterinary education; communication; complaint management; medical skills; medical expense; attitudes of stakeholders

1. Introduction

In modern society, veterinarians encounter heightened risks of malpractice claims and medical disputes, primarily driven by deepening client–animal bonds [1] and an increased awareness of legal rights [2,3]. Perceived or real malpractice can result in medical disputes where the unsatisfactory outcomes of improper treatment may lead to litigation against veterinarians [2,4,5]. These disputes can profoundly affect veterinarians, heightening their concern about client complaints and litigation fears. For example, a 2021 survey by the British Veterinary Association revealed that 57% of veterinary staff felt intimidated by their clients' behavior in the previous year, marking a 10% increase from 2019 [6]. This intimidation contributed to adverse mental stress, strained relationships with future clients, increased work pressure, and even career burnout [7,8].

Intriguingly, the pivotal factor influencing a client's decision to instigate a malpractice claim or medical disagreement is not necessarily anchored to the caliber of veterinary healthcare provided. Rather, it is frequently caused by communication failures that act as the crucial catalyst [4,6,9–12]. These disputes can be induced by client dissatisfaction with the care process or clients' inability to accept unexpected prognoses. For example, clients anticipate veterinarians to provide accurate diagnoses and compassionately explain their patients' conditions [4,11,13]. Additionally, complaints can precipitate medical disputes when clients feel neglected or receive insufficient explanations regarding medical expenses [14–18].

A considerable body of research underscores the increased work stress experienced by veterinary professionals, primarily due to suboptimal communication [7,14,19,20]. Veterinarians frequently express discontent or agitation from medical disputes due to communication breakdowns with clients. These negative experiences can exacerbate physical and mental health issues, emotional fatigue, and professional burnout, leading to suicide [14,19–22]. Some studies have assessed the impact of complaints on veterinarians or support staff [14,19,23], while others have explored the underlying causes of grievances in veterinary practice. For instance, the thematic analysis of numerous veterinary medical disputes initially attributed to technical failures revealed that they mainly resulted from professional conduct deficiencies [9]. The key concerns included shortcomings in stakeholders' attitudes (trustworthiness and honesty), medical skills (high-quality care), effective client communication (appropriate methods and complaint management), and equitable medical expenses charged to clients [10,14,24].

Conversely, effective client communication can mitigate dissatisfaction and enhance satisfaction. Prior research has demonstrated that fulfilling clients' expectations and cultivating a positive rapport offer considerable benefits [4,25–27]. Notably, clients are less inclined to file formal complaints or initiate malpractice litigation against veterinarians with whom they have developed amicable relationships [11]. The most efficient approach to managing unfavorable veterinary outcomes includes minimizing the associated risks, proactively addressing clients' frustrations to prevent escalation, and devising practical methods to identify and rectify pre-existing disappointments. Consequently, veterinarians have advocated enhancing their abilities to meet clients' expectations [4,11,28–30]. Although it has traditionally been undervalued, the significance of communication and interpersonal skills is increasingly acknowledged in veterinary medicine, which may better equip veterinarians to confront anticipated challenges [6,7,24,31,32].

Nonetheless, skillful communication necessitates a thorough understanding of the expectations of the veterinarian and the clients. To date, a limited number of studies have attempted to contrast the perspectives of veterinarians and clients regarding communication and the factors contributing to medical disputes [4,7,24,33,34]. Consequently, it is crucial to devote more research efforts to enhance our comprehension. This study, therefore, examines the factors contributing to medical disputes from the differing viewpoints of veterinarians and clients. It compares their perceptions to pinpoint disparities that warrant remedial actions to prevent medical disputes and their associated risks. This research aims to understand better clients' and veterinarians' perceptions of selected interactions in veterinary practice. The outcome should promote improved veterinarian–client relationships and decrease dissatisfaction and disappointment, thus reducing medical dispute risks and work stress.

2. Materials and Methods

2.1. Study Design and Questionnaire

This study was conducted in November of 2022 and investigated the perceptions of inducing medical dispute risk factors and reducing medical dispute possible solutions between veterinarians and clients in Taiwan. The study adopted the validity- and reliability-tested, semi-structured questionnaire developed by Hsu (2014) [33], which was modified using a literature review, and then by focus groups of experts, professors, and experienced veterinarians. Furthermore, this study shares thematic continuity with the research published by Chen et al. [24]. Consequently, elements of their questionnaire have been incorporated, serving as a portion of the questionnaire content in the current investigation.

There are three parts to the questionnaire: the first part was about demographic characteristics, including age, gender, stakeholders (veterinarian or client), the experience of medical disputes, and the outcomes of medical disputes. The second part focused on assessing the perceptions of risk factors for inducing medical disputes, comprising twenty-three risk factor questions that belong to six dimensions [24]: medical skills, modes of communication, the attitudes of stakeholders during interactions, medical expenses, complaints management, and clients' perspectives (see Table 1). The third part was about the measures of perceptions of possible solutions to reduce medical dispute risks, including fifteen solutions and one open-ended question.

In the questionnaire's subsequent segment, respondents were solicited to assess, based on their prior experiences, their perceptions of each risk factor that potentially instigates a medical dispute. This evaluation employed a Likert scale of 5 points spanning from 1 to 5: "Very unlikely, unlikely, neutral, likely, very likely", respectively. In the last part, they were asked to evaluate their perceptions of the likelihood that each possible solution reduces the medical dispute risk based on their prior experiences using a Likert scale of five points spanning from 1 to 5: "Very unlikely, unlikely, neutral, likely, very likely", respectively. The Likert scale represents a prevalently utilized instrument for the quantification of phenomena within the realm of medical science [35]. Previous studies have employed various analytical approaches for Likert scales [36–38]. The assessment derived from Likert scales can be analyzed as either ordinal or interval data [36–38], a feature that leads to differing opinions among researchers. Certain scholars advocate for the mean as a superior measure of central tendency, rather than the median [38–41]; yet, others propose a contrary viewpoint [36,37]. This investigation received approval from the Research Ethics Committee of National Taiwan University (NTU-REC No.: 202209HS024).

Table 1. Six questionnaire dimensions for measures of perceptions of risk factors for inducing medical disputes.

Dimensions	Risk Factors That Might Induce Medical Disputes
Medical skills	Misdiagnosis that results in the deterioration of the patient's condition. Inadequate or unsuitable hospital care or treatment protocols.
Modes of communication	The elucidations offered by veterinarians to clients are overly simplified. The use of excessive medical terminology during explanations without providing comprehensive clarifications. Clients harbor uncertainties about the treatment yet either neglect to seek clarification or receive unsatisfactory responses from the veterinarians before the treatment. A disparity between clients' anticipated and actual treatment outcomes, attributable to an information deficit impeding decision-making before treatment. The absence of decisive action from the clients' families during discussions about further treatment procedures with the veterinarian. The veterinarians do not furnish additional written resources to clients to enhance their understanding of the treatment.
The attitudes of stakeholders during interactions	Veterinarians endeavor to induce clients into reluctant acceptance of the proposed diagnosis and treatments. Veterinarians fail to respond suitably or implement effective measures to address clients' concerns. Veterinarians do not convey feelings of support and encouragement during client interactions, thereby leading to the perception that they may be indifferent to the wellbeing of the afflicted animals. In instances where the perspectives of clients and veterinarians diverge on the animal's condition, the client tends to adhere to their subjective perception.
Medical expenses	Veterinarians fail to communicate potential comprehensive medical expenses to clients beforehand. Veterinarians do not explicitly elucidate the possible medical costs of each treatment procedure. The divergence between clients' anticipated and actual medical expenditures.
Complaints management	Veterinarians exhibit no initiative in promptly addressing the complaints. There is an absence of senior personnel attending to the complaints. The complaint resolution process is conducted with inappropriate attitudes and improper methods. Staff members lack the relevant professional training necessary for managing the complaints.
Client's perceptions	Clients rely on self-acquired information. Clients possess numerous inquiries regarding treatment and manifest a deficiency of trust in the interaction. Clients harbor misconceptions about their pets being attended to by the veterinarian. Clients might potentially harbor ulterior motives of extortion.

2.2. Respondents

Within the scope of this study, two principal stakeholder groups were the subjects of surveying: veterinarians and clients. An online Google Form platform was used to disseminate the anonymous, self-executed, semi-structured questionnaire. The distribution of this questionnaire was facilitated via multiple channels, encompassing academic institutions, professional associations, and various social media platforms, such as Facebook and LINE. Veterinarians were invited to participate through email or social networks connected to veterinary medical associations and animal hospitals.

The questionnaire was distributed through social media, such as Facebook groups and Line groups. The responses from veterinarians and clients were anonymously collected. Before responding, respondents were presented with an informed consent statement outlining the survey details, including estimated completion time and confidentiality measures. Respondents proceeded to complete the questionnaire upon giving informed consent. Due to the anonymous nature of the online Google Form, the response rate is not reported.

2.3. Analysis

Demographic attributes, including age, gender, experiences of medical disputes, and the outcomes of these disputes, were synthesized by employing descriptive statistical methodologies. These encompassed quantitative measures such as counts, averages, and percentages. The perceptions of potential risk factors leading to medical disputes and possible solutions to reduce such disputes were quantified across six dimensions using a five-point Likert scale. These responses were treated as continuous variables and subjected to statistical analysis, specifically determining their means and standard deviations.. The t-test was utilized to compare the perceptions of inducing medical dispute risk factors between stakeholders, genders, and experiences of medical disputes. t-test statistical analyses were executed using SPSS statistical software, maintaining a significance level of $p < 0.05$. In the questionnaire, we added an open-ended question for collecting veterinarians' and clients' perspectives of approaches to reducing medical risks. The gathered responses were carefully organized, categorized, and investigated to reveal underlying implications.

3. Results

A total of 253 respondents took part in the survey, consisting of 125 veterinarians and 128 clients. However, the analysis ultimately excluded eight respondents due to several factors, including being below 20 years of age, finishing the survey in an implausibly short time (less than 1 min), or providing an excessive number of incomplete responses. As a result, the final analysis included data from 125 veterinarians and 120 clients.

3.1. Demographic Characteristics

A total of 245 individuals participated in the questionnaire, which included 125 veterinarians and 120 clients. In terms of age distribution, both veterinarians and clients were primarily concentrated in the 30–39 and 40–49 age groups (see Table 2). These groups accounted for 71.2% of veterinarians and 71.66% of clients. Only 8 veterinarians (6.4%) were over 50, while 14 clients (11.7%) were in this age group. Regarding gender distribution (see Table 2), most veterinarians and clients were female, with 56% of veterinarians and 95.8% of clients being women. Male clients only made up 4.2%. In the experiences of medical disputes category (see Table 2), a high percentage (90.4%) of veterinarians had experienced medical disputes. In contrast, only 33 clients (27.5%) reported having these experiences. When examining the outcomes of medical disputes experienced by respondents (see Table 2), it was found that nearly 50 veterinarians (40%) resolved disputes through simple communication. An additional 53 veterinarians (42.4%) resolved disputes through communication combined with financial compensation or reduced medical fees, totaling 82.4%. Of clients, 14 were unclear about the outcomes, while roughly 60% of disputes were resolved through simple communication or financial compensation/reduced fees. Concerning third-party intervention in dispute resolution, 22 veterinarians (17.6%) and 34 clients (28.3%) endeavored to resolve conflicts utilizing this approach. In most instances involving third-party participation, approximately sixteen veterinarians and eight clients reached agreements through mediation and financial compensation. In addition, one veterinarian and two clients settled medical disputes through third-party intervention and straightforward communication. Out of the 125 veterinarians surveyed, only 4% resorted to legal proceedings. Conversely, the clients demonstrated a higher propensity (20%) to pursue legal recourse even after engaging in third-party mediation.

Table 2. Demographic characteristics distribution of veterinarians and clients.

Characteristics	Veterinarians ($n = 125$)		Clients ($n = 120$)	
	N	%	N	%
Age				
20–29 years old	28	22.40%	20	16.67%
30–39 years old	55	44.00%	46	38.33%
40–49 years old	34	27.20%	40	33.33%
50–years old	8	6.40%	14	11.67%
Gender				
Male	55	44.00%	5	4.17%
Female	70	56.00%	115	95.83%
Experiences of medical disputes				
Experienced	113	90.40%	33	27.50%
Did not experience	12	9.60%	87	72.50%
Outcomes of medical disputes				
No idea	0	0.00%	14	11.67%
Resolved by simple communication.	50	40.00%	37	30.83%
Resolved by communication and reconciliation via money compensation or medical fee reduction.	53	42.40%	35	29.17%
Resolved/unresolved by third-party involvement/mediation.	22	17.60%	34	28.34%
-Resolved by third-party involvement/ mediation and simple communication.	1	0.80%	2	1.67%
-Resolved by third-party involvement/ mediation and reconciliation via money compensation or medical fee reduction.	16	12.80%	8	6.67%
-Unresolved even with third-party involvement and the complaint was filed in the court.	5	4.00%	24	20.00%

Veterinarians with medical dispute experience had an average age of 36.88 (SD = 8.31). In contrast, those without dispute experience had an average age of 31.50 years (SD = 7.99), which represents a statistically significant difference ($p = 0.03$). For clients, those with medical dispute experience had an average age of 37.76 years (SD = 8.63), while those without dispute experience had an average age of 38.98 years (SD = 9.28); however, no statistically significant difference was observed (see Table 3).

Table 3. Comparison of age differences between the subgroups of the stakeholder with and without medical dispute experience: the cases of veterinarians and clients.

Subgroups	Veterinarians' Age				Clients' Age			
	N (%)	Mean	SD	p	N (%)	Mean	SD	p
Experiences of medical disputes	113 (90.4%)	36.88	8.31	0.03 *	33 (27.5%)	37.76	8.67	0.05
Without experiences of medical disputes	12 (9.6%)	31.5	7.99		87 (72.5%)	38.98	9.28	

p value < 0.05 *.

3.2. Ranking of the Perceptions of Risk Factors for Inducing Medical Disputes in Six Dimensions

This study evaluated the respondents' perceptions of inducing medical dispute risk factors using a five-point Likert scale. The subsequent analysis involved the calculation of mean and standard deviation. Higher scores indicated a greater likelihood of a specific risk factor contributing to medical disputes. The six dimensions of risk factors for inducing medical disputes were arranged in descending order based on their mean scores (refer to Table 4). For example, veterinarians with medical dispute experience identified the attitudes of stakeholders during interactions, complaint management, and medical expenses as the top three contributing factors to the risk of medical disputes. In contrast, clients considered medical skills, complaints management, and medical expenses as the top three factors.

Table 4. Ranking of the perceptions of risk factors for inducing medical disputes in six dimensions for veterinarians and clients.

Dimensions of Risk Factors for Inducing Medical Disputes	Veterinarians						Clients					
	All		With Experiences of Medical Disputes				All		With Experiences of Medical Disputes			
	$n = 125$		Yes ($n = 113$)		No ($n = 12$)		$n = 120$		Yes ($n = 33$)		No ($n = 87$)	
	Mean	Rank [1]	Mean	Rank	Mean	Rank	Mean	Rank	Mean	Rank	Mean	Rank
Attitudes of stakeholders during interactions	4.26	1	4.27	1	4.23	4	4.09	4	4.12	4	4.08	3
Complaints management	4.20	2	4.19	2	4.25	3	4.45	2	4.6	2	4.39	2
Medical expenses	4.18	3	4.17	3	4.28	2	4.10	3	4.23	3	4.05	4
Medical skills	4.13	4	4.12	4	4.29	1	4.64	1	4.71	1	4.61	1
Clients' perspectives	4.07	5	4.06	5	4.17	5	3.88	6	3.89	6	3.88	6
Modes of communication	3.98	6	3.98	6	4.01	6	3.99	5	3.98	5	3.99	5

[1] Rank by the mean from highest to lowest.

Meaningful comparisons were observed between the top risk factors for inducing medical disputes recognized by veterinarians and clients. Veterinarians regarded attitudes during interactions between veterinarians and clients as the primary risk factor leading to medical disputes, while clients identified medical skills as the main factor (see Table 4). Interestingly, younger veterinarians without medical dispute experience exhibited views similar to those of clients concerning the risk levels associated with factors contributing to medical disputes (see Table 4).

3.3. Differences in Perception of Risk Factors for Inducing Medical Disputes between Veterinarians and Clients

Veterinarians and clients demonstrated statistically significant differences in the perceptions of four risk factor dimensions induced by medical disputes (see Table 5). For instance, clients assigned noticeably higher scores in specific dimensions of inducing medical dispute risk factors, such as medical skills (clients: 4.64 ± 0.55; veterinarians: 4.13 ± 0.84, $p < 0.001$) and complaints management (clients: 4.45 ± 0.61; veterinarians: 4.20 ± 0.60, $p = 0.002$). Conversely, veterinarians perceived the risk level of stakeholders' attitudes during interactions leading to medical disputes to be significantly higher than that of clients (veterinarians: 4.26 ± 0.57, clients: 4.09 ± 0.70, $p = 0.038$), and also, believed that clients' perspectives posed a significantly higher risk of medical disputes than the clients themselves acknowledged (veterinarians: 4.07 ± 0.65, clients: 3.88 ± 0.67, $p = 0.04$) (see Table 5).

Upon further analysis, by comparing perspectives based on medical dispute experience, both veterinarians and clients exhibited similar perceptions of the risk factor dimensions leading to medical disputes (see Table 5), particularly in the areas of medical skills (clients: 4.71 ± 0.48; veterinarians: 4.12 ± 0.85, $p < 0.001$) and complaints management (clients: 4.60 ± 0.53; veterinarians: 4.19 ± 0.6, $p < 0.001$). Clients assigned significantly higher scores in these two dimensions seemed to agree on the risk level associated with these factors. Although veterinarians' scores for complaints management appeared lower than those of the clients, experienced veterinarians ranked it as the second-highest risk factor for medical disputes, suggesting that they also placed considerable importance on this aspect (see Table 5). However, the medical dispute risk factor of medical skills was ranked fourth by veterinarians. Despite this, the dimension's score was still above four (likely to induce medical disputes), indicating that veterinarians recognized its importance, but held a different view than that of the clients regarding ranking and evaluation (see Table 5).

Table 5. Differences in perception of risk factors for inducing medical disputes between veterinarians and clients by experiences of medical disputes.

Dimensions of Risk Factors for Inducing Medical Disputes	All					With Experiences of Medical Disputes				
	Veterinarians n = 125		Clients n = 120		p	Veterinarians n = 113		Clients n = 33		p
	Mean	SD	Mean	SD		Mean	SD	Mean	SD	
Attitudes of stakeholders during interactions	4.26	0.57	4.09	0.70	0.038 *	4.27	0.59	4.12	0.68	0.229
Complaints management	4.20	0.6	4.45	0.61	0.002 **	4.19	0.6	4.6	0.53	0.001 **
Medical expenses	4.18	0.67	4.10	0.83	0.414	4.17	0.68	4.23	0.81	0.648
Medical skills	4.13	0.84	4.64	0.55	<0.001 ***	4.12	0.85	4.71	0.48	<0.001 ***
Clients' perspectives	4.07	0.65	3.88	0.76	0.04 *	4.06	0.64	3.89	0.72	0.204
Modes of communication	3.98	0.56	3.99	0.67	0.909	3.98	0.56	3.98	0.74	0.953

p value < 0.05 *; p value < 0.01 **; p value < 0.001 ***.

3.4. The Perceptions of Veterinarians and Clients on Possible Solutions to Reduce the Medical Disputes Risk

In the third section of the questionnaire, utilizing a five-point Likert scale, this study assessed the perceptions of veterinarians and clients of fifteen potential solutions for reducing the risk of medical disputes (see Table 6). Table 6 lists the potential solutions and the dimensions they belong to and the abbreviations of the solutions. In addition, the fifteen possible solutions for reducing medical disputes could be grouped into six dimensions: medical skills, modes of communication, the attitudes of stakeholders during interactions, medical expenses, complaints management, and training and education.

Table 6. The abbreviation of possible solutions for medical disputes.

Dimensions	Possible Solutions for Reducing the Medical Dispute Risks	Abbreviations
Medical skill	Encourage veterinarians to improve their medical skills through on-the-job training and seminars.	Impr_MS
	Use checklists during the diagnostic and treatment to avoid overlooking details and mistakes.	Use_CL
	To prevent errors and disputes, encourage veterinarians to use forms or records and provide clear instructions during patient handoffs.	Handoffs
Modes of communication	Design educational materials like pamphlets or brochures with disease-related information to increase clients' understanding, reduce misunderstandings, and avoid negligence.	Des_Mate
	Inform clients of the potential risks and treatment outcomes related to patients' diseases, enabling them to make informed decisions.	Info_OC
	Explain the risks and have clients sign a consent form before performing surgical procedures or treating critically ill patients.	Cons_Form
	Ensure mutual confirmation and agreement on subsequent treatment and provide written information to clients, even for non-surgical or non-critical incidents.	Writ_Info

Table 6. *Cont.*

Dimensions	Possible Solutions for Reducing the Medical Dispute Risks	Abbreviations
Attitudes of stakeholders during interactions	Encourage veterinarians to express empathy and compassion during interactions with clients.	Emp_Compa
	Encourage clients to express their concerns and questions clearly, allowing veterinarians to address them promptly, thereby increasing trust.	Ques_Expres
Medical expenses	Provide clients with a possible cost range estimate before starting treatment and explain it clearly.	Cost_Esti
Complaints management	Offer continuing education courses for colleagues, such as clinical communication, handling customer complaints, and medical disputes.	CC_Course
	Address complaints promptly to reduce negative impacts.	Addr_CC
Education and training	Organize public education seminars by the clinic or veterinary organizations to educate clients on proper pet care practices and effective communication with veterinarians.	Edu_Client
	Organize in-house employee training to improve communication skills, such as practical discussions and case study.	In_House
	Add education courses related to medical disputes and customer complaints, such as communication skills and handling customer complaints, to the veterinary curriculum at universities.	Uni_Course

The subsequent analysis involved calculating the mean and standard deviation, with higher scores signifying a greater likelihood of a solution effectively reducing the medical dispute risks evaluated by veterinarians and clients. The top five solutions were then arranged in descending order based on their mean scores for veterinarians and clients (see Table 7).

Table 7. Ranking of the perceptions of possible solutions for veterinarians and clients.

Rank [1]	Veterinarians			Clients		
	All $n = 125$	With Experiences of Medical Disputes		All $n = 120$	With Experiences of Medical Disputes	
		Yes ($n = 113$)	No ($n = 12$)		Yes ($n = 33$)	No ($n = 87$)
Top 1 (Mean)	Cost_Esti (4.42)	Cost_Esti (4.40)	Cost_Esti (4.67)	Cons_Form (4.76)	Cons_Form (4.88)	Cons_Form (4.71)
Top 2 (Mean)	Emp_Compa (4.39)	Info_OC (4.39)	Emp_Compa (4.58)	Ques_Expres (4.73)	Info_OC (4.88)	Ques_Expres (4.70)
Top 3 (Mean)	Ques_Expres (4.38)	Emp_Compa (4.37)	Ques_Expres (4.42)	Info_OC (4.71)	Writ_Info (4.88)	Cost_Esti (4.68)
Top 4 (Mean)	Info_OC (4.36)	Ques_Expres (4.37)	Addr_CC (4.42)	Handoffs (4.68)	Addr_CC (4.82)	Handoffs (4.66)
Top 5 (Mean)	Addr_CC (4.31)	Addr_CC (4.30)	Writ_Info (4.42)	Addr_CC (4.67)	Ques_Expres (4.79)	Emp_Compa (4.66)

[1] Rank by the mean from highest to lowest.

For instance, veterinarians regarded "Providing clients with a possible cost range estimate before starting treatment and explaining it clearly (Cost_Esti)" as the most effective solution (see Table 7), followed by "Encouraging veterinarians to express empathy and compassion during interactions with clients (Emp_Compa)" and "Urging clients to articulate their concerns and questions clearly, allowing veterinarians to address them promptly and thereby increasing trust (Ques_Expres)". Additionally, veterinarians with medical dispute experience ranked "Informing clients of potential risks and treatment outcomes related to patients' diseases, enabling them to make informed decisions (Info_OC)" as the second most effective solution. However, different from the viewpoints of veterinarians, clients identified "Explaining risks and having clients sign a consent form before performing surgical procedures or treating critically ill patients (Cons_Fo)" as the most effective solution (see Table 7).

The study also included one open-ended question to gather other potential solutions. Thirty-two respondents (13%) provided valuable insights, with sixteen veterinarians and sixteen clients, summarized as three key points:

Point 1: The importance of communication courses and training. As mentioned by ten veterinarians and ten clients, the main suggestions were as follows: "Offer communication skills, empathy-related courses, or psychology-related courses to hospital staff, veterinarians, and future veterinary students to develop empathy and communication skills" (38-year-old, female client), "Enhance the cooperative relationship between medical personnel and clients through regular training and health education, fostering mutual trust and achieving a win-win situation" (36-year-old, female client), and "Emphasize the importance of empathy among veterinarians and staff, as pets are considered family members by their owners" (56-year-old, female client).

Point 2: Having enough time and information for communication and decision making. As mentioned by five veterinarians and seven clients, the main suggestions were as follows: "Implement an appointment system to provide sufficient communication time for both parties" (36-year-old, male veterinarian) and "Involve clients in medical decision-making (Shared Decision Making) to encourage informed decision-making and shared responsibility" (43-year-old, male veterinarian).

Point 3: Surveillance video systems. As mentioned by two veterinarians and one clients, the main suggestion was as follows: "Install surveillance video systems in clinics to document treatment procedures." (51-year-old, female veterinarian).

These suggestions were condensed into three possible solutions: "Time Management and Appointment Control", "Install Surveillance Systems in Clinics to Document Treatment Procedures", and "Involve Clients in Decision-Making (Shared Decision Making)". We summarized these potential solutions recommendations with valuable insights into critical facets/items according to six dimensions and presented them in Table 8.

Table 8. Modified possible solutions to reduce the medical dispute risks.

Dimensions	Possible Solutions for Reducing the Medical Dispute Risks
Medical skill	Encourage veterinarians to improve their medical skills through on-the-job training and seminars.
	Use checklists during the diagnostic and treatment to avoid overlooking details and mistakes.
	To prevent errors and disputes, encourage veterinarians to use forms or records, and provide clear instructions during patient handoffs.
Modes of communication	Design educational materials, such as pamphlets or brochures with disease-related information, to increase clients' understanding, reduce misunderstandings, and avoid negligence.
	Inform clients of the potential risks and treatment outcomes related to patients' diseases, enabling them to make informed decisions.
	Explain the risks and have clients sign a consent form before performing surgical procedures or treating critically ill patients.
	Ensure mutual confirmation and agreement on subsequent treatment and provide written information to clients, even for non-surgical or non-critical incidents.
	Control appointment times and allow enough time for communication between veterinarians and clients. (Newly added,)
	Involve clients in decision-making to increase trust and collaboration (shared decision making). (Newly added.)
	Install surveillance systems in clinics to document treatment procedures for records. (Newly added.)

Table 8. *Cont.*

Dimensions	Possible Solutions for Reducing the Medical Dispute Risks
Attitudes of stakeholders during interactions	Encourage veterinarians to express empathy and compassion during interactions with clients.
	Encourage clients to express their concerns and questions clearly, allowing veterinarians to address them promptly, thereby increasing trust.
Medical expenses	Provide clients with a possible cost range estimate before starting treatment and explain it clearly.
Complaints management	Offer continuing education courses for colleagues, such as clinical communication, handling customer complaints, and medical disputes.
	Address complaints promptly to reduce negative impacts.
Education and training	Organize public education seminars by the clinic or veterinary organizations to educate clients on proper pet care practices and effective communication with veterinarians.
	Organize in-house employee training to improve communication skills, such as practical discussions and case study.
	Add education courses related to medical disputes and customer complaints, such as communication skills and handling customer complaints, to veterinary curriculums at universities.

4. Discussion

The present study examined the perceptions of risk factors and possible solutions for medical disputes between veterinarians and clients, revealing several noteworthy findings. The results noted shared perspectives between the two groups on certain elements, yet there were marked differences in their perceptions regarding the risk factors that could instigate medical disputes and potential solutions to alleviate them.

4.1. Age and Medical Dispute Experience

One interesting observation was the significant difference in age between veterinarians with and without medical dispute experience. This observation might be explained by the fact that older veterinarians are more likely to have encountered many more cases. Therefore, the risk of conflicts is much higher due to the number of cases handled.

Previous research has indicated that older physicians may possess more clinical experience. Those with more years of practice may encounter more medical disputes due to their exposure to more cases [29,42]. According to the findings by Hickson et al., there was no significant difference in the risk of complaints between physicians aged 26–35 and those aged ≤25. However, older practitioners faced a 1.5-to-2.1-times-higher risk of receiving complaints, which generally increases with age [29]. Nevertheless, veterinarians with more years of practice may have more medical skills experience, enabling them to identify risks of complaints earlier and address them promptly, potentially reducing their likelihood of encountering medical disputes [18,28,43].

Fortunately, to mitigate the risk of medical disputes, relying solely on age or years of practice to accumulate skills and experience handling these issues is unnecessary. Through practical training and sharing case experiences, understanding clients' needs and expectations can effectively reduce complaints and medical disputes. Veterinarians with continuous education can significantly improve their abilities in preventing disputes and managing complaints [11,22,31,32,43].

4.2. Perceptions of Risk Factors for Inducing Medical Dispute Risks

Veterinarians and clients exhibited differing perceptions of risk factors for inducing medical disputes. Veterinarians emphasized the attitudes of stakeholders during interactions, while the clients were more concerned about medical skills. Intriguingly, younger veterinarians without medical dispute experience shared similar perspectives to those of clients regarding the risk levels associated with factors contributing to medical disputes. A cross-sectional study conducted between 2014 and 2022 found that young veterinarians and veterinary students with no dispute experience often perceive medical skills as the primary risk factor for medical disputes [24]. This divergence in perspectives might stem from experienced veterinarians' professional knowledge and experience, making them consider the importance of communication in maintaining positive relationships with clients [2,6,23]. Moreover, a 1995 study in Taiwan by Yang et al. investigated the perspectives of 99 clients to determine the criteria for a "good veterinarian". The main factors identified were "accurate diagnosis" and "detailed explanation". These findings imply that clients generally lack medical expertise and might prioritize veterinarians' technical competence in treating their pet patients [34]. Interestingly, these results coincide with the findings of the current study. However, numerous studies highlight that although a lack of medical expertise contributes to the risk of medical disputes, ineffective communication with clients represents the most significant factor. Poor communication can undermine trust and hinder establishing a robust collaborative relationship, ultimately leading to clients' complaints and potential medical disputes [6,9,10,14,22,23].

4.3. Perceptions of Possible Solutions to Reduce Medical Dispute Risks

Both veterinarians and clients identified potential solutions for reducing medical dispute risks, with similarities and differences in their preferences. For instance, providing cost estimates and fostering empathy and compassion were highly valued by veterinarians, while obtaining informed consent and providing written information were considered to be crucial by clients [23,34].

Studies concerning reducing the number of client complaints and medical dispute risks have emphasized explaining medical costs. Communication skills and training methods in human medicine and veterinary medicine are similar, as both aim to improve the interactions between healthcare providers and professionals dedicated to enhancing patients' health [30].

Empathy, a fundamental communication skill, is particularly relevant when one is discussing medical costs. Providing detailed explanations of costs ensures that clients understand the expenses and prognosis, allowing them to accept the proposed treatment's financial implications [10,17,18,23,30]. Moreover, research on increasing client satisfaction indicates that when veterinarians establish trust with clients, client satisfaction improves, as does job satisfaction and the sense of accomplishment for veterinarians [44].

The open-ended responses provided additional insights into potential strategies for reducing medical disputes, such as time management and appointment control, installing surveillance systems in clinics [2,9], and involving clients in decision making [6,23,45]. However, research has shown that the duration of each visit may not necessarily be related to client satisfaction with the veterinarian. Instead, open-ended questions during communication allow the clients to express their concerns and doubts [4,6,23]. In addition, effective communication and time management in appointment systems can be achieved through the expertise and experience of veterinarians [44]. Lastly, veterinary-related research on shared decision making often stems from the significant knowledge gap between veterinarians and clients. Veterinarians must provide relevant knowledge and specific advice, express support, and enable clients to make informed decisions [6,45].

These preferences may reflect each group's priorities and concerns, with veterinarians being focusing on clear communication and compassionate care, and clients emphasizing transparency and shared decision making in their pets' treatment. These suggestions underscore the importance of improving communication between veterinarians and clients, enhancing the transparency of treatment procedures and fostering a collaborative approach to healthcare.

4.4. Limitations and Implications for Future Research

The findings of this study have important implications for veterinary practice, as they emphasize the need for effective communication, empathy, and shared decision making in the prevention and resolution of medical disputes. Veterinary professionals should be aware of these factors and consider implementing strategies to address them, such as providing cost estimates, obtaining informed consent, and offering written information to clients.

Despite its valuable insights, the study bears several constraints that warrant consideration. Initially, the investigation was conducted in Taiwan, characterized by a comparatively diminutive veterinarian population relative to those of other nations. Consequently, the applicability of the findings to countries with divergent healthcare frameworks and cultural contexts might be limited. Secondly, the study hinged on self-reported data, potentially rendering it susceptible to social desirability bias. This might have led participants to furnish responses that are perceived to be socially acceptable, rather than those that genuinely mirror their authentic perceptions. Alternatively, exploring human psycho-social and emotional contexts presents considerable challenges. Nonetheless, undertaking comparative analyses in these domains could be of significant importance. The same sentiment could not be expected from clients who lost their companion animals and someone whose animals only spent a long time hospitalized due to a medical error. Gaining insights into these factors could provide a valuable understanding of the reasons behind evolving perceptions.

As a result, this method precluded the extraction of more profound insights from the study. Ultimately, despite the frequent use of the Likert scale to obtain interval data within medical research, it is intrinsically ordinal. Consequently, the data were analyzed according to the median rather than the mean, a factor that could potentially impact the interpretation of the findings.

Despite these constraints, the study offers invaluable perspectives into the understanding of risk factors instigating medical disputes between veterinarians and clients. Future investigations may delve into the elements contributing to the risk perception among diverse stakeholders, compare the perception of risk factors inciting medical disputes across different countries, and scrutinize the efficacy of potential solutions aimed at mitigating the risk of medical disputes. Furthermore, a future study could be designed that selects participants who have previously handled or were involved in medical disputes and excludes non-experienced participants. Future investigations could additionally explore the effectiveness of various continuing education programs in cultivating practical communication competencies and complaint management techniques among emerging veterinarians. In conclusion, an understanding of clients' perceptions can foster enhanced relationships and elevate the quality of care provided to companion animals, diminish the likelihood of medical disputes, and improve the expertise of veterinary practitioners.

In conclusion, this study offers valuable insights into the perceptions of risk factors and possible solutions for medical disputes between veterinarians and clients. The findings highlight the importance of communication, empathy, and shared decision making in preventing and resolving medical disputes and suggest potential avenues for further research and practical interventions to enhance the quality of care in veterinary practice. Collaborative efforts between veterinarians and clients can contribute to more effective communication, greater transparency, and improved client satisfaction, ultimately leading to decreased medical disputes and a better overall experience for both parties. By fostering a strong partnership between veterinarians and clients, it is possible to achieve high-quality care and better outcomes for companion animals.

Author Contributions: Conceptualization, Z.-F.C., Y.-H.E.H., J.-J.L. and C.-H.C.; data curation, Z.-F.C. and Y.-H.E.H.; investigation, Z.-F.C.; methodology, Z.-F.C., Y.-H.E.H., J.-J.L. and C.-H.C.; project administration, Z.-F.C.; resources, Y.-H.E.H. and C.-H.C.; supervision, Y.-H.E.H., J.-J.L. and C.-H.C.; validation, Y.-H.E.H. and C.-H.C.; writing—original draft, Z.-F.C.; writing—review and editing, Y.-H.E.H., J.-J.L. and C.-H.C. All authors have read and agreed to the published version of the manuscript.

Funding: This research received no external funding.

Institutional Review Board Statement: The protocol was approved by Research Ethics Committee of National Taiwan University. The committee is organized under and operates in accordance with

Social and Behavioral Research Ethical Principles and Regulations of National Taiwan University and government laws and regulations (NTU-REC No.: 202209HS024 and date of approval: from 11 October 2022 to 31 July 2023).

Informed Consent Statement: Informed consent was obtained from all subjects involved in the study.

Data Availability Statement: Not applicable.

Conflicts of Interest: The authors declare no conflict of interest.

References

1. Milani, M. Client-animal relationship-based communication. *Can. Vet. J.* **2016**, *57*, 1293–1294. [PubMed]
2. Gibson, J.; White, K.; Mossop, L.; Oxtoby, C.; Brennan, M. 'We're gonna end up scared to do anything': A qualitative exploration of how client complaints are experienced by UK veterinary practitioners. *Vet. Rec.* **2022**, *191*, e1737. [CrossRef] [PubMed]
3. Quartarone, V.; Russo, M.; Fazio, A.; Passantino, A. Mediation for medical malpractice actions: An efficient approach to the law and veterinary care. *Open J. Anim. Sci.* **2011**, *1*, 61–64. [CrossRef]
4. Gregório, H.; Santos, P.; Pires, I.; Prada, J.; Queiroga, F.L. Comparison of veterinary health services expectations and perceptions between oncologic pet owners, non-oncologic pet owners and veterinary staff using the SERVQUAL methodology. *Vet. World* **2016**, *9*, 1275. [CrossRef] [PubMed]
5. Lyu, S.Y.; Liao, C.K.; Chang, K.P.; Tsai, S.T.; Lee, M.B.; Tsai, F.C. Analysis of medical litigation among patients with medical disputes in cosmetic surgery in Taiwan. *Aesthetic Plast. Surg.* **2011**, *35*, 764–772. [CrossRef]
6. Stansfield, E. Using interpersonal skills to manage challenging client behaviour. *Companion Anim.* **2023**, *28*, 2–7. [CrossRef]
7. Wojtacka, J.; Grudzień, W.; Wysok, B.; Szarek, J. Causes of stress and conflict in the veterinary professional workplace—A perspective from Poland. *Ir. Vet. J.* **2020**, *73*, 23. [CrossRef]
8. Gardner, D.H.; Hini, D. Work-related stress in the veterinary profession in New Zealand. *N. Z. Vet. J.* **2006**, *54*, 119–124. [CrossRef]
9. Russell, E.; Mossop, L.; Forbes, E.; Oxtoby, C. Uncovering the 'messy details' of veterinary communication: An analysis of communication problems in cases of alleged professional negligence. *Vet. Rec.* **2022**, *190*, e1068. [CrossRef]
10. Gordon, S.J.G.; Gardner, D.H.; Weston, J.F.; Bolwell, C.F.; Benschop, J.; Parkinson, T.J. Quantitative and thematic analysis of complaints by clients against clinical veterinary practitioners in New Zealand. *NZVJ* **2019**, *67*, 117–125. [CrossRef]
11. O'Connell, D.; Bonvicini, K.A. Addressing disappointment in veterinary practice. *Vet. Clin.* **2007**, *37*, 135–149. [CrossRef]
12. Shaw, J.R.; Adams, C.L.; Bonnett, B.N. What can veterinarians learn from studies of physician-patient communication about veterinarian-client-patient communication? *J. Am. Vet. Med. Assoc.* **2004**, *224*, 676–684. [CrossRef]
13. Levinson, W.; Roter, D.L.; Mullooly, J.P.; Dull, V.T.; Frankel, R.M. Physician-patient communication: The relationship with malpractice claims among primary care physicians and surgeons. *JAMA* **1997**, *277*, 553–559. [CrossRef]
14. Rogers, C.W.; Murphy, L.A.; Murphy, R.A.; Malouf, K.A.; Natsume, R.E.; Ward, B.D.; Tansey, C.; Nakamura, R.K. An analysis of client complaints and their effects on veterinary support staff. *Vet. Med. Sci.* **2022**, *8*, 925–934. [CrossRef]
15. Park, R.M.; Gruen, M.E.; Royal, K. Association between Dog Owner Demographics and Decision to Seek Veterinary Care. *Vet. Sci.* **2021**, *8*, 7. [CrossRef]
16. Chen, Z.-F.; Hsu, Y.-H.E.; Lee, J.-J.; Chou, C.-H. Bibliometric Analysis of Veterinary Communication Education Research over the Last Two Decades: Rare Yet Essential. *Vet. Sci.* **2022**, *9*, 256. [CrossRef]
17. Kipperman, B.S.; Kass, P.H.; Rishniw, M. Factors that influence small animal veterinarians' opinions and actions regarding cost of care and effects of economic limitations on patient care and outcome and professional career satisfaction and burnout. *J. Am. Vet. Med. Assoc.* **2017**, *250*, 785–794. [CrossRef]
18. Coe, J.B.; Adams, C.L.; Bonnett, B.N. A focus group study of veterinarians' and pet owners' perceptions of the monetary aspects of veterinary care. *J. Am. Vet. Med. Assoc.* **2007**, *231*, 1510–1518. [CrossRef]
19. Bryce, A.R.; Rossi, T.A.; Tansey, C.; Murphy, R.A.; Murphy, L.A.; Nakamura, R.K. Effect of client complaints on small animal veterinary internists. *J. Small Anim. Pract.* **2019**, *60*, 167–172. [CrossRef]
20. Wu, Y.; Jiang, F.; Ma, J.; Tang, Y.L.; Wang, M.; Liu, Y. Experience of medical disputes, medical disturbances, verbal and physical violence, and burnout among physicians in China. *Front. Psychol.* **2021**, *11*, 556517. [CrossRef]
21. Wan, S.-Y.; Tsai, P.-Y.; Lo, L.-J. Quantifying Perceived Facial Asymmetry to Enhance Physician–Patient Communications. *Appl. Sci.* **2021**, *11*, 8398. [CrossRef]
22. Shaw, J.R.; Barley, G.E.; Hill, A.E.; Larson, S.; Roter, D.L. Communication skills education onsite in a veterinary practice. *Patient Educ. Couns.* **2010**, *80*, 337–344. [CrossRef] [PubMed]
23. Coe, J.B.; Adams, C.L.; Bonnett, B.N. A focus group study of veterinarians' and pet owners' perceptions of veterinarian-client communication in companion animal practice. *J. Am. Vet. Med. Assoc.* **2008**, *233*, 1072–1080. [CrossRef] [PubMed]
24. Chen, Z.-F.; Hsu, Y.-H.E.; Lee, J.-J.; Chou, C.-H. Perceptions of Veterinarians and Veterinary Students on What Risk Factors Constitute Medical Disputes and Comparisons between 2014 and 2022. *Vet. Sci.* **2023**, *10*, 200. [CrossRef]
25. Pun, J.K. An integrated review of the role of communication in veterinary clinical practice. *BMC Vet. Res.* **2020**, *16*, 394. [CrossRef]
26. Garforth, C.J.; Bailey, A.P.; Tranter, R.B. Farmers' attitudes to disease risk management in England: A comparative analysis of sheep and pig farmers. *Prev. Vet. Med.* **2013**, *110*, 456–466. [CrossRef]

27. Jansen, J.; Steuten, C.D.M.; Renes, R.J.; Aarts, N.; Lam, T.J.G.M. Debunking the myth of the hard-to-reach farmer: Effective communication on udder health. *J. Dairy Sci.* **2010**, *93*, 1296–1306. [CrossRef]
28. Irwin, A. Managing client complaints: Identifying and mitigating their detrimental impacts on veterinary practitioners. *Vet. Rec.* **2022**, *191*, 157–159. [CrossRef]
29. Spittal, M.J.; Bismark, M.M.; Studdert, D.M. Identification of practitioners at high risk of complaints to health profession regulators. *BMC Health Serv. Res.* **2019**, *19*, 380. [CrossRef]
30. Hamood, W.J.; Chur-Hansen, A.; McArthur, M.L. A qualitative study to explore communication skills in veterinary medical education. *Int. J. Med. Educ.* **2014**, *5*, 193–198. [CrossRef]
31. Duijn, C.; Bok, H.; Kremer, W. Qualified but not yet fully competent: Perceptions of recent veterinary graduates on their day-one skills. *Vet. Rec.* **2020**, *186*, 216. [CrossRef]
32. Latham, C.E.; Morris, A. Effects of formal training in communication skills on the ability of veterinary students to communicate with clients. *Vet. Rec.* **2007**, *160*, 181–186. [CrossRef]
33. Hsu, Y.-H.E. Innovation Communication Education in Veterinary Medicine: A Client-Centered Model. In *NSTC Medical Education Conference*, 1st ed.; Government Research Bulletin; National Science and Technology Council: Tainan, Taiwan, 2014; pp. 125–130. Available online: https://www.grb.gov.tw/search/planDetail?id=3170065&docId=426656 (accessed on 13 July 2022).
34. Yang, H.L.; Huang, H.P.; Liang, S.L.; Chen, H.Y.; Lai, S.S. Studies of the Owner-Pet and Veterinarian-Client Relationships in Taipei Area: A Survey in National Taiwan University Veterinary Hospital. *Taiwan Vet. J.* **1995**, *21*, 316–325. [CrossRef]
35. May, T.W.; Pfäfflin, M.; Bien, C.G.; Hamer, H.M.; Holtkamp, M.; Rating, D.; Schulze-Bonhage, A.; Straub, H.B.; Strzelczyk, A.; Thorbecke, R. Attitudes toward epilepsy assessed by the SAPE questionnaire in Germany—Comparison of its psychometric properties and results in a web-based vs. face-to-face survey. *Epilepsy Behav.* **2022**, *130*, 108665. [CrossRef]
36. Jakobsson, U. Statistical presentation and analysis of ordinal data in nursing research. *Scand. J. Caring Sci.* **2004**, *18*, 437–440. [CrossRef]
37. South, L.; Saffo, D.; Vitek, O.; Dunne, C.; Borkin, M.A. Effective use of Likert scales in visualization evaluations: A systematic review. *Comput. Graph Forum.* **2022**, *41*, 43–55. [CrossRef]
38. Lewis, J.R. Multipoint scales: Mean and median differences and observed significance levels. *Int. J. Hum. Comput. Int.* **1993**, *5*, 383–392. [CrossRef]
39. Bentley, H.; Lee, J.; Supersad, A.; Yu, H.; Dobson, J.L.; Wong, S.A.; Stewart, M.; Vatturi, S.S.; Lebel, K.; Crivellaro, P.; et al. Preparedness of residents and medical students for the transition to competence by design in diagnostic radiology post-graduate medical education. *Can. Assoc. Radiol. J.* **2023**, *74*, 241–250. [CrossRef]
40. Senos, R.; Leite, C.A.R.; dos Santos Tolezano, F.; Roberto-Rodrigues, M.; Pérez, W. Using videos in active learning: An experience in veterinary anatomy. *Anat. Histol. Embryol.* **2022**, *52*, 50–54. [CrossRef]
41. Schoenfeld-Tacher, R.M.; Dorman, D.C. Effect of Delivery Format on Student Outcomes and Perceptions of a Veterinary Medicine Course: Synchronous versus Asynchronous Learning. *Vet. Sci.* **2021**, *8*, 13. [CrossRef]
42. Hickson, G.B.; Federspiel, C.F.; Pichert, J.W.; Miller, C.S.; Gauld-Jaeger, J.; Bost, P. Patient Complaints and Malpractice Risk. *JAMA* **2002**, *287*, 2951–2957. [CrossRef] [PubMed]
43. Mellanby, R.J.; Herrtage, M.E. Survey of mistakes made by recent veterinary graduates. *Vet. Rec.* **2004**, *11*, 761–765.
44. Shaw, J.R.; Adams, C.L.; Bonnett, B.N.; Larson, S.; Roter, D.L. Veterinarian satisfaction with companion animal visits. *J. Am. Vet. Med. Assoc.* **2012**, *240*, 832–841. [CrossRef] [PubMed]
45. Christiansen, S.B.; Kristensen, A.T.; Lassen, J.; Sandøe, P. Veterinarians' role in clients' decision-making regarding seriously ill companion animal patients. *Acta Vet. Scand.* **2015**, *58*, 30. [CrossRef]

Disclaimer/Publisher's Note: The statements, opinions and data contained in all publications are solely those of the individual author(s) and contributor(s) and not of MDPI and/or the editor(s). MDPI and/or the editor(s) disclaim responsibility for any injury to people or property resulting from any ideas, methods, instructions or products referred to in the content.

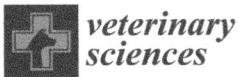

Article

The Current State of Veterinary Toxicology Education at AAVMC Member Veterinary Schools

David C. Dorman [1], Robert H. Poppenga [2] and Regina M. Schoenfeld-Tacher [1,*]

[1] Department of Molecular Biosciences, College of Veterinary Medicine, North Carolina State University, Raleigh, NC 27607, USA
[2] California Animal Health and Food Safety Laboratory, School of Veterinary Medicine, University of California, Davis, CA 95616, USA
* Correspondence: regina_schoenfeld@ncsu.edu

Simple Summary: Veterinary student education in toxicology is important. This study surveyed individuals affiliated with veterinary schools that are members of the Association of American Veterinary Medical Colleges. The online survey was designed to collect information about the credentials of the faculty that teach toxicology at veterinary schools, the topics that they include in their coursework, and faculty assessments regarding how prepared new graduates are at performing professional activities related to clinical toxicology. Nearly half of all schools provided a response to our survey. We found that toxicology was included as part of all veterinary school coursework. Toxicology classes across the different programs shared similar content. Most respondents to our survey felt that most of their students were prepared to perform professional activities related to veterinary toxicology.

Abstract: This study assessed the depth, breadth, and perception of toxicology education in curricula at Association of American Veterinary Medical Colleges (AAVMC) member veterinary schools. An online questionnaire was sent twice to all 54 AAVMC members and sent once to a veterinary toxicology list serve. The survey covered areas related to instructor demographics, the depth and extent of toxicology taught, and the respondent's perceptions of their student's ability to perform entrustable professional activities (EPA). Results were analyzed using descriptive statistics. Our survey resulted in a 44% response rate. All responding schools included toxicology in their curriculum, and it was a required course in 23 programs. Contact hours in stand-alone veterinary toxicology courses ranged from 14 to 45 h. Most respondents indicated that the current time allotted for toxicology was inadequate, despite indicating that most of their students could perform most EPAs autonomously. One exception related to the ability of students to analyze toxicology data. We found small variations in teaching methods and curriculum content. The results of our study can assist veterinary schools in evaluating their curricula to better prepare new graduates for the management of toxicology issues they may face in their veterinary careers.

Keywords: curriculum; veterinary; toxicology; competency-based veterinary education; entrustable professional activities

Citation: Dorman, D.C.; Poppenga, R.H.; Schoenfeld-Tacher, R.M. The Current State of Veterinary Toxicology Education at AAVMC Member Veterinary Schools. *Vet. Sci.* **2022**, *9*, 652. https://doi.org/10.3390/vetsci9120652

Academic Editors: Simona Sacchini and Ayoze Castro-Alonso

Received: 27 October 2022
Accepted: 17 November 2022
Published: 22 November 2022

Publisher's Note: MDPI stays neutral with regard to jurisdictional claims in published maps and institutional affiliations.

Copyright: © 2022 by the authors. Licensee MDPI, Basel, Switzerland. This article is an open access article distributed under the terms and conditions of the Creative Commons Attribution (CC BY) license (https:// creativecommons.org/licenses/by/ 4.0/).

1. Introduction

Toxicology is an experimental science that investigates the fate of chemicals in the body, the mode of action of chemicals, and the adverse effects they induce. Veterinary toxicology has both basic (e.g., comparative toxicology) and clinical (e.g., veterinary clinical toxicology) science components. In many veterinary school curricula, students initially focus on the basic sciences, while later in their training, the focus shifts to clinical sciences. Thus, toxicology instruction, like training in pharmacology [1], should span these stages of veterinary education.

Domestic animals and wildlife can be exposed to a vast array of potential toxicants, including human and veterinary medications; illicit drugs; toxic plants, mycotoxins, algal toxins, and microbial toxins; pesticides; toxic metals and metalloids; and a variety of household products and industrial chemicals. The effects of toxicants can vary amongst different animal species. For example, exposure to the mycotoxin fumonisin is associated with equine leukoencephalomalacia and a pulmonary edema syndrome in swine [2]. The diversity of animal species that may be exposed to these agents and important species differences in response distinguishes veterinary from human toxicology.

Core concepts in toxicology as well as the diverse set of potentially toxic agents and animal species of interest to veterinarians make the design of a curriculum in veterinary toxicology challenging. Information regarding the current state of the toxicology curricula in professional veterinary programs in the United States and elsewhere is scarce. Toxicologists engaged in education and affiliated with either the American Board of Veterinary Toxicology (ABVT) or the American Academy of Veterinary and Comparative Toxicology developed a priority listing of fundamental concepts and knowledge that entry-level veterinarians should possess [3]. This included nine concepts (e.g., biotransformation, diagnosis, dose–response) and 73 agents (e.g., acetaminophen, botulism, lead) or classes of agents (e.g., cardiac glycoside-containing plants, ionophores, mycotoxins) with various effects in different animal species. The methods used in identifying and prioritizing these agents were not provided. This proposed curriculum did not consider the amount of time needed for delivery. A conservative estimate that each core concept could require one hour of instruction and each agent or agent class another 15 min yields a total of approximately 27 h of instruction. Development of toxicology curricula at veterinary schools could also be informed by efforts in human toxicology. Consensus-based lists of core topics that should be included in curricula for medical toxicology clerkships in medical schools have been proposed [4–6]. One proposed curriculum includes over 200 agents or classes of agents in addition to an extensive consideration of core concepts [5].

Veterinary education is increasingly focusing on assessing essential competencies in which trainees must become proficient before undertaking them independently [7]. To that end, a team of educators has proposed eight entrustable professional activities (EPAs) for the assessment of workplace activities deemed essential for veterinary practice [8,9]. These have been proposed as a practical framework for the implementation of competency-based education. An EPA is defined as "an essential task of a discipline that a learner can be trusted to perform with limited supervision in a given context and regulatory requirements, once sufficient competence has been demonstrated" [9]. The core EPAs help define Day One practice expectations for every veterinary graduate.

The ABVT recently formed an Education Committee to better inform the specialty on ways that veterinary toxicology is currently being taught at Association of American Veterinary Medical Colleges (AAVMC) member veterinary schools. Colleges and schools of veterinary medicine that seek to join the AAVMC must be accredited by the American Veterinary Medical Association (AVMA) Council on Education (COE). There are currently 54 AAVMC members, including all 33 veterinary colleges in the United States. This study helps address current gaps in our knowledge and provides an updated report on veterinary toxicology education in the United States and elsewhere.

2. Materials and Methods

An online survey consisting of 34 items was created to assess the extent and depth of toxicology education in veterinary programs at AAVMC member schools. The survey was reviewed and approved by both the North Carolina State University Institutional Review Board (IRB) and the AAVMC Survey Committee. The survey was developed by the authors and tested by several individuals prior to distribution to determine completion time and identify components that needed revision or clarification. The complete survey is provided in Appendix A. Participation in the study was voluntary, and all participants received descriptive information regarding the study along with a link to the survey. All invitees were informed that their information would be kept confidential.

The survey was distributed twice (on 6 July 2021 and 16 November 2021) by the AAVMC Survey Committee via email to the Associate Deans of Academic Affairs at member institutions. Distribution occurred using a web-based Qualtrics survey tool. The solicitation email to the Associate Deans requested them to forward the survey invitation to the faculty member most involved in teaching toxicology in their veterinary curriculum. The survey was also distributed (on 28 July 2022) to individuals that participate in the ABVT email listserv. The survey was kept open for approximately 13 months and was closed on 16 September 2022.

The first survey question addressed informed consent. An affirmative response was required to proceed with the rest of the questionnaire. Survey questions were divided into distinct sections, including portions focused on consent, instructor data, veterinary curriculum, veterinary courses, opinions, curricular change, and syllabi. Instructor data collected demographic information about the program and the credentials of individuals providing instruction in veterinary toxicology. The section on the toxicology curriculum asked respondents to estimate the amount of toxicology instruction provided by different types of individuals (e.g., faculty members, trainees, adjunct faculty). Data sought about veterinary courses included course titles, methods of instruction, whether courses were required or electives, resources used, and course content. This section also asked the respondent's perception of how prepared their veterinary students would be at the time of graduation to perform the seven entrustable professional activities (EPAs) pertaining to a case involving toxicant exposure. It also asked respondents whether they would use peer-reviewed online materials to either teach or assess these EPAs. Respondent opinions regarding the adequacy of the toxicology curriculum were collected. The next section addressed veterinary curriculum changes at the respondent's institution and student interests in toxicology as a career. The final section provided respondents with the opportunity to upload syllabi for their required or elective toxicology courses. All results were analyzed using descriptive statistics. Mean ($\pm$standard deviations) have been provided for some response data.

3. Results

A total of 29 surveys were received. Three invalid surveys (incomplete demographic data including identification of the institution) were excluded from our study. One completed survey came from an institution that was not a member of the AAVMC, and data from this survey were excluded from most analyses. This survey response did provide a toxicology course syllabus that contributed to the list of agents presented in Appendix B. Of the 54 schools and colleges eligible for the study, 24 unique institutions responded to the survey, resulting in an overall 44% response rate. Most ($n = 18/24$) responses were from academic institutions based in the United States. Three responses were obtained from institutions in Australia, England, or New Zealand, two responses were received by Canadian schools, and one response was obtained from a school based in the Caribbean. Two responses were received from faculty at one veterinary school based in the United States. These individuals were responsible for different facets of the toxicology curriculum, and their individual responses were retained as appropriate, resulting in 25 respondents to the survey. Most ($n = 16/18$) of the veterinary schools based in the United States and Canada were affiliated with academic institutions that also had a diagnostic laboratory accredited by the American Association of Veterinary Laboratory Diagnosticians (AAVLD). Most ($n = 23/25$) of the respondents personally teach toxicology to veterinary students at their home institution. The mean ($\pm$SD) number of years that the respondents had taught toxicology at their home institution and the total number of years they had taught toxicology across all locations were 12.7 $\pm$ 9.9 and 20.1 $\pm$ 10.3 years, respectively.

Of the 23 participants reporting their credentials, most ($n = 20$) respondents held a veterinary degree (DVM or equivalent). Other degrees held by respondents included a Master's degree (n = 1) or Ph.D. or equivalent (n = 15). Board certification was common among the respondents. Eleven individuals were certified by the ABVT, four by the American Board of Toxicology, two by the American College of Veterinary Pathologists, one by the American College of Theriogenology, one by the American College of Veterinary Internal Medicine, one by the American College of Veterinary Emergency Critical Care, and one European Registered Toxicologist. Most (n = 18/24) of the AAVMC member schools relied on a single individual to teach the majority of the toxicology in the curriculum. However, most of the veterinary programs had additional individuals teach more than two hours of contact time in the veterinary toxicology curriculum. The mean number of instructors involved in teaching toxicology at AAVMC member institutions was 3.6 ± 2.8 (range 1–10). Most of the toxicology curriculum was provided by faculty members at the home institution. Trainees or staff provided some instruction at four schools (1–45% of the contact time in toxicology). Two veterinary schools relied almost entirely (>90% instruction time) on either adjunct/locum instructors or guest lecturers. A third institution indicated that 35% of the instruction in toxicology was provided by an adjunct/locum instructor.

Table 1 provides a summary of the method of instruction used prior to the COVID-19 pandemic and the types of educational resources that are currently used to teach toxicology to veterinary students. Only 25% (n = 6/24) of the respondents indicated that recent changes in teaching format due to the COVID-19 pandemic would cause a permanent alteration in the way toxicology was taught in the future. Most respondents (n = 16/24) indicated that a permanent change was possible because of recent changes in teaching format due to the COVID-19 pandemic. Most respondents (n = 19/24) indicated that a curriculum change had occurred within the past ten years at their home institution. No change in contact time because of a curriculum change was reported by most of the respondents (n = 16/23). Only one respondent indicated that contact time in toxicology increased following a curriculum change at their institution. Fifteen respondents provided comments regarding how they would use additional time to teach toxicology. The most frequently mentioned ways additional time dedicated to toxicology would be used by these 15 respondents included increased time allocated to cases (66.7%), enhanced discussion of the management of poisoned animals (33.3%), increased coverage of poisonous plants (33.3%), and discussion of topics related to environmental and ecotoxicology (20%).

Table 1. Current didactic resources and primary method of instruction provided in toxicology courses between 2018 and 2019 at AAVMC member institutions (n = 24). Percentage of institutions.

Method of Instruction	%	Didactic Resources	%
In-person lecture	100.0	Printouts of instructor-created PowerPoints	100
In-person discussion/small group activities	62.5	Optional textbook(s)	79.2
In-person laboratory	37.5	Case-based materials	75.0
Asynchronous online instruction	12.5	Instructor-generated text-based notes	58.3
Field investigations	12.5	Practice quizzes	54.2
Synchronous online instruction	8.3	Problem sets	37.5
		Required textbook(s)	4.2

Information about toxicology courses was provided for 22 institutions. All survey respondents indicated toxicology instruction is provided within their veterinary curriculum. Toxicology as a stand-alone course or as part of a broader course (e.g., veterinary pharmacology and toxicology, pathobiology) was required at nearly all programs (n = 21/22). Additional elective or selective courses in toxicology were available at some (n = 7/22) of the responding institutions. Mean contact hours in stand-alone veterinary toxicology courses was 30.5 ± 10.7 h (range: 14–45 h, n = 12). Most respondents (n = 17/24) felt that more time was needed to prepare students for day-one competency.

Our survey found that toxicology as a career option is considered by some veterinary students. The percentage of students in each class indicating an interest in toxicology, however, varies between institutions. Most (17/23) respondents indicated that fewer than 5% of their veterinary students expressed an interest in toxicology as a career choice. Two respondents however indicated that over 20% of their students expressed an interest in toxicology as a career.

Toxicology topics taught at AAVMC member institutions are reported in Table 2. Most topics were taught using a comparative approach that considered multiple species. Because veterinary toxicology is often taught in multiple courses, many toxicology topics were also included in courses that focused on either small animals, horses, large animals, or wildlife and exotics. One topic that appears less frequently is environmental toxicology. Likewise, toxicology in wildlife and exotic species is also less commonly included in existing veterinary curricula. This observation was also borne out by comments made by several respondents.

Table 2. Basic veterinary toxicology concepts and topics taught at AAVMC member institutions (n = 24).

Domain	% of Respondents				
	All Species Comparative Perspective	Small Animal	Equine	Food Animal	Wildlife and/or Exotics
Clinical and diagnostic toxicology	87.0	17.4	17.4	17.4	8.7
Drugs	87.5	20.8	12.5	12.5	8.3
Environmental toxicology	65.0	10.0	10.0	15.0	35.0
Feed and water contaminants	72.7	22.7	18.2	27.3	18.2
Household chemicals	69.6	39.1	4.4	4.4	0
Metals and micronutrients	82.6	26.1	13.0	26.1	13.0
Mycotoxins	79.2	25.0	20.8	25.0	4.2
Pesticides	78.3	30.4	21.7	30.4	17.4
Poisonous plants	81.8	27.3	22.7	27.3	4.6
Principles of toxicology	95.7	8.7	8.7	8.7	0
Therapeutic measures	90.9	18.2	18.2	18.2	4.6
Toxic gases	76.5	5.9	5.9	23.5	5.9
Zootoxins	85.0	15.0	15.0	20.0	0

Respondent assessment of the competency of their students to perform entrustable professional activities (EPA) is provided in Table 3. In most cases, respondents felt that > 80% of their students could perform most toxicology-related EPAs autonomously and in some cases could mentor others in an activity. One exception related to the ability of students to analyze toxicology data where only 50% of respondents felt their students could perform this activity without supervision. A related question queried the confidence of the respondents in their ability to evaluate students' preparation to perform an EPA. Approximately 10 to 20% of respondents indicated that they lacked confidence in their ability to evaluate their student's ability to perform one or more EPAs.

Table 3. Respondent perceptions regarding entrustable professional activities associated with toxicology (number of responses varies per question).

Entrustable Professional Activity (EPA)	Respondent's Assessment of Their Confidence in Their Students' Ability to Perform an EPA at Graduation (%)				Respondent's Confidence in Their Ability to Evaluate Students' Preparation to Perform an EPA (%)		
	Not Competent	Can Perform with Support from a Mentor	Can Perform Autonomously	Can Mentor Others in Developing the Skill	Not Confident	Somewhat Confident	Very Confident
Recognize a patient requiring urgent or emergent care and initiate evaluation and management (n = 23)	0.0	13.0	82.6	4.4	12.5	33.3	54.2
Interpret toxicology data (n = 22)	9.1	40.9	50.0	0	16.7	50.0	33.3

Table 3. *Cont.*

Entrustable Professional Activity (EPA)	Respondent's Assessment of Their Confidence in Their Students' Ability to Perform an EPA at Graduation (%)				Respondent's Confidence in Their Ability to Evaluate Students' Preparation to Perform an EPA (%)		
	Not Competent	Can Perform with Support from a Mentor	Can Perform Autonomously	Can Mentor Others in Developing the Skill	Not Confident	Somewhat Confident	Very Confident
Gather a toxicologic history, perform an examination, and create a prioritized differential diagnosis list ($n = 23$)	4.4	8.7	78.3	8.7	16.7	37.5	45.8
Formulate relevant questions and retrieve evidence to advance care ($n = 23$)	0	13.0	82.6	4.4	8.3	50.0	41.7
Formulate recommendations for preventive healthcare ($n = 21$)	4.8	14.3	66.7	14.3	20.8	45.8	33.3
Develop and implement a management/treatment plan ($n = 23$)	4.4	13.0	78.3	4.4	16.7	37.5	45.8
Develop a diagnostic plan and interpret results ($n = 22$)	4.6	13.6	72.7	9.1	12.5	33.3	54.2

Respondents were generally receptive to using online, peer-reviewed materials to either teach or assess EPAs (Table 4).

Table 4. Respondent's likely use of online, peer-reviewed materials to either teach or assess EPAs (number of responses varies per question).

Entrustable Professional Activity (EPA)	Teach EPAs (%)			Assess EPAs (%)		
	Likely	May or May not	Unlikely	Likely	May or May not	Unlikely
Recognize a patient requiring urgent or emergent care and initiate evaluation and management ($n = 23$)	54.2	41.7	4.2	54.2	41.7	4.2
Interpret toxicology data ($n = 22$)	54.2	41.7	4.2	54.2	37.5	8.3
Gather a toxicologic history, perform an examination, and create a prioritized differential diagnosis list ($n = 23$)	62.5	25.0	12.5	54.2	37.5	8.3
Formulate relevant questions and retrieve evidence to advance care ($n = 23$)	58.3	33.3	8.3	50.0	45.8	4.2
Formulate recommendations for preventive healthcare ($n = 21$)	50.0	45.8	4.2	54.2	41.7	4.2
Develop and implement a management/treatment plan ($n = 23$)	66.7	20.8	12.5	58.4	33.3	8.3
Develop a diagnostic plan and interpret results ($n = 22$)	62.5	25.0	12.5	54.2	37.5	8.3

A total of 22 respondents provided comments related to perceived strengths and weaknesses in their institution's toxicology curriculum. Multiple respondents reported similar strengths in their curriculum, including broad coverage of agents and general principles of toxicology in the curriculum (54.5%), use of a case- or problem-based approach to presenting the curriculum (27.3%), toxicology was taught by one or more experienced veterinary toxicologists (18.5%), and availability of a toxic plant garden (13.6%). Several respondents viewed a stand-alone toxicology course as a strength of the program. These respondents also provided comments related to programmatic gaps or weaknesses. Overall, these responses varied between institutions with fewer common concerns. Several of the 22 respondents (18.2%) were concerned about the lack of integration of toxicology in the overall curriculum, including an overall lack of knowledge of how toxicology may be taught by others in the curriculum. Likewise, 18.2% of respondents noted a lack of time dedicated to the teaching of toxicology. Two instructors with specialization in critical care or pathology indicated that they may not have the background needed to teach toxicology. There was also a concern by several respondents that topics related to forensics or large animal toxicology may not be adequately covered in the toxicology curriculum.

Syllabi for one or more courses were provided by 11 institutions. These included syllabi for required as well as elective courses. All required toxicology courses included one or more lectures on basic concepts (e.g., terminology, decontamination procedures, pharmacokinetics). Most syllabi also provided learning objectives. A summary of basic concepts and learning objectives found in multiple syllabi is provided in Appendix C. The remainder of the required courses often focused on toxicologic syndromes associated with toxic agents or classes of agents. Presentation of this material varied amongst institutions. Several syllabi used a systems approach (e.g., neurotoxicants) to organize the course, while others used an agent-based approach.

4. Discussion

Despite concerns about the demise of toxicology as a theme in the professional veterinary medical curriculum, all survey respondents indicated toxicology instruction is provided within their veterinary curriculum. Indeed, many AAVMC member institutions provide students with both required and elective courses in toxicology. The teaching of veterinary toxicology is generally provided by veterinarians, many of whom also hold advanced graduate degrees and additional board specialization. Nearly half of all institutions provide a stand-alone course in toxicology. This finding differs from that seen in United States and Canadian medical schools, where less than 5% had formal courses in toxicology [10]. Dedicated veterinary toxicology courses at AAVMC member institutions had between 14 and 45 contact hours. Mean contact hours devoted to toxicology training in American and Canadian medical schools were 5 and 6 h, respectively [10].

Based on our results, veterinary toxicology is often offered through a team-based education effort provided by multiple instructors. In fewer cases, the veterinary curriculum rests on the efforts of a single instructor. Prior to the COVID-19 pandemic, most instruction occurred in person with less reliance on online instruction. We examined this timeframe since the COVID-19 pandemic prompted instruction at many veterinary schools to switch to remote teaching formats. Most respondents thought that recent changes in teaching format due to COVID-19 could possibly change the way toxicology was taught. A recent study found student performance in a veterinary toxicology course delivered online asynchronously during the pandemic was similar to achievement during the prior, in-person course [11]. All respondents presented didactic lectures and provided students with copies of their PowerPoint presentations, suggesting this remains the primary means of instruction in veterinary toxicology. Case-based materials and problem sets were also used by many instructors. Our perception is that novel educational strategies, including flipped classroom techniques, are less commonly used in veterinary student instruction in toxicology. Approaches like flipping the classroom have been associated with improved academic performance in medical students [12].

Our survey explored the respondent's assessment of their students' ability to perform EPAs at graduation. The seven EPAs included in our study were modified from those developed by the AAVMC Competency-Based Veterinary Education Working Group [13].

These EPAs describe the most relevant activities a veterinarian carries out in private veterinary practice [14]. The EPAs provide an insight into what newly graduated veterinarians should be able to do and how much supervision may be required as they start professional practice [15]. Our data indicate that most (>80%) respondents felt their graduates could autonomously perform five of the seven EPAs included in our study. Approximately 25% of the respondents indicated that their graduates would require support to formulate recommendations for preventive healthcare. In retrospect, interpretation of this EPA could vary between respondents. For example, some individuals may perceive this to mean client communication regarding toxicologic hazards. Other respondents may have assumed this related to the initial management of an exposed animal. Mentorship was also needed for students to analyze toxicology data. This later finding is not unexpected since this represents an activity often associated with working toxicologists [16]. Interestingly, nearly one-quarter of all respondents lacked the confidence to assess their student's ability to perform this EPA. Most (>80%) respondents were somewhat confident or very confident in their ability to assess the ability of their students to perform the remaining EPAs. Nearly 45% of all respondents indicated their graduates would require guidance to interpret toxicology data. The majority (>50%) of respondents indicated that they would be likely to use online, peer-reviewed materials to either teach EPAs or assess their students' ability to perform an EPA. Less than 10% of all respondents indicated that they were unlikely to use these resources if they were available.

Based on our results, the majority of respondents used a comparative approach to teaching veterinary toxicology to their students. With few exceptions, there were common topics incorporated into veterinary curricula across responding institutions. One such exception related to wildlife and ecotoxicology was mentioned several times as a weakness of the toxicology curriculum. Our finding that major concepts and topics are often shared across different academic disciplines suggests that a next step could involve the definition of an agreed-upon set of core concepts for veterinary toxicology curricula. Similar approaches have occurred for pharmacology [17–19] and toxicology [20] programs within human health professions education, as well as for farm animal medicine [21] within veterinary medicine. Evidence from biology and pharmacology education indicates that core concepts are useful and effective structures around which such a curriculum can be designed to facilitate student learning [22,23]. Subsequent efforts could focus on the selection and development of specific assessment instruments to measure students' ability to perform the EPAs to demonstrate ability to manage cases of toxicant ingestion, building on the efforts of Duijin and coworkers [24]. A group of veterinary educators under the auspices of the CBVE Working Group have proposed a draft Competency-Based Veterinary Education Toolkit, outlining recommended assessment formats for each CBVE Domain of Competency [25]. Among these, Script Concordance Tests (SCTs) stand out as a method faculty could use to assess their students' ability to analyze toxicology data [26,27]. Since these examinations are challenging and time consuming to develop and validate, the fact that most curricula include similar toxicology content and teaching methods paves the way for a consortium effort to develop assessment tools.

There are methodological limitations to our study. Our data are often derived from a single individual at each school and may be biased because either the respondents have vested interests in the survey outcome, or they interpret the questions differently. Another major limitation of this investigation is the response rate. Acceptable response rates for web-based surveys remain poorly defined. Our response rate (44%) is qualitatively similar to that seen in a meta-analysis that reported a mean response rate for web surveys was 39.6% [28]. It remains uncertain if those who responded to our survey have similar views regarding veterinary toxicology as those who did not respond. Despite our effort to increase the response rate by careful consideration of the number of survey questions, using an easily accessible web-based survey, and sending an email reminder, the response rate was still only moderate. We believe that many factors contributed to our low rate, including survey fatigue, time constraints, and the time required to finish the survey. These factors have been noted by others [29]. Distribution of the survey relied on Associate Deans of Academic Affairs forwarding the email they received from the AAVMC. Associate Deans and recipient faculty may have missed these email communications resulting in decreased response rates. An additional plausible explanation is that some survey recipients may not have had the appropriate knowledge about toxicology instruction status at their institution. Despite the moderate response rate, our study provides valuable information on the current perception of the respondents regarding toxicology instruction in veterinary programs.

5. Conclusions

In conclusion, this study describes the current depth and breadth of toxicology instruction in a sample of veterinary programs at AAVMC member schools. There was a general agreement among the respondents that veterinary schools and colleges devote curricular space to toxicology instruction. The depth and the extent of toxicology topics coverage varied among institutions.

Author Contributions: Conceptualization, R.H.P. and R.M.S.-T.; methodology, R.M.S.-T. and D.C.D.; formal analysis, R.M.S.-T. and D.C.D.; original draft preparation, D.C.D.; writing—review and editing, R.H.P. and R.M.S.-T. All authors have read and agreed to the published version of the manuscript.

Funding: This research received no external funding.

Institutional Review Board Statement: The study was conducted in accordance with the Declaration of Helsinki, and approved by the Institutional Review Board of North Carolina State University (Protocol Code 24020 and 12 May 2021).

Informed Consent Statement: Informed consent was obtained from all subjects involved in the study.

Data Availability Statement: Data is contained within the article or Appendix.

Acknowledgments: The authors thank the respondents to the survey for their contributions to this study. We also acknowledge the support of the AAVMC Survey Committee for assistance with distribution of the survey.

Conflicts of Interest: The authors declare no conflict of interest.

Appendix A Survey Elements

Consent Form

Q1.1. You are being asked to complete a survey for research purposes.
- I currently reside in North America, South America, Asia, Africa, or Australia
- I currently reside in the European Economic Area, including the United Kingdom

Instructor Data

Q2.1. Name of your institution:
Q2.2. Does your institution have an AAVLD-accredited diagnostic laboratory?
Q2.3. Do you personally teach toxicology to veterinary students at your home institution?
Q2.4. How many years have you taught toxicology at your home institution?
Q2.5. How many years have you taught toxicology overall?
Q2.6. What are your academic credentials? (select all that apply)
- Ph.D., Sc.D. or equivalent
- DVM, VMD, BVSc, or equivalent
- Board-certified toxicologist (ABVT)
- Board-certified toxicologist (ABT)
- European Registered Toxicologist (ERT)
- Other (specify)

Q2.7. Does your institution rely on a single person to teach the majority of the toxicology content to veterinary students?
Q2.8. What are that individual's academic credentials? (select all that apply)

- Ph.D., Sc.D. or equivalent
- DVM, VMD, BVSc, or equivalent
- Board-certified toxicologist (ABVT)
- Board-certified toxicologist (ABT)
- European Registered Toxicologist (ERT)
- Other (specify)

Q2.9. Do other instructors teach significant (over 2 h of contact time per instructor) portions of the course?

Q2.10. How many of these other instructors provide over 2 h of contact time in the veterinary toxicology course?

Q2.11. How many of them are certified by the American Board of Veterinary Toxicology (ABVT)?

Veterinary Curriculum

Q3.1. When thinking about your entire veterinary curriculum (DVM, VMD, BVSc or equivalent), please estimate the amount of toxicology instruction provided by each of the following (number of instructors and Percentage of veterinary toxicology instruction across all curriculum years):
- CVM/SVM faculty members
- CVM/SVM trainee or staff
- Locum/adjunct instructor
- Guest lecturers
- Other: (specify)

Veterinary Courses

Q4.1. Please list all toxicology and poisonous plants learning opportunities (courses, labs, rotations, etc) available to students in your program. Data collected includes course title, year in curriculum, primary delivery method (e.g., lecture, lab, rotation, etc), total number of contact hours, required or elective, and percentage of students completing.

Q4.2. How was this instruction provided in 2018–2019 (pre-COVID). Check all that apply:
- In-person lecture
- In-person laboratory
- In-person discussion/small group activities
- Synchronous online instruction
- Asynchronous online instruction
- Other: please specify

Q4.3. Which (if any) of these didactic resources are used in the courses? Check all that apply:
- Required textbook (specify author/title)
- Optional textbooks (author/title)
- Instructor-generated text-based notes
- Instructor-created PowerPoints and printouts of these presentations
- Case-based materials
- Problem sets or quizzes

Q4.4. Which of these textbooks are required for the course(s)? Select all that apply (10 titles provided).

Q4.5. Which of these textbooks are optional for the course(s)? Select all that apply (10 titles provided).

Q4.6. Please indicate which of the following content areas are covered in the toxicology curriculum at your institution, and in what species (options included: all species/comparative perspective, small animal, equine, food animal, and wildlife and/or exotics):

- Clinical and diagnostic toxicology
- Drugs
- Environmental toxicology
- Feed and water contaminants
- Household chemicals
- Metals and micronutrients
- Mycotoxins
- Pesticides
- Poisonous plants
- Principles of toxicology
- Therapeutic measures
- Toxic gases
- Zootoxins

Q4.7. To what extent do you perceive that your DVM students are prepared to perform the following activities at the time of graduation from your institution, for a case involving toxicant exposure (options included: not competent, can perform with support from a mentor, can perform autonomously, can mentor others in developing the skill, don't know/not applicable):
- Interpret toxicology data
- Gather a toxicologic history, perform an examination, and create a prioritized differential diagnosis list
- Develop a diagnostic plan and interpret results
- Develop and implement a management/treatment plan
- Recognize a patient requiring urgent or emergent care and initiate evaluation and management
- Formulate relevant questions and retrieve evidence to advance care
- Formulate recommendations for preventive healthcare

Q4.8. How confident are you in your current ability to evaluate students' preparation to perform each of the following entrustable professional activities (EPAs)? (options included: not confident, somewhat confident, very confident):
- Interpret toxicology data
- Gather a toxicologic history, perform an examination, and create a prioritized differential diagnosis list
- Develop a diagnostic plan and interpret results
- Develop and implement a management/treatment plan
- Recognize a patient requiring urgent or emergent care and initiate evaluation and management
- Formulate relevant questions and retrieve evidence to advance care
- Formulate recommendations for preventive healthcare

Q4.9. How likely would you be to use online, peer-reviewed materials to teach these skills? (options included: likely, may or may not, unlikely):
- Interpret toxicology data
- Gather a toxicologic history, perform an examination, and create a prioritized differential diagnosis list
- Develop a diagnostic plan and interpret results
- Develop and implement a management/treatment plan
- Recognize a patient requiring urgent or emergent care and initiate evaluation and management
- Formulate relevant questions and retrieve evidence to advance care
- Formulate recommendations for preventive healthcare

Q4.10. How likely would you be to use online, peer-reviewed materials to assess these skills? (options included: likely, may or may not, unlikely):

- Interpret toxicology data
- Gather a toxicologic history, perform an examination, and create a prioritized differential diagnosis list
- Develop a diagnostic plan and interpret results
- Develop and implement a management/treatment plan
- Recognize a patient requiring urgent or emergent care and initiate evaluation and management
- Formulate relevant questions and retrieve evidence to advance care
- Formulate recommendations for preventive healthcare

Opinions

Q5.1. In your opinion, is the contact time currently allotted to teaching veterinary toxicology adequate to prepare students for day-one competency? (Options included: yes, no—need more time, no we have too much time to fill)

Q5.2. If you were allotted more contact time, what additional topics or concepts would you add to the toxicology curriculum?

Q5.3. What are the greatest strengths of your current toxicology curriculum?

Q5.4. What do you see as the biggest gaps or weaknesses in your current toxicology curriculum? *Curricular Change*

Q6.1. When was the most recent veterinary curricular change implemented at your institution?

Q6.2. What effect did this change have on how toxicology is taught in your program?

Q6.3. What approximate percentage increase in contact time occurred due to the most recent change in your institution's veterinary curriculum?

Q6.4. What approximate percentage decrease in contact time occurred due to the most recent change in your institution's veterinary curriculum?

Q6.5. Are recent changes in teaching format due to COVID-19 likely to cause permanent alterations in the way you teach toxicology in the future? (options included: yes, possibly, no)

Q6.6. Over the past five years, approximately what percentage of students in each class indicate an interest in toxicology as it pertains to their career goals (e.g., pursuing a graduate or residency program in toxicology, emergency and critical care medicine, government, or industry).

Syllabi

Q7.1. Finally, would you be willing to share syllabi for core or elective toxicology courses? Please upload each file individually, using as many of the spaces on the next page as needed (option provided to upload up to five files).

Appendix B

Table A1. Toxic agents covered in one or more veterinary toxicology courses.

Algal Toxins	Household Toxins	Plants (Common Names)
- Anatoxin-a(s)	- Alcohols (methanol, ethanol, isopropyl)	- Black locust
- Microcystin	- Corrosive, caustics, and detergents	- Black walnut
Bacterial toxins/zootoxins	- Ethylene glycol	- Bracken fern
- Black widow spiders	- Fertilizer	- Buckwheat
- Blister beetles	- Petroleum distillates	- Buttercup
- Brown recluse spiders	- Polyurethane glue	- Butternut
- Bufo toads	- Silica gel	- Calcium oxalate plants

Table A1. *Cont.*

Algal Toxins	Household Toxins	Plants (Common Names)
• Botulism	**Minerals and Metals**	• Castor bean
• Coral snakes	• Arsenic	• Cocklebur
• Fireflies	• Copper	• Cotton seed (gossypol)
• Pit vipers	• Copper chrome arsenic (CCA)	• Cyanogenic glycosides
• Tick paralysis	• Fluoride	• Fescue
Drugs	• Lead	• Grayanotoxin plants
• Acetaminophen	• Selenium	• Horsetail
• Albuterol	• Sodium	• Hops
• Amitraz	• Zinc	• Lantana
• Amphetamines	**Mushrooms**	• Larkspur
• Atropine	• Amanita muscaria	• Lilies
• Avermectins	**Mycotoxins**	• Locoweeds
• Barbiturates	• Aflatoxins	• Marijuana
• Benzodiazepines	• Deoxynivalenol (DON)/Vomitoxin	• Oaks
• Drugs of abuse	• Fumonisins	• Oleander
• Nonsteroidal anti-inflammatory drug (NSAID)	• Ochratoxin A	• Perilla mint-ABPEE
• Opiates and opioids	• Slaframine	• Pine needle abortion
• Phenylpropanolamine	• Tremorgenic	• Poison hemlock
• Salicylates	**Pesticides**	• Pyrrolizidine alkaloids
• Scopolamine	**Fumigants**	• Red maple
• Serotonin syndrome	• Sulfuryl fluoride	• Redroot pigweed
• Tetracyclines	• Chloropicrin	• Rosary pea
Feed toxicants/foods	**Herbicides**	• Russian knapweed
• Avocado	• Chlorophenoxy herbicides (2,4-D)	• Sago palms
• Chocolate	**Insecticides**	• Saponin plants
• Grapes and raisins	• Carbamates	• Solanaceous plants
• Ionophores	• Organophosphates	• Sorghum
• Macadamia nuts	• Pyrethrins and pyrethroids	• Spurges
• Nitrate-nitrite	**Rodenticides**	• St. John's Wort
• Nonprotein nitrogen/urea	• Anticoagulant rodenticides	• Sweet clover
• Onion	• 5-Fluorouracil	• Tobacco
• Thiaminases (fish)	• Bromethalin	• Tropane alkaloids
• Xylitol	• Cholecalciferol	• Veratrum
Gases	• Strychnine	• Water hemlock
• Carbon monoxide	• Zinc phosphide	• White snakeroot
• Cyanide		• Yellow star-thistle
• Hydrogen sulfide		• Yesterday-today-and-tomorrow
• Teflon		• Yew
		Radiation

Appendix C

Table A2. Learning objectives shared by multiple veterinary toxicology courses.

Clinical Toxicology
- Correctly obtain historical information to support a toxicology diagnosis.
- Describe and understand differences between the major treatment modalities in toxicology, including decontamination, direct and indirect countering of toxicant effects, and supportive treatment.
- Be able to describe the uses, contraindications, and side effects associated with common therapies (e.g., emetics, activated charcoal) used to decrease animal exposure to poisons.
- Describe general approaches to poisoning prevention and risk management.
- List the sources of a toxicant of interest and the factors that contribute to exposure risk
- Recognize the clinical signs of poisoning with a toxicant of interest and be able to create a list of possible intoxicants from a description of clinical signs.
- List the treatment options and generate treatment plans based on the degree of exposure, stage, and severity of poisoning.
- Correctly read and interpret case histories.

Dose–Response Relationships
- Identify, explain, and know toxicant examples that fit the following dose–response models: threshold; linear; hermetic; hysteretic.
- Define and use dose–response graphs to identify NOAEL, LOAEL, and ED50 or LD50.
- Interpret dose–response graphs and derived toxicity parameters in terms of relative toxicant potency and poisoning risk in an individual patient.
- Interpret dose–response relationships including threshold response, non-threshold response, LD50 response, and quantal responses.

Forensics
- Describe and explain principles and approaches used to make a toxicological diagnosis and relate the diagnostic process to realistic poisoning scenarios.
- Describe and/or recognize from a photograph or written description the pathological lesions associated with a toxicant of interest.
- Describe the basics of performing a toxicological investigation.
- Describe sampling procedures for diagnostic toxicology cases including common test assays, necropsy procedures, and field investigations.
- Correctly order suitable tests using ideal samples of choice.
- Correctly interpret test results and come up with a proper interpretive summary.

General Concepts
- Understand and apply common toxicological terminology
- Poison, toxin, toxicant, toxicity, toxicosis, LD50, relay toxicosis;
- Concentration, dose, dosage;
- Hazard, risk, standard safety margin, and chronicity factor;
- Exposure;
- Dose–response relationship.
- Understand and explain the basic theory of poisoning.
- Know and understand major physical–chemical toxicant properties that influence environmental distribution and exposure to toxicants.
- Know and understand the mechanisms of mixture effects that influence poisoning risk and severity, including major chemical interactions, pharmacokinetic interactions, and pharmacodynamic interactions.
- Describe physiologic, pathophysiologic, and toxicologic factors that could influence an animal's response to a chemical. Given an animal species and exposure to a specified toxicant, identify factors that could increase or reduce expected effects on the animal.
- Describe the mechanism of action of a toxicant of interest.
- Identify species differences that affect response to common toxicants.

Plant Identification
- Recognize (from a photograph or plant specimens) the toxic plant(s) that might be responsible for a particular set of clinical signs or lesions (from a photograph or written description).

Toxicology Calculations
- Perform calculations to determine the amount of toxin in feed or to which an animal might have been exposed.

Toxicology Information Resources
- List where to find reliable toxicological information.
- Learn how to access and use established and reliable print and electronic resources to characterize a suspected toxicant.

References

1. Gilliland, W.R.; Waechter, D.M. A curricular divide: Basic pharmacology vs. clinical pharmacology. *Clin. Pharmacol. Ther.* **2011**, *89*, 24–26. [CrossRef] [PubMed]
2. Ross, P.F.; Nelson, P.E.; Richard, J.L.; Osweiler, G.D.; Rice, L.G.; Plattner, R.D.; Wilson, T.M. Production of fumonisins by Fusarium moniliforme and Fusarium proliferatum isolates associated with equine leukoencephalomalacia and a pulmonary edema syndrome in swine. *Appl. Environ. Microbiol.* **1990**, *56*, 3225–3226. [CrossRef] [PubMed]

3. Anonymous. News from the American Board of Veterinary Toxicology: Core content for veterinary toxicology. *Vet. Hum. Toxicol.* **1996**, *38*, 393.
4. Goldfine, C.; Lung, D.; Beauchamp, G.; O'Connor, A.; Stolbach, A.; Kao, L.; Judge, B.; Wax, P.; Patwari, R.; Kazzi, Z. Consensus development of a core content for a standardized medical toxicology curriculum for medical students. *J. Med. Toxicol.* **2022**, *18*, 139–144. [CrossRef] [PubMed]
5. Hendrickson, R.G.; Bania, T.C.; Baum, C.R.; Greenberg, M.I.; Joldersma, K.B.; Keehbauch, J.N. The 2021 core content of medical toxicology. *J. Med. Toxicol.* **2021**, *17*, 425–436. [CrossRef] [PubMed]
6. Nelson, L.S.; Baker, B.A.; Osterhoudt, K.C.; Snook, C.P.; Medical Toxicology Core Content Task Force for the Medical Toxicology Subboard; Keehbauch, J.N.; American Board of Emergency Medicine. The 2012 core content of medical toxicology. *J. Med. Toxicol.* **2012**, *8*, 183–191. [CrossRef]
7. Hodgson, J.L.; Pelzer, J.M.; Inzana, K.D. Beyond NAVMEC: Competency-based veterinary education and assessment of the professional competencies. *J. Vet. Med. Educ.* **2013**, *40*, 102–118. [CrossRef] [PubMed]
8. Matthew, S.M.; Bok, H.G.J.; Chaney, K.P.; Read, E.K.; Hodgson, J.L.; Rush, B.R.; May, S.A.; Salisbury, S.K.; Ilkiw, J.E.; Frost, J.S.; et al. Collaborative development of a shared framework for competency-based veterinary education. *J. Vet. Med. Educ.* **2020**, *47*, 578–593. [CrossRef]
9. Salisbury, S.K.; Rush, B.R.; Ilkiw, J.E.; Matthew, S.M.; Chaney, K.P.; Molgaard, L.K.; May, S.A.; Bok, H.G.J.; Hodgson, J.L.; Frost, J.S.; et al. Collaborative development of core entrustable professional activities for veterinary education. *J. Vet. Med. Educ.* **2020**, *47*, 607–618. [CrossRef]
10. Hays, E.P., Jr.; Schumacher, C.; Ferrario, C.G.; Vazzana, T.; Erickson, T.; Hryhorczuk, D.O.; Leikin, J.B. Toxicology training in US and Canadian medical schools. *Am. J. Emerg. Med.* **1992**, *10*, 121–123. [CrossRef] [PubMed]
11. Schoenfeld-Tacher, R.M.; Dorman, D.C. Effect of delivery format on student outcomes and perceptions of a veterinary medicine course: Synchronous versus asynchronous learning. *Vet. Sci.* **2021**, *20*, 13. [CrossRef] [PubMed]
12. Tahir, F.; Hafiz, B.; Alnajjar, T.; Almehmadi, B.; Besharah, B.; Gari, A.; Katib, Y. Comparison of performance of medical students between two teaching modalities "Flip the classroom" and traditional lectures: A single center educational interventional study. *Pak. J. Med. Sci.* **2020**, *36*, 958–964. [CrossRef] [PubMed]
13. AAVMC Working Group on Competency-Based Veterinary Education; Molgaard, L.K.; Hodgson, J.L.; Bok, H.G.J.; Chaney, K.P.; Ilkiw, J.E.; Matthew, S.M.; May, S.A.; Read, E.K.; Rush, B.R.; et al. *Competency-Based Veterinary Education: Part 2—Entrustable Professional Activities*; Association of American Veterinary Medical Colleges: Washington, DC, USA, 2018; Available online: https://www.aavmc.org/wp-content/uploads/2020/10/CBVE-Publication-2-EPA.pdf (accessed on 30 September 2022).
14. Molgaard, L.K.; Chaney, K.P.; Bok, H.G.J.; Read, E.K.; Hodgson, J.L.; Salisbury, S.K.; Rush, B.R.; Ilkiw, J.E.; May, S.A.; Danielson, J.A.; et al. Development of core entrustable professional activities linked to a competency-based veterinary education framework. *Med. Teach.* **2019**, *41*, 1404–1410. [CrossRef] [PubMed]
15. Favier, R.P.; Ten Cate, O.; Duijn, C.; Bok, H.G.J. Bridging the gap between undergraduate veterinary training and veterinary practice with entrustable professional activities. *J. Vet. Med. Educ.* **2021**, *48*, 136–138. [CrossRef] [PubMed]
16. Wood, C.S.; Weis, C.P.; Caro, C.M.; Roe, A. A practice analysis of toxicology. *Regul. Toxicol. Pharmacol.* **2016**, *82*, 140–146. [CrossRef] [PubMed]
17. Lloyd, H.; Hinton, T.; Bullock, S.; Babey, A.M.; Davis, E.; Fernandes, L.; Hart, J.; Musgrave, I.; Ziogas, J. An evaluation of pharmacology curricula in Australian science and health-related degree programs. *BMC Med. Educ.* **2013**, *13*, 153. [CrossRef] [PubMed]
18. Midlöv, P.; Höglund, P.; Eriksson, T.; Diehl, A.; Edgren, G. Developing a competency-based curriculum in Basic and Clinical pharmacology–A Delphi study among physicians. *Basic Clin. Pharmacol. Toxicol.* **2015**, *117*, 413–420. [CrossRef]
19. O'Shaughnessy, L.; Haq, I.; Maxwell, S.; Llewelyn, M. Teaching of clinical pharmacology and therapeutics in UK medical schools: Current status in 2009. *Br. J. Clin. Pharmacol.* **2010**, *70*, 143–148. [CrossRef]
20. Gray, J.P.; Curran, C.P.; Fitsanakis, V.A.; Ray, S.D.; Stine, K.E.; Eidemiller, B.J. Society of Toxicology develops learning framework for undergraduate toxicology courses following the vision and change core Concepts model. *Toxicol. Sci.* **2019**, *170*, 20–24. [CrossRef]
21. Duijn, C.C.; Ten Cate, O.; Kremer, W.D.; Bok, H.G. The development of entrustable professional activities for competency-based veterinary education in farm animal health. *J. Vet. Med. Educ.* **2019**, *46*, 218–224. [CrossRef]
22. American Association for the Advancement of Science (AAAS). *Vision and Change in Undergraduate Biology Education: A Call to Action*; American Association for the Advancement of Science: Washington, DC, USA, 2011; Available online: https://visionandchange.org/wp-content/uploads/2011/03/Revised-Vision-and-Change-Final-Report.pdf (accessed on 30 September 2022).
23. White, P.J.; Davis, E.A.; Santiago, M.; Angelo, T.; Shield, A.; Babey, A.M.; Kemp-Harper, B.; Maynard, G.; Al-Sallami, H.S.; Musgrave, I.F.; et al. Identifying the core concepts of pharmacology education. *Pharmacol. Res. Perspect.* **2021**, *9*, e00836. [CrossRef]
24. Duijn, C.C.; Dijk, E.J.; Mandoki, M.; Bok, H.G.; Cate, O.T. Assessment tools for feedback and entrustment decisions in the clinical workplace: A systematic review. *J. Vet. Med. Educ.* **2019**, *46*, 340–352. [CrossRef] [PubMed]
25. Foreman, J.H.; Danielson, J.A.; Fogelberg, K.; Frost, J.; Gates, C.; Hodgson, J.; Matthew, S.; Read, E.; Schoenfeld-Tacher, R. *Competency Based Veterinary Education (CBVE) Assessment Toolkit*; Association of American Veterinary Medical Colleges:

26. Washington, DC, USA, 2022; Available online: https://static1.squarespace.com/static/5fd7ed081606b00a310bbbf5/t/62be04b3e353830d9d309f82/1656620213228/CBVE.Assessment.Toolkit.pdf (accessed on 4 October 2022).
26. Dufour, S.; Latour, S.; Chicoine, Y.; Fecteau, G.; Forget, S.; Moreau, J.; Trépanier, A. Use of the script concordance approach to evaluate clinical reasoning in food-ruminant practitioners. *J. Vet. Med. Educ.* **2012**, *39*, 267–275. [CrossRef] [PubMed]
27. Tayce, J.D.; Saunders, A.B. The use of a modified script concordance test in clinical rounds to foster and assess clinical reasoning skills. *J. Vet. Med. Educ.* **2021**, *16*, e20210090; Epub ahead of print. [CrossRef] [PubMed]
28. Cook, C.; Heath, F.; Thompson, R.L. A meta-analysis of response rates in web- or internet-based surveys. *Educ. Psychol. Meas.* **2000**, *60*, 821–836. [CrossRef]
29. Sammut, R.; Griscti, O.; Norman, I.J. Strategies to improve response rates to web surveys: A literature review. *Int. J. Nurs. Stud.* **2021**, *123*, 104058. [CrossRef] [PubMed]

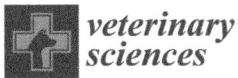

Article

The Evaluation of a High-Fidelity Simulation Model and Video Instruction Used to Teach Canine Dental Skills to Pre-Clinical Veterinary Students

James Fairs [1,*], Anne Conan [2], Kathleen Yvorchuk-St. Jean [1], Wade Gingerich [3], Nicole Abramo [1], Diane Stahl [1,†], Carly Walters [1,†] and Elpida Artemiou [4]

[1] Department of Clinical Sciences, Ross University School of Veterinary Medicine, Basseterre P.O. Box 334, Saint Kitts and Nevis; kstejan@gmail.com (K.Y.-S.J.); nabramo@rossvet.edu.kn (N.A.); dstahl@rossvet.edu.kn (D.S.); cwalters@rossvet.edu.kn (C.W.)
[2] Centre for Applied One Health Research and Policy Advice, City University of Hong Kong, 31 To Yuen Street, Kowloon, Hong Kong SAR 999077, China; ayconan@cityu.edu.hk
[3] Pet Dental Center, 9252 Corkscrew, STE 18, Estero, FL 33928, USA; wadeging@yahoo.com
[4] Texas Tech University School of Veterinary Medicine, 7671 Evans Dr., Amarillo, TX 79106, USA; elpida.artemiou@ttu.edu
* Correspondence: jfairs@rossvet.edu.kn
† These authors contributed equally to this work.

Simple Summary: Dental disease is the most diagnosed disease in small-animal general practice and has a significant impact on the health and welfare of patients. Despite the prevalence of dental disease, there is a recognized gap between the dental skill training veterinary students receive and the expectations of employers regarding the competencies of new graduates in this field. Furthermore, there is a lack of published research reporting on veterinary dental skill training. This study evaluates the models and videos used to teach canine dental core skills. Dental skill acquisition and confidence were found to be higher in students who were trained using models rather than videos. However, there was no significant difference in perceptions related to small-animal dentistry between students trained using the different modalities. The authors recommend using both models and videos to train veterinary students in order to optimize skill acquisition in this field. The conclusions drawn from this research can be used to improve student training so that new graduates may enter the profession better prepared to demonstrate these skills.

Abstract: In recent years, there has been an increased focus on the teaching of small-animal dentistry to veterinary students in order to address the recognized gap between dental skill training and the expectations of employers regarding the competencies of new graduates in this field. In this study, third-year veterinary students were trained in three canine dental core skills using either a high-fidelity model (Group A) or video instruction (Group B). An objective structured clinical examination was used to assess skill acquisition and questionnaires were distributed in order to assess student confidence and perceptions related to small-animal dentistry practice and related skills before and after the training. All results were compared between the two groups. Group A outperformed Group B in skill acquisition ($p < 0.001$) and there was greater improvement in skill confidence for Group A than Group B ($p < 0.001$). There was no statistical difference in perceptions related to small-animal dentistry between the two groups after the training ($p \geq 0.1$). Group A rated their training experience more highly than Group B ($p < 0.001$). Although dental skill acquisition shows greater improvement when training is provided by models rather than video instruction, a blended approach to teaching dental skills is likely to be the best approach to optimizing dental skill acquisition.

Keywords: veterinary dentistry skills; veterinary dental education; veterinary clinical skills; simulation; high-fidelity dental model

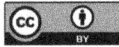

1. Introduction

Periodontitis is the most frequently diagnosed disease in small-animal medicine [1], affecting over 87 percent of dogs over two years of age [2]. This is a disease that can cause bacteremia and which has been linked to several systemic diseases [3–5]. Pain associated with periodontitis and other dental diseases is well established in human patients and is one of the most common reasons patients seek dental treatment [6]. However, animals rarely display overt signs of oral pain associated with mild-to-moderate dental disease [7]. The lack of clinical signs in small-animal patients leads to dental disease progression and compromises health and welfare without the knowledge of even the most attentive of owners [7]. Therefore, the provision of dental services i.e., the prevention, diagnosis, and treatment of periodontitis and other dental diseases, is a paramount responsibility of the primary-care veterinary practitioner [8].

Unequivocally, small-animal dentistry knowledge and skills are highly sought by employers and are considered day-one competencies [8,9]. Small-animal practitioners have recognized the importance of new graduates having skills in dental prophylaxis, tooth extraction, and routine periodontal treatment [10]. New graduates are expected to perform these skills on an average of once per week with proficiency and minimal supervision [10]. However, the current curricula specific to veterinary dental education appear insufficient and limited. Specifically, a large survey of veterinary schools across the USA and the Caribbean found that, in pre-clinical years (years 1–3), small-animal veterinary dentistry was only taught as core course content in 30 percent of veterinary schools, and only as an elective in 23 percent of schools, while 17 percent of schools did not include it in the curriculum [8]. Furthermore, the same study reported that veterinary schools offered a mode of only one to four hours of lecture- and laboratory-based instruction, further illustrating the limited dentistry training opportunities provided to pre-clinical veterinary students [8]. The time students spend practicing dental skills in their clinical year (year 4) was unclear [8].

In recognizing the gap that exists between veterinary dental service demands and skills and in ensuring the adequacy of the small-animal dentistry skills of new graduates, there has been an increased focus in recent years on the teaching of small-animal dentistry to veterinary students. Outside of the lecture-based teaching of canine dentistry, the hands-on, deliberate practice of dental skills is fundamental to ensure graduates are practice-ready in this field [8,9]. In 2020, the teaching of dentistry was acknowledged as a requirement by the American Veterinary Medical Association (AVMA) [11]; this was further supported by the recommendations given by the World Small Animal Veterinary Association (WSAVA) [12].

To bridge the gap in dental skill instruction, models can be utilized to facilitate the acquisition of essential skills, such as those used to teach teeth cleaning skills, be they high-fidelity, mid-fidelity or low-fidelity [13]. Evidence supports the use of simulation as an essential part of modern medical curricula. Simulations are used to facilitate the acquisition of essential clinical skills and competencies through repetition and feedback within currently accepted learning theory frameworks. Mannequins have been used in human dental simulation training since the 1960s [14]. More recently, 3D-printed model teeth manufactured for use in simulation were found to be realistic and cost-effective [15]. A recent publication assessed student perceptions of four different modalities used to teach anatomy: natural teeth, 3D-printed teeth, a 3D virtual model and augmented reality (AR) [16]. The results showed that the natural teeth were of the highest educational value, the 3D-printed teeth were the easiest to use, and the AR model was the most interesting. However, the AR model scored the lowest rating for ease of use and educational value [16]. The paper concluded that there are limitations associated with AR, but that it is an area of significant ongoing development with potential for use in future dental training [16]. This example underscores that, in order to understand the benefits of models, validation of their use is essential, regardless of the level of fidelity, before their implementation in a curriculum.

As advances are made in simulation development, the impact on trainee skill acquisition, or competency, must also be studied in order to provide an understanding of training outcomes. The assessment of competency is essential from both an educational and a financial perspective when the costs associated with model development and the management of simulation laboratories are considered. The human dental field is far more advanced than the veterinary field, with the use of haptic and virtual reality (VR) simulations having transformed the modern dental world [17]. While recognizing that additional studies are needed to further evaluate the use of VR systems in dental skill acquisition, it is important to acknowledge that VR simulators can collect, summarize and analyze all of an operator's work to provide an objective assessment with real-time feedback, and that this assessment can be considered to be more appropriate than human expert assessment [17]. However, faculty feedback provides insight into weaknesses in student technique and provides context to procedural errors; more studies are needed to further evaluate the use of VR systems used in dental skill acquisition [18,19].

In contrast to the human field, the use of only a small number of dental models has been validated in veterinary medical education. A rudimentary model has been found to be an effective way of teaching dental cleaning when compared to the use of video instruction [20]. This same study also reported that all participating students agreed that training on a model would be beneficial to their skill acquisition and that all those who learnt using the model acknowledged improvements in their confidence [20]. In 2021, a study compared the use of three modes in teaching and practicing dental cleaning [13]. This study found that low-fidelity models are as effective as mid-fidelity and high-fidelity models for teaching cleaning. However, students were more accepting of the higher-fidelity models in the study [13]. Although low-fidelity models performed well in terms of instruction, experts recommended the use of higher-fidelity models for skill assessment [13]. In 2022, a published study investigated the use of 3D models to teach scaling and dental charting and found that students gained more confidence if models were used in advance of a cadaver laboratory [21].

There is no uniformity in how useful alternate fidelity simulation modalities are in terms of ensuring skill acquisition. As with veterinary dental skills, the positive effectiveness of low-fidelity models has been reported for veterinary surgical skills [22,23] and in human dentistry [24]. The appropriate validation and assessment of the use of veterinary models is essential; this is especially true in the field of small-animal veterinary dentistry, given the minimal available literature on this subject.

The aim of this study was to evaluate the use of a high-fidelity model (HFM) and video instruction to teach three canine dental core skills to pre-clinical veterinary students: radiographic positioning; cleaning (scaling and polishing); and extractions. Students' skill acquisition was assessed using an objective standardized clinical examination (OSCE) and students' performance was compared between the two groups. Questionnaires were utilized to assess potential changes in the confidence of the students and their perceptions related to small-animal dentistry before and after receiving the training. The results were compared between the two groups. We adopted the hypothesis that students who practiced skills using different modalities, whether HFM or video instruction, would perform differently in the OSCE and have differing levels of confidence when applying skills. A secondary hypothesis was that exposing students to a novel modality, i.e., HFMs, would change their perception of and interest in small-animal dentistry.

2. Materials and Methods

This study was conducted at the Ross University School of Veterinary Medicine (RUSVM), an American Veterinary Medical Association (AVMA)-accredited international veterinary school that provides an intensive pre-clinical course of seven semesters over two years and four months. RUSVM students complete their one year (three semesters) of clinical training at an affiliated AVMA-accredited veterinary school.

At the time this study was conducted, small-animal dentistry instruction at RUSVM was delivered in (i) eight hours of didactic lectures in semester five, (ii) a one-hour self-directed online laboratory in semester six, and (iii) a three-hour elective canine live-animal laboratory in semester seven. The didactic lectures covered the pathology, diagnosis, treatment and prevention of common dental diseases and the core skills of radiology, cleaning, and extractions. The online laboratory focused on instrument identification and use, as well as the charting, and recognition and grading of pathology. The live-animal elective included dental radiography interpretation, probing, charting, and cleaning, with students performing supragingival and subgingival scaling and the polishing of all teeth in one quadrant of a dog's mouth.

Students in semester seven (third year) were invited to participate in this study. Participants were excluded if they were certified veterinary technicians (CVTs) (or international equivalent qualification) or if they had already participated in the seventh-semester elective live-animal laboratory. The study was conducted between January 2020 and January 2021 with three cohorts of students, with each cohort drawn from a different seventh semester. Over the duration of the three cohorts, 105 students enrolled in this study. An administrative colleague independent of the study applied the RAND formula in Microsoft Excel™ to a list of participating students for each cohort to randomly assign them into one of two instructional groups: one group trained using HFMs in a laboratory setting (group A), $n = 52$, and one group trained via video instruction (group B), $n = 53$. All study participants completed a written consent form. This study was approved by RUSVM's Institutional Review Board (IRB), protocol number: 19-03-XP.

The primary author developed a concise skill sheet, which was reviewed and approved by a Diplomate of the American Veterinary Dental College (AVDC) (fourth author). The skill sheet described (i) dental anatomy; (ii) equipment, instruments, and consumables; (iii) personal protective equipment (PPE); and (iv) the three skill sets: radiographic positioning, cleaning (scaling and polishing), and extractions. All participating students within each cohort received a copy of a skill sheet by email on the same day, providing them with a resource to complement their training. The skill sheet was used as the script in the video instruction and HFM laboratories and participants were encouraged to read it as many times as they preferred prior to watching the video or attending the HFM laboratory, as well as in advance of the OSCE. Additionally, the skill sheet was sent to the video instruction group in an email with a link to the video; these students were also informed that they could watch the video as many times as they felt appropriate. The HFM laboratories took place within one to four days of sending the skill sheet. All participants completed a dental skills OSCE two weeks after the HFM laboratories.

The 38 min video included a canine skull to present anatomy and a cadaverous head to demonstrate the skills, describing each element as they were presented or performed (Figure 1).

The HFMs used in this study were made of silicone, plastic, and rubber. They were manufactured by Veterinary Simulators Industries Limited (VSI) (Figure 2). The HFMs had lips that could be reflected, as well as a tongue, an epiglottis, an esophagus, and a trachea. The maxillae and mandibles could be replaced with simulated teeth, bone, and soft rubber gingiva. The HFMs were provided with an arm and clamp that could be employed to secure the model to a tabletop, but these were not used in this study.

At the time the study was conducted, three sets of jaws were available for use to teach different skillsets. (i) One set was used to teach scaling and polishing that included simulated calculus painted onto the teeth. Once dry, an ultrasonic scaler could be used to remove the simulated calculus as in a live patient. (ii) A second set with radiodense teeth was used to teach radiographic positioning (Figure 3). (iii) A third set was used to teach extractions, which included a simulated periodontal ligament. These techniques were used to perform gingival flap creation, alveolar bone removal, tooth elevation and tooth extraction (Figure 4). Components were colored in a realistic fashion to allow for the identification of different simulated tissues.

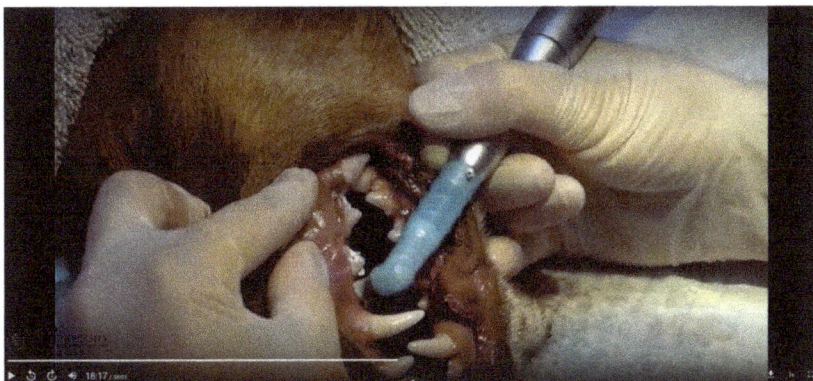

Figure 1. Video Screenshot Demonstrating Polishing.

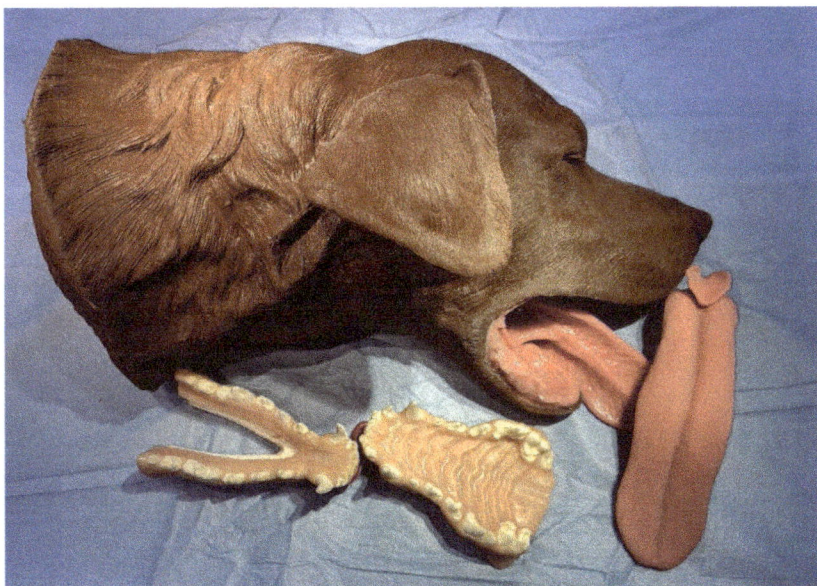

Figure 2. Constituent Parts of the High-Fidelity Model (HFM): head, maxilla, mandible, and tongue.

This study asked three veterinarians to provide face validation for the models prior to their use in laboratories. We asked two diplomates of AVDC (one of them being the fourth author) and an experienced primary care clinician with an interest in small-animal veterinary dentistry (fifth author) to participate. They identified that the teeth of the radiology models had poor contrast. In response, VSI improved the contrast of the models. A subsequent assessment by the same veterinarians identified that the improved models included a variety of teeth that were found not to be strictly anatomically correct, and that some tooth roots had hollow appearances. However, the models were deemed to be appropriate for use in teaching radiographic positioning. In conclusion, the models were deemed to be appropriate for use to practice cleaning, radiographic positioning, and extraction skills, and were considered especially useful for learning instrument-handling skills and gaining familiarity with oral anatomy.

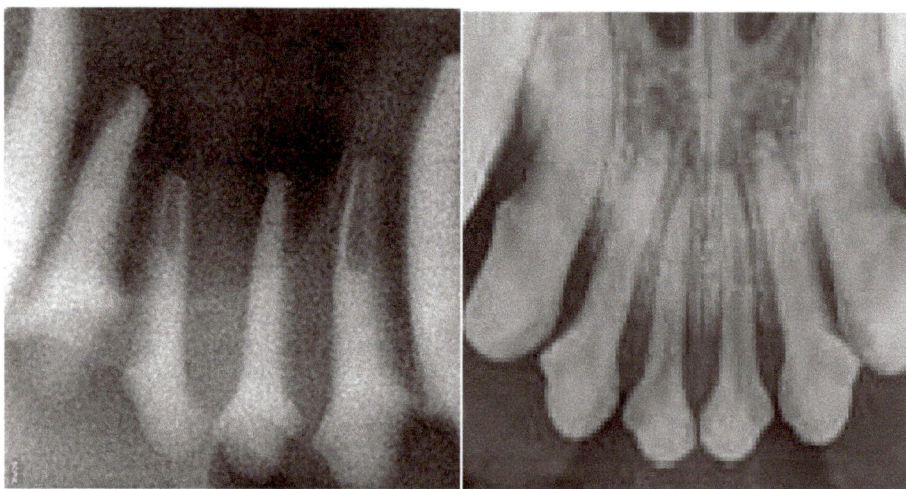

Figure 3. Radiographs of the Maxillary Incisors of the HFM (**left**) and a Live Patient (**right**).

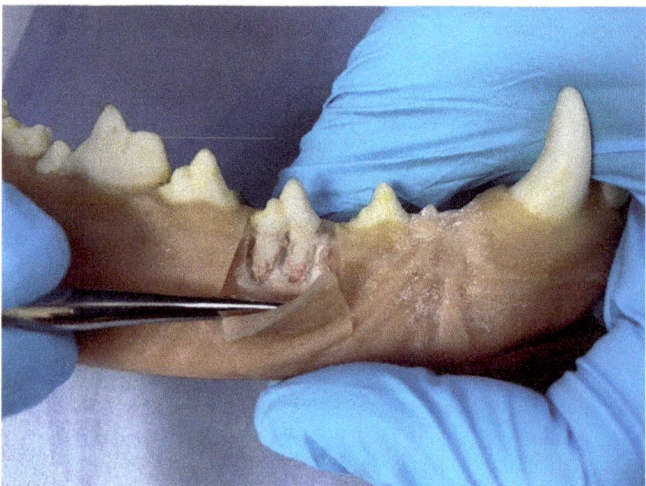

Figure 4. HFM Mandible Demonstrating Gingival Flap and Surgical Extraction Technique.

One veterinarian (first author), one CVT (sixth author) and one certified veterinary technologist (seventh author) facilitated the training in the HFM laboratory and used the same script as that used in the video to present and guide the students through the skills. No additional information was provided to the students. All equipment, instruments and consumables used in the video were identical to those used in all laboratories and assessments. The HFM laboratories were delivered over three one-hour stations, one for each skill set: radiographic positioning; cleaning (scaling and polishing); and extraction. Small groups of students, n = 3–4, rotated through the stations. The HFM laboratories engaged students in performing the skills under supervision, receiving in-the-moment trainer feedback. The trainers in the HFM laboratories were the same individuals who developed the video and they were consistent in the delivery of content through all laboratories and cohorts.

Skill acquisition was assessed using a five-station, 13-item OSCE, and skills were assessed using a five-point Likert scale checklist: 1: below expectations, 2: novice, 3: advanced beginner, 4: competent, 5: proficient (Appendix A.1). The rubric was developed by the primary author and reviewed by the third author, who had significant experience in OSCE design, as well as by a diplomate of AVDC (fourth author). All stations were allocated 5 min to complete the tasks, with a 30 s inter-station change set aside.

Veterinarians and CVTs (or international equivalent) who were independent of the study rated student performance. Rater recruitment required individuals to have a minimum of five years of professional small-animal practice experience. Limited rater availability required the recruitment of raters of varied small-animal dental experience. Raters were provided with detailed guidance about their station and checklist prior to the start of the OSCE. Students were randomly scheduled for their OSCE times using Excel™ and raters were blinded to the training each student had received.

Participating students completed online pre-training and post-OSCE questionnaires to assess their dental skill confidence and their perceptions related to small-animal dentistry (Appendices A.2 and A.3). The questionnaires consisted of 10 questions and required input on the basis of five-point Likert-scale response categories (e.g., not at all confident, slightly confident, somewhat confident, moderately confident, extremely confident). The pre-training questionnaire was completed before any training took place and before the skill sheet was shared. Pre-training questionnaires also included two binary response exclusion questions regarding participant qualifications and participation in the semester seven live-animal laboratory, as discussed earlier. The post-OSCE questionnaire included a Likert-scale response question regarding students' opinions of the training they had received and an open-ended question asking students to provide feedback on the experience of the training they had received. Questionnaire answers were anonymous and collected through the Qualtrics online survey tool to ensure data protection.

All descriptive statistics include median and interquartile ranges. The Wilcoxon rank-sum test was used to compare each OSCE item score and the overall OSCE score between the two groups. Cronbach's α was calculated in order to determine OSCE reliability. The impact of individual stations and items on the reliability of the OSCE was evaluated by comparing Cronbach's α with or without each station or item.

To test the initial randomization, responses of the pre-training questionnaire were compared between the two groups using a Wilcoxon rank-sum test. The responses of the pre-training questionnaire were compared with the post-OSCE questionnaire using the Wilcoxon signed-rank test (paired by student) in order to determine if student confidence and perceptions improved throughout the study in both groups. Furthermore, the difference (subtraction) in the scores between pre-training and post-OSCE questionnaires was compared. In particular, we used the Wilcoxon rank-sum test to assess the level of change in confidence and perceptions between the two groups. Differences were considered significant for p value ≤ 0.05.

3. Results

Out of a total of 105 students, 52 attended the HFM laboratory, 53 completed the video instruction, and all 105 completed the OSCE. Student participation took place in January 2020 ($n = 18$); October 2020 ($n = 21$); and January 2021 ($n = 66$). There was no statistical difference in the baseline confidence or perceptions between the two groups before any training had taken place, $p \geq 0.2$, confirming the random selection of groups (Appendix A.4).

Overall, group A outperformed group B, $p < 0.001$ (Table 1). Group A significantly outperformed group B for 7 of the 13 OSCE items. Group B did not outperform group A for any OSCE item. Station 4 reported that group A outperformed group B by the greatest degree, and Station 4 was the only station for which all items in a station produced a statistically significant difference in performance between the groups.

Table 1. Comparison of OSCE Results Between Video Instruction and HFM Laboratory Groups.

	Grade HFM Laboratory Group A	Grade Video Instruction Group B	Wilcoxon Rank-Sum Test p Value
	Median (IQR)	Median (IQR)	
Overall OSCE (denominator = 100)	80.6 (72.4–85.8)	67.1 (56.7–71.3)	<0.001 *
Station 1			
Put on the necessary personal protective equipment to obtain dental radiographs.	4 (3–4)	2 (2–4)	0.008 *
Prepare the digital radiography sensor to obtain dental radiographs.	4 (2–4)	3 (2–4)	0.2
Place the canine head on the table and in the correct position to obtain a dental radiograph of the mandible. Indicate verbally to the examiner once you have completed this task.	3 (1–4)	2 (1–4)	0.6
Station 2			
Position the radiography sensor and the tube head of the radiograph generator to obtain a radiograph of the mandibular incisors at 45°. Indicate verbally to the examiner once you have completed the task.	3 (2–4)	3 (2–4)	0.8
Position the radiography sensor and the tube head of the radiograph generator to obtain a radiograph of mandibular premolar tooth 4 and molar tooth 1 in quadrant 3. Indicate verbally to the examiner once you have completed the task.	2 (1–3)	1 (1–2)	0.006 *
Station 3			
Put on the necessary personal protective equipment to perform a canine cleaning and polishing procedure.	4 (4–4)	4 (3–4)	0.3
Switch on the ultrasonic scaler machine and verify that it is working correctly.	4 (2–4)	2 (2–3)	<0.001 *
Switch on the air-driven dental unit and verify the three-in-one syringe handpiece is working correctly.	4 (4–4)	4 (4–4)	0.5
Station 4			
All teeth in the cadaver head have had all tartar removed. Demonstrate a scaling procedure on the left mandibular canine tooth.	3.5 (3–4)	2 (2–4)	0.001 *
Assemble the polisher handpiece so that it is ready for use and then polish the left mandibular canine tooth.	4 (3–4)	3 (2–4)	0.003 *
Station 5			
Select the necessary items to perform an incisor extraction. Place on Card A.	3.5 (3–4)	3 (2–4)	0.052
Select any elevator and use it to demonstrate how to hold this tool correctly when in use.	4 (4–4)	3 (2–4)	<0.001 *
Select the necessary instruments to perform a gingival flap—instruments for suturing are not necessary. Place on Card B.	3 (1–4)	1 (1–3)	0.03 *
Assemble the high-speed handpiece so that it is ready to remove alveolar bone from around a tooth root.	4 (3.75–4)	3 (1–3)	<0.001 *

IQR: interquartile range; grade for item: 1–5. * Statistically significant p values. Each item was scored using a five-point Likert scale checklist.

The OSCE had an overall reliability of $\alpha = 0.66$ (95% confidence interval: 0.64–0.69) (Appendix A.5). Reliability varied significantly between stations, $\alpha = 0.003$–0.59, and between raters, $\alpha =< 0$–0.85 (Appendix A.5). Some items have more impact on reliability than others, and the overall OSCE reliability would increase, $\alpha > 0.66$, if these items were removed from the analysis. This is true for all items in Station 1 and Item 1 in Station 3 (Appendix A.6).

A total of 84 students completed the pre-training and post-OSCE questionnaires, with 40 drawn from group A and 44 from group B. Group A had significantly greater confidence post-OSCE than pre-training in all six related questions, $p < 0.001$ (Appendix A.4). Group B had significantly greater confidence post-OSCE than pre-training in five of the six related questions, $p \leq 0.01$ (Appendix A.4). There was no statistically significant improvement for any of the perception-related questions for either group, $p \geq 0.1$ (Appendix A.4).

Group A had significantly greater improvements in confidence than the group B after the training and OSCE, with $p < 0.001$ for all related questions (Appendix A.4). In the post-OSCE questionnaire, group A rated their training experience to be better than group B's, $p < 0.001$ (Appendix A.4). A total of 63 participants provided comments on their training experience in the post-OSCE questionnaire, $n = 38$ from group A, and $n = 25$ from group B. The primary author has summarized and purposely selected some of these comments in Table 2 to provide an overview of the students' experience.

Table 2. Selection of Participant Comments.

Comments from Group A
The high-fidelity models were really nice to learn on. I enjoyed getting the feel of how it is actually done on a live patient. I am amazed at what stuck with me after learning about it once for three hours two weeks ago.
As someone who has never been exposed to dentistry, I believe the lab helped me out a tremendous amount, I feel much more confident than I did prior to the in-person labs. I hope every vet student gets the chance to learn using the models, my confidence in dentistry has significantly improved after only one day of training.
I really enjoyed the models, I felt like it was a really good experience to feel and handle a model that's similar to real life. The models were very helpful for getting a good understanding of accurate canine dental anatomy.
The high-fidelity models were extremely helpful for me because I could visualize and assess all procedures with all my senses. It was a great learning experience. I got very interested in dentistry because of the models.
Comments from Group B
Being assigned to the videos, I like the fact that I could review the material prior to the OSCE and rewatch them. However, I don't think they are as helpful as a hands-on lab. There are many questions I wish I could have asked and even with watching the videos multiple times I don't feel prepared to perform these skills on a live patient by myself.
I felt like I learned a lot watching the videos but not nearly as much as if I had done the lab in person. It's hard to assess your understanding without being able to do something with direct instruction and immediate feedback.
I did not find the videos very helpful in learning how to perform the tasks demonstrated. However, I do feel that they would be a good to refer to after completing the lab on the models, should any questions come up after the lab.
Felt videos were good quality. However, online was able to slack off. There is also no feedback or possible corrections made to your skills with online videos and no live instructor.

4. Discussion

To the authors' knowledge, this is the first published work that studies veterinary dental radiographic positioning and tooth extraction skill acquisition. In this study, the use of the HFMs to teach dental skills was shown to be of significant benefit when compared to video instruction, with the HFM group outperforming the video instruction group in the OSCE. Both video instruction and HFM laboratories improved skill confidence. However, there was a significantly greater increase for the HFM laboratory group, and the HFMs were rated as being better resources than the video. Neither training experience significantly affected perceptions.

The positive impact of video resources on enhancing teaching and skill acquisition in human medical and dental education, as well as veterinary education, is widely reported [25–29], with the results of this study further supporting this. Although the HFM group outperformed the video instruction group in the OSCE, there was no statistical difference in improvement between the two groups for 6 of the 14 items. In total, 3 of these items were related to radiology skills, 2 items were related to cleaning, and 1 item was related to extractions. There are several possible explanations for the similarity in the acquisition of these skills between the two groups. Firstly, the complexity of these skills may have been such that the hands-on practice with HFM instruction was insignificant in terms of improving skill acquisition when compared to video instruction. Specifically, these skills could be considered easy to learn and can be taught through observation using video instruction. Secondly, students may have drawn from skills learnt elsewhere in the curriculum such as radiology laboratories and lectures, therefore bringing bias to the analysis. Thirdly, the potential of the HFMs may not have been realized due to an absence of the opportunity for deliberate practice, acknowledging that the use of deliberate practice in simulation-based medical education increases the success of clinical skill acquisition [30–32]. It is reasonable to surmise that the performance of the skills in question could have been influenced by the ease of developing an understanding via video instruction and the absence of opportunity for deliberate practice with the HFMs. The authors hypothesize that both video instructions and HFMs are valuable resources to teach dental veterinary skills and the level of difficulty can guide the approach. Varied teaching strategies can be employed to improve learning experiences, which is of particular interest to disciplines that may struggle to garner interest from students. A recent study investigated the use of a flipped classroom and peer-assisted learning to teach equine nutrition, a subject which most post-graduation veterinarians lack knowledge of and skills in [33]. Despite half of the students questioned in the study reporting to be uninterested in the subject matter, most expressed positive attitudes towards the teaching methods used [33]. Providing diverse learning opportunities has the potential to engage students with unpopular disciplines, which could raise the profile of under-resourced areas of study and ultimately improve animal welfare.

The results of the post-OSCE questionnaire report that there was no significant overall increase in practical experience for the video instruction group; this is to be expected, as these students were not provided with any practical experience. However, the video did significantly improve confidence for all specific skill sets, and the OSCE results supported the notion that the video had a positive impact on skill acquisition. Although the HFM lab experience was rated higher than the video instruction in terms of improving skill acquisition, the video was also favorably rated. This result aligns with other research reports that find the use of video resources to be beneficial in terms of improving preparedness for assessments and reducing stress [34]. Students were less accepting of the notion that video instruction increased confidence in comparison with their relationship to HFM. This was potentially due to: (i) Students not spending sufficient time watching the video or doing so with due attention. Indeed, students reported varied, consumption of videos with peak viewing one or two days before assessment [34]. (ii) The length of the video being 38 min, considering that videos longer than 6 min have been found to have poor student engagement [35]. (iii) An absence of feedback and expert supervision, which are important in skill acquisition [22,36].

In the future, the authors recommend a blended approach to veterinary dental skill training, whereby videos lasting a maximum of 6 min are used in conjunction with the HFMs. Blended learning has well-documented benefits in terms of clinical skills development in the human and veterinary fields [37,38]. The use of technology provides students with the flexibility, convenience, and independence required for an individualized approach to learning [37,38]. The videos can be shared in advance of labs, used in lectures, and used as a resource for study outside of the classroom and laboratory. Veterinary students have been found to use online resources to prepare for practical classes [39]; further work on how veterinary students use videos to supplement their dental skill training would be beneficial to efforts to guide their use.

The HFM group in this study reported a greater improvement in confidence post-OSCE than the video instruction group. Indeed, an increase in confidence with skills learned using HFMs over lower-fidelity models is well reported in medical education [39–41]. Feedback and individualized learning with the active participation of the trainee are also very important to the success of simulation skill labs and are accepted in improving outcomes [39,40]. When considering the outcomes of this study, it is reasonable to conclude that the greater increase in confidence for the HFM group can be attributed to both the fidelity of the models and the training group size, $N = 3$–4, which allows for students to receive real-time individualized feedback from both instructors and peers.

Neither training experience significantly affected perceptions. Students' backgrounds and interests in career choice have been reported positive influences on the outcome of associated clinical skill acquisition [42]. If an interest in a chosen career path is associated with success in clinical skill acquisition, it could also reinforce perceptions of skills, hence the lack of significant change from pre-training to post-OSCE.

This study does not consider other knowledge and skills students may be gaining when using the HFMs such as anatomy, patient handling, and personal posture, and practicing skills with water and a tongue in the simulated patient's mouth. Simulation enhances psychomotor skills and hand–eye coordination, which are especially important for surgery [43]. Some of these experiences are difficult to achieve with lower-fidelity models, which is another area worthy of future consideration and study. The classification of simulation model fidelity is subjective and encompasses an array of features [39,44]; when compared with other veterinary models documented in the published literature, the authors consider their classification as high to be reasonable and in agreement with another published study [13]. However, if they are compared with models used in the human field, this would not be the case [18]. The lack of a standardized method of classification of simulated models creates challenges when comparisons and validation are sought [39]. Further consideration should be given to standardizing the classification of model fidelity between and within professions.

The overall reliability of the OSCE would be considered low, indicating differences in rating between raters. Raters A and E were CVTs with considerable experience of small-animal dentistry practice, and rater B was a CVT with little experience of small-animal dentistry. No CVT raters had experience of OSCE rating. Raters C, F, G and H were veterinarians with considerable experience of small-animal dentistry practice and rater D was a veterinarian with no experience of small-animal dentistry practice. All veterinarian raters had experience of OSCE rating. Reliability as raters varied considerably between raters and stations. However, it is notable that the raters with $\alpha < 0$ were the CVT and the veterinarian with no significant small-animal dentistry practice experience. The results suggest that CVTs and veterinarians can assess pre-clinical veterinary students' dentistry skills with a similar degree of reliability, and similarly, that both CVTs and veterinarians should be recruited as raters based on sound clinical dentistry experience and be provided with robust training in advance of performing an OSCE. Furthermore, acknowledging that rubric wording is important and is reported to impact assessors and pass/fail decisions [45], validity could be improved by increasing expert input to OSCE station and rubric design, robust rater training, and running pilots of the OSCE and rubric. There is additionally value in analyzing the results of specialists, experienced practitioners and new graduates whose skills have been assessed using the OSCE and rubric and comparing them with student results [46,47]. With investment in OSCE and rubric design and by analyzing the assessment results of different groups, over time the items could be refined and the reliability of these assessments improved.

There are significant costs associated with the use of HFMs. Radiology jaw sets can be used with minimal wear over time but do eventually need replacement. The teeth of the models used for cleaning wear down after several uses and the cleaning procedures also cause wear to the model heads. Therefore, these models have a higher rate of turnover than radiology sets. The teeth of the extraction jaw sets cannot be replaced, each tooth is single-use, and extraction procedures cause wear to the model heads, meaning that judicious use of these models is warranted. In the HFM laboratories used for this study, each student extracted one incisor and one two-rooted tooth. The availability and storage of cadavers and other means of teaching, as well as budgets, will influence investment in the HFMs. Simulation models can only be as good as the educational environment in which they are used [44]. Therefore, these HFMs should be implemented into a curriculum with careful planning, and further assessment of their use is warranted. The models can also be used to teach nerve blocks and endotracheal intubation. Future positive validation of their use to teach these skills may influence laboratory investment.

5. Study Limitations

This study presents several limitations. Raters were assigned based on their availability. As such, there were limitations in maintaining rater–station continuity. Indeed, examiner cohorts are reported to have a significant and replicable influence on OSCE scores [48]. There are numerous possible factors that could be influencing the differences in rater assessment: rater experience of practicing small-animal dentistry, rater experience of assessing small-animal dentistry and rater experience of assessing the use of an OSCE. Additionally, numerous types of rater errors are recognized in medical assessments. Some of these errors are the most significant threats to assessment validity [49,50]. In the human dental field, rater training has been found to improve the inter-rater reliability of performance assessment, with rater training workshops and encouraging rater involvement with OSCE development used to facilitate these improvements [46,51]. Similarly, rater training has been recommended as a means to improve assessment validity in veterinary education [50]. Rater training could have been used in this study to improve reliability. However, rater impact is unlikely to have altered the results as they were blinded to the experimental group (HFM or video instruction) and participant order in the OSCE was randomly assigned.

Students in the video instruction group could not have been expected to safely use a high-speed handpiece in the OSCE as they had not received in-person training to ensure that each student fully understood the necessary health and safety requirements of this handpiece, thus limiting the assessment of associated extraction skills. Further assessment of the acquisition of extraction skills is necessary.

6. Conclusions

Students greatly appreciated the opportunity to learn on HFMs and core dental skill acquisition showed greater improvement when training was provided with HFMs than video instruction. The use of HFMs to teach dentistry skills did not change students' preference for small-animal dentistry over video instruction. The authors recommend the use of small-group simulation laboratory learning in rotation to facilitate the acquisition of multiple skills, this can be carried out for large cohorts if planned well. The primary author also recommends using appropriately trained and experienced CVTs as instructors in some clinical skills. CVTs and veterinarians can assess pre-clinical veterinary students' dentistry skills with a similar degree of reliability. CVTs and veterinarians should be recruited based on sound clinical dentistry experience. Further work to assess the use of HFMs in a blended learning course, in comparison to cadavers and lower-fidelity models, and the transferability of acquired skills to the live patient should be conducted. In the future, a dental skills course that includes the use of videos lasting no longer than 6 min, and models of varied fidelity, may achieve similar outcomes to a course using HFMs alone and be preferable from a budgetary standpoint.

Author Contributions: Conceptualization, J.F. and E.A.; methodology, J.F. and E.A.; validation, K.Y.-S.J., W.G. and N.A.; formal analysis, A.C.; investigation, J.F., D.S. and C.W.; resources, J.F., D.S. and C.W.; data curation, J.F., writing—original draft preparation, J.F.; writing—review and editing, A.C., K.Y.-S.J. and E.A.; visualization, J.F. and A.C.; supervision, E.A.; project administration, J.F.; funding acquisition, J.F. All authors have read and agreed to the published version of the manuscript.

Funding: Funding for this study was provided by an intramural grant from Ross University School of Veterinary Medicine, Center for Research and Innovation in Veterinary Medical Education, grant number 44001-2019.

Institutional Review Board Statement: The study was conducted in accordance with the Declaration of Helsinki and approved by the Institutional Review Board of Ross University School of Veterinary Medicine (protocol code 19-03-XP, 26 July 2019).

Informed Consent Statement: Informed consent was obtained from all subjects involved in the study.

Data Availability Statement: All data is contained within this article or Appendix A.

Acknowledgments: We thank Kevin Stepaniuk for his role in face validation of the HFMs; Juliette Bouillon, Renata de Rosayro, Louise Dowd, Stephanie Jackson, Kurt Roman, Olivia Shelley, Nigel Smith, Jemma Thorogood, and Matthew Valentine for their role as raters in the OSCEs; Alexandra Fontanetta, Damiana Gumiran, and Kaylin Stewart for assistance in OSCE management; Antoine Laws for his assistance in data collection; and Cleon Bradshaw and Kazzi Heath for their assistance in creating the video.

Conflicts of Interest: The authors declare no conflict of interest.

Appendix A.

Appendix A.1. OSCE Rubric

Station One

Item 1: Put on the necessary personal protective equipment to obtain dental radiographs.

1. Does not choose a lead gown or a thyroid protector.
2. Chooses lead gown and thyroid protector but puts them on incorrectly with/without disposable gloves.
3. Chooses lead gown and thyroid protector and puts them on correctly. Does not choose disposable gloves.
4. Chooses lead gown, thyroid protector, and disposable gloves. Hesitates to put them on correctly.
5. Chooses a lead gown, thyroid protector and disposable gloves and puts them on correctly and confidently.

Item 2: Prepare the digital radiography sensor to obtain dental radiographs.

1. Does not choose the plastic sheath and/or the cohesive wrapping bandage tape and/or does not identify the sensor.
2. Correctly chooses plastic sheath and cohesive bandage but applies them in the wrong order.
3. Applies the plastic sheath and cohesive bandage in the correct order but poorly so that the sensor is insecurely or incompletely covered.
4. Correctly chooses a disposable plastic sheath and cohesive wrapping bandage tape. Applies them correctly but hesitantly.
5. Correctly chooses disposable plastic sheath and cohesive wrapping bandage tape. Confidently applies them to the radiography sensor with the wrap over the sheath so that the sensor is completely and securely covered.

Item 3: Place the canine head on the table and in the correct position to obtain a dental radiograph of the mandible. Indicate verbally to the examiner once you have completed this task.

1. The head is not placed in dorsal recumbency.
2. The head is placed in dorsal recumbency. The mandible is not parallel with the table because towels, or any other form of support, are not used.
3. The head is placed in dorsal recumbency. Towels, or other forms of support, are used to position the head, but the mandible is not parallel with the table.
4. The head is placed in dorsal recumbency. Towels or other forms of support are used to position the head. The mandible is parallel with the table. This is performed hesitantly.
5. The head is placed in dorsal recumbency. Towels or other forms of support are used to position the head. The mandible is parallel with the table. This is performed confidently.

Station Two

Item 1: Position the radiography sensor and the tube head of the radiograph generator to obtain a radiograph of the mandibular incisors at 45°. Indicate verbally to the examiner once you have completed the task.

1. The sensor is not placed against the crowns of the incisors and/or the X-ray tube is remote from the mandibular incisors.
2. The sensor is not in the correct orientation but is placed against the crowns of the incisors AND the tube is not placed at 45° but is directed at the mandibular incisors.
3. The sensor is not in the correct orientation but is placed against the crowns of the incisors OR the tube is not placed at 45° but is directed at the mandibular incisors.
4. The sensor is correctly placed and in the correct orientation but the student struggles to support it well and/or the X-ray tube is directed at the mandibular incisors at 45° but is touching the head.
5. The sensor is placed in the mouth, resting against the crowns of the mandibular incisors and lingual mucosa, in the correct orientation. The sensor is supported appropriately with gauze/bandage material/props. The X-ray tube is directed at the mandibular incisors, positioned at 45° and close to the mandible but not touching it.

Item 2: Position the radiography sensor and the tube head of the radiograph generator to obtain a radiograph of the mandibular premolar tooth 4 and molar tooth 1 in quadrant 3. Indicate verbally to the examiner once you have completed the task.

1. The sensor is not placed against the crowns of the correct teeth and/or the X-ray tube is remote from the correct teeth.
2. The sensor is not in the correct orientation but is placed against the crowns of the correct teeth AND the tube is not in parallel with the sensor but is directed at the correct teeth.
3. The sensor is not in the correct orientation but is placed against the crowns of the correct teeth OR the tube is not in parallel with the sensor but is directed at the correct teeth.
4. The sensor is correctly placed and in the correct orientation but the student struggles to support it well and/or the X-ray tube is directed in parallel to the sensor, but it is touching the head.
5. The sensor is placed in the mouth, resting against the crowns of the teeth and lingual mucosa in the correct orientation. The sensor is supported appropriately with gauze/bandage material/props. The X-ray tube is directed in parallel to the sensor; close to the mandible, but not touching it.

Station Three

Item 1: Put on the necessary personal protective equipment to perform a canine cleaning and polishing procedure.

1. Only chooses goggles OR only chooses a mask without visor OR only chooses gloves.
2. Chooses disposable gloves and a mask without visor or goggles.

3. Does not choose disposable gloves but does choose a mask with visor or a mask with goggles.
4. Chooses disposable gloves and a mask with visor or mask with goggles. Struggles to put them on correctly.
5. Chooses disposable gloves and a mask with visor or mask with goggles and puts them on correctly and confidently.

Item 2: Switch on the ultrasonic scaler machine and verify that it is working correctly.
1. Does not identify the correct machine and/or does not identify the correct handpiece.
2. Is unable to switch the machine on.
3. Does not apply the tip to a metal surface.
4. Does not identify the correct machine and/or the handpiece initially.
5. Confidently identifies the ultrasonic scaler machine and switches it on. Holds the handpiece in the dominant hand, pushes the metal ring on the handpiece to verify that water is flowing from the scaler tip and applies the tip to a metal surface to verify it's working correctly.

Item 3: Switch on the air-driven dental unit and verify the three-in-one syringe handpiece is working correctly.
1. Does not identify the correct machine and/or does not identify the correct handpiece.
2. Is unable to switch the machine on.
3. Does not demonstrate water and air flow separately and together.
4. Does not identify the correct machine and/or handpiece initially.
5. Confidently identifies the air-driven dental unit and switches it on. Holds the three-in-one syringe in the dominant hand using a palm grip and verifies that it is operating correctly by pressing each of the two buttons separately and together to demonstrate water and air can be delivered at the appropriate pressure, whether separately or together.

Station Four

Item 1: All teeth in the cadaver head have had all tartar removed. Demonstrate a scaling procedure on the left mandibular canine tooth.
1. Fails to engage the metal ring and/or fails to identify the correct machine or handpiece.
2. Regardless of how the handpiece is held and what areas are de-scaled, the student uses the scaler for longer than 10 s on the tooth and/or does not move the scaler constantly.
3. Regardless of how the handpiece is held, the student does not de-scale all these areas: the buccal, mesial, distal aspects and subgingival area.
4. Does not use a modified pen grasp and/or uses excessive force and/or is not confident with the action.
5. Confidently holds the handpiece with a modified pen grasp. Uses a constant sweeping motion with a light touch to scale the tooth. Scales the buccal, mesial, and distal aspects of the tooth (lingual not essential) and the subgingival area. Does not keep the scaler in contact with the tooth for longer than 10 s.

Item 2: Assemble the polisher handpiece so that it is ready to use and then polish the left mandibular canine tooth.
1. Fails to identify the correct handpiece or fails to use the foot pedal.
2. Fails to attach a polishing head to the body of the handpiece and/or does not keep the cup in constant motion and/or does not polish the correct tooth.
3. Does not polish all these areas: buccal, mesial, distal aspects and subgingival area.
4. Does not use a modified pen grasp and/or uses excessive force and/or is not confident with the action. Does not identify the correct handpiece to start with and/or does not assemble the handpiece confidently.
5. Confidently identifies and assembles the polisher handpiece by attaching the polishing head. Applies paste to the head. Holds the handpiece with a modified pen grasp.

Uses a light touch and keeps the cup in constant motion. Polishes the buccal, mesial, and distal aspects of the tooth (lingual not essential) and the subgingival area.

Station Five.

Item 1: Select the necessary instruments to perform an incisor extraction. Place on Card A.

1. Does not select an elevator AND does not select a scalpel blade.
2. Does not select an elevator OR does not select a scalpel blade.
3. Chooses an elevator over 3 mm and/or chooses a scalpel blade that is not a 15.
4. Does not choose a scalpel handle and/or chooses a 1 mm or 3 mm elevator.
5. Selects all the following: 15-scalpel blade, scalpel handle, 2 mm elevator.

Item 2: Select any elevator and use it to demonstrate how to hold this instrument correctly when in use.

1. Does not select an elevator.
2. Does not use a palm grasp.
3. The elevator is held in a palm grasp. The index finger is on the stem of the elevator but not close to the tip.
4. The elevator is held in a palm grasp. The index finger is on the stem of the elevator and close, but not at, the tip.
5. The elevator is held in a palm grasp. The index finger is on the stem of the elevator and close, but not at, the tip.

Item 3: Select the necessary instruments to perform a gingival flap, instruments for suturing are not necessary. Place on Card B.

1. Does not select a periosteal elevator AND does not select a scalpel blade.
2. Does not select a periosteal elevator OR does not select a scalpel blade.
3. Regardless of whether a scalpel handle is selected. Selects a periosteal elevator and a scalpel blade that is not a 15.
4. Does not select a scalpel handle.
5. Selects all the following: 15-scalpel blade, scalpel handle, periosteal elevator.

Item 4: Assemble the high-speed handpiece so that it is ready to remove alveolar bone from around a tooth root.

1. Does not select a bur AND does not select the correct handpiece.
2. Does not select a bur OR does not select the correct handpiece.
3. Is unable to insert any bur to the handpiece.
4. Does not select the correct bur but inserts a bur correctly and/or does not verify that the bur is secure.
5. Selects the high-speed handpiece and a #2 or #4 round bur and inserts the bur to the turbine correctly. Verifies that the bur is secure.

Appendix A.2. Pre-Training Questionnaire

Canine Dental Skills: Questionnaire A

This questionnaire includes 2 demographics questions, followed by 11 self-evaluation questions on dental clinical skills competencies. Questionnaire must be completed before any learning has started and before the distribution of any supporting documents.

Demographic questions:

1. Are you a certified/licensed/registered veterinary technician/technologist/nurse?
   Yes
   No
2. Have you completed the elective live animal dental lab in Ross University Veterinary Clinic (RUVC)?
   Yes

No

If you have answered 'Yes' to either question 1 or 2 do not continue, you are excluded from this study.

Dental Skills Assessment:

1. How do you rate your level of practical experience of canine dentistry skills?

    1 = not at all experienced; 2 = slightly experienced; 3 = somewhat experienced; 4 = moderately experienced, 5 = extremely experienced.

2. How do you rate your confidence with regards to canine teeth polishing skills?

    1 = not at all confident; 2 = slightly confident; 3 = somewhat confident; 4 = moderately confident; 5 = extremely confident.

3. How do you rate your confidence with regards to canine teeth de-scaling skills?

    1 = not at all confident; 2 = slightly confident; 3 = somewhat confident; 4 = moderately confident; 5 = extremely confident.

4. How do you rate your confidence with regards to canine dental radiographic positioning skills?

    1 = not at all confident; 2 = slightly confident; 3 = somewhat confident; 4 = moderately confident; 5 = extremely confident.

5. How do you rate your confidence with regards to canine single-rooted tooth extractions?

    1 = not at all confident; 2 = slightly confident; 3 = somewhat confident; 4 = moderately confident; 5 = extremely confident.

6. How do you rate your confidence with regards to canine two-rooted tooth extractions?

    1 = not at all confident; 2 = slightly confident; 3 = somewhat confident; 4 = moderately confident; 5 = extremely confident.

7. How do you rate your level of interest in canine dentistry skills?

    1 = not at all interested; 2 = slightly interested; 3 = neutral; 4 = interested; 5 = very interested.

8. How important do you think canine dentistry skills are to your pre-clinical learning?

    1 = not at all important; 2 = slightly important; 3 = neutral; 4 = important; 5 = very important.

9. How important do you think canine dentistry skills are to a new graduate?

    1 = not at all important; 2 = slightly important; 3 = neutral; 4 = important; 5 = very important.

10. How likely are you to pursue a career in veterinary dentistry?

    1 = extremely unlikely; 2 = unlikely; 3 = neutral; 4 = likely; 5 = extremely likely.

11. How likely are to pursue a career in small-animal practice?

    1 = extremely unlikely; 2 = unlikely; 3 = neutral; 4 = likely; 5 = extremely likely.

Appendix A.3. Post-OSCE Questionnaire

Canine Dental Skills: Questionnaire B

This questionnaire includes 14 self-evaluation questions on dental clinical skills competencies and your experience of the skills lab. This questionnaire must be completed once all training has been completed.

1. How do you rate your level of practical experience of canine dentistry skills?

    1 = not at all experienced; 2 = slightly experienced; 3 = somewhat experienced; 4 = moderately experienced; 5 = extremely experienced.

2. How do you rate your confidence with regards to canine teeth de-scaling skills?

    1 = not at all confident; 2 = slightly confident; 3 = somewhat confident; 4 = moderately confident; 5 = extremely confident.

3. How do you rate your confidence with regards to canine teeth polishing skills?

4. How do you rate your confidence with regards to canine dental radiographic positioning skills?

    1 = not at all confident; 2 = slightly confident; 3 = somewhat confident; 4 = moderately confident; 5 = extremely confident.

5. How do you rate your confidence with regards to canine single-rooted tooth extractions?

    1 = not at all confident; 2 = slightly confident; 3 = somewhat confident; 4 = moderately confident; 5 = extremely confident.

6. How do you rate your confidence with regards to canine two-rooted tooth extractions?

    1 = not at all confident; 2 = slightly confident; 3 = somewhat confident; 4 = moderately confident; 5 = extremely confident.

7. How do you rate your level of interest in canine dentistry skills?

    1 = not at all interested; 2 = slightly interested; 3 = neutral; 4 = interested; 5 = very interested.

8. How important do you think canine dentistry skills are to your pre-clinical learning?

    1 = not at all important; 2 = slightly important; 3 = neutral; 4 = important; 5 = very important.

9. How important do you think canine dentistry skills are to a new graduate?

    1 = not at all important; 2 = slightly important; 3 = neutral; 4 = important; 5 = very important.

10. How useful do you think the lab was in improving the acquisition of canine dentistry

    1 = not at all useful; 2 = slightly useful; 3 = neutral; 4 = useful; 5 = very useful.

11. How likely are you to pursue a career in veterinary dentistry?

    1 = extremely unlikely; 2 = unlikely; 3 = neutral; 4 = likely; 5 = extremely likely.

12. How likely are to pursue a career in small-animal practice?

    1 = extremely unlikely; 2 = unlikely; 3 = neutral; 4 = likely; 5 = extremely likely.

13. Which dental laboratory did you participate in?

    1. Videos.
    2. High-fidelity models.

14. Please provide further details regarding your experience of the lab:

Appendix A.4. Questionnaire Statistical Analysis

	Group A (HFM)			Group B (Video Instruction)			p Value Baseline between Groups [2]	p Value Evolution between Groups [2]
	Before	After	p Value [1]	Before	After	p Value [1]		
How do you rate your level of practical experience of canine dentistry skills?	1 (1–2)	3 (2–4)	<0.001 *	1 (1–2)	1.5 (1–2)	0.4	0.8	<0.001 *
How do you rate your confidence with regards to canine teeth de-scaling skills?	1 (1–1)	4 (3–4)	<0.001 *	1 (1–2)	2 (1–3)	0.008 *	0.4	<0.001 *
How do you rate your confidence with regards to canine teeth polishing skills?	1 (1–1)	4 (4–4.25)	<0.001 *	1 (1–2)	2 (1.75–3)	<0.001 *	0.4	<0.001 *
How do you rate your confidence with regards to canine dental radiographic positioning skills?	1 (1–2)	3 (2–3)	<0.001 *	1 (1–2)	2 (1–2.25)	0.01 *	0.7	<0.001 *

	Group A (HFM)			Group B (Video Instruction)			p Value Baseline between Groups [2]	p Value Evolution between Groups [2]
	Before	After	p Value [1]	Before	After	p Value [1]		
How do you rate your confidence with regards to canine single-rooted tooth extractions?	1 (1–1)	3 (2.75–4)	<0.001 *	1 (1–1)	2 (1–2)	<0.001 *	0.4	<0.001 *
How do you rate your confidence with regards to canine two-rooted tooth extractions?	1 (1–1)	3 (2–3)	<0.001 *	1 (1–1)	1 (1–2)	0.01 *	0.2	<0.001 *
How do you rate your level of interest in canine dentistry skills?	4 (4–4.25)	4 (3–5)	0.5	4 (3–5)	4 (3–4)	0.7	0.7	0.7
How important do you think canine dentistry skills are to your pre-clinical learning?	5 (5–5)	5 (5–5)	0.2	5 (4.75–5)	5 (5–5)	0.6	0.8	0.7
How important do you think canine dentistry skills are to a new graduate?	5 (5–5)	5 (5–5)	0.1	5 (5–5)	5 (5–5)	0.6	0.7	0.2
How likely are you to pursue a career in veterinary dentistry?	3 (2–3)	3 (2.75–3)	0.4	3 (2–3)	3 (2–3)	0.9	0.7	0.7
How likely are to pursue a career in small-animal practice?	5 (4–5)	5 (4–5)	0.8	5 (4–5)	5 (5–5)	1	0.6	0.4
How useful do you think the lab was in improving the acquisition of canine dentistry skills?		5 (5–5)			3.5 (2–5)		-	<0.001 *

[1] Wilcoxon Signed-Rank Test (paired). [2] Wilcoxon Rank-Sum Test. * Statistically significant p values. N = 84.

Appendix A.5. Cronbach α by Station, Cohort and Rater

	Cohort 1	Cohort 2	Cohort 3	All Cohorts
Station 1 (3 Items)	0.52 (Rater A)	<0 (Rater B)	0.03 (Mixed Raters)	0.003
Station 2 (2 Items)		0.51 (Rater C)		0.51
Station 3 (3 Items)	<0 (Rater D)		0.24 (Mixed Raters)	0.19
Station 4 (2 Items)	0.63 (Rater E)	0.85 (Rater F)	0.47 (Mixed Raters)	0.59
Station 5 (4 Items)	0.59 (Rater G)		0.55 (Rater H)	0.56
All stations	0.74	0.64	0.64	0.66

Cohort 1: January 2020, $n = 18$; Cohort 2: October 2020, $n = 21$; Cohort 3: January 2021, $n = 66$.

Appendix A.6. Sensitivity Analysis: Cronbach α Calculated without each Station or Item

	Cronbach α
Station 1	**0.69**
Put on the necessary personal protective equipment to obtain dental radiographs.	0.67
Prepare the digital radiography sensor to obtain dental radiographs.	0.67
Place the canine head on the table and in the correct position to obtain a dental radiograph of the mandible. Indicate verbally to the examiner once you have completed this task.	0.67
Station 2	**0.62**
Position the radiography sensor and the tube head of the radiograph generator to obtain a radiograph of the mandibular incisors at 45°. Indicate verbally to the examiner once you have completed the task.	0.65
Position the radiography sensor and the tube head of the radiograph generator to obtain a radiograph of the mandibular premolar tooth 4 and molar tooth 1 in quadrant 3. Indicate verbally to the examiner once you have completed the task.	0.62

	Cronbach α
Station 3	**0.64**
Put on the necessary personal protective equipment to perform a canine cleaning and polishing procedure.	0.67
Switch on the ultrasonic scaler machine and verify that it is working correctly.	0.62
Switch on the air-driven dental unit and verify the three-in-one syringe handpiece is working correctly.	0.66
Station 4	**0.58**
All teeth in the cadaver head have had all tartar removed. Demonstrate a scaling procedure on the left mandibular canine tooth.	0.63
Assemble the polisher handpiece so that it is ready to use and then polish the left mandibular canine tooth.	0.62
Station 5	**0.53**
Select the necessary items to perform an incisor extraction. Place on Card A.	0.66
Select any elevator and use it to demonstrate how to hold this tool correctly when in use.	0.63
Select the necessary instruments to perform a gingival flap, instruments for suturing are not necessary. Place on Card B.	0.65
Assemble the high-speed handpiece so that it is ready to remove alveolar bone from around a tooth root.	0.61

References

1. Niemiec, B.A. Periodontal disease. *Top. Companion Anim. Med.* **2008**, *23*, 72–80. [CrossRef]
2. Wiggs, R.; Lobprise, H. Periodontology. In *Veterinary Dentistry, Principles and Practice*, 1st ed.; Wiggs, R., Lobprise, H., Eds.; Lippincott Raven: Philadelphia, PA, USA, 1997; pp. 186–231.
3. Pereira dos Santos, J.D.; Cunha, E.; Nunes, T.; Tavares, L.; Oliveira, M. Relation between periodontal disease and systemic diseases in dogs. *Res. Vet. Sci.* **2019**, *125*, 136–140. [CrossRef] [PubMed]
4. Glickman, L.T.; Glickman, N.W.; Moore, G.E.; Lund, E.M.; Lantz, G.C.; Pressler, B.M. Association between chronic azotemic kidney disease and the severity of periodontal disease in dogs. *Prev. Vet. Med.* **2011**, *99*, 193–200. [CrossRef]
5. Glickman, L.T.; Glickman, N.W.; Moore, G.E.; Goldstein, G.S.; Lewis, H.B. Evaluation of the risk of endocarditis and other cardiovascular events on the basis of the severity of periodontal disease in dogs. *J. Am. Vet. Med. Assoc.* **2009**, *234*, 486–494. [CrossRef] [PubMed]
6. Hargreaves, K.; Abbott, P.V. Drugs for pain management in dentistry. *Aust. Dent. J.* **2005**, *50* (Suppl. S2), S14–S22. [CrossRef] [PubMed]
7. Holmstrom, S.; Frost, P.; Eisner, E. *Veterinary Dental Techniques for the Small Animal Practitioner*, 2nd ed.; W. B. Saunders: Philadelphia, PA, USA, 1998; pp. 255–318.
8. Anderson, J.G.; Goldstein, G.; Boudreaux, K.; Ilkiw, J.E. The State of Veterinary Dental Education in North America, Canada, and the Caribbean: A Descriptive Study. *J. Vet. Med. Educ.* **2017**, *44*, 358–363. [CrossRef] [PubMed]
9. Clark, W.T.; Kane, L.; Arnold, P.K.; Robertson, I.D. Clinical skills and knowledge used by veterinary graduates during their first year in small animal practice. *Aust. Vet. J.* **2002**, *80*, 37–40. [CrossRef]
10. Greenfield, C.L.; Johnson, A.L.; Schaeffer, D.J. Frequency of use of various procedures, skills, and areas of knowledge among veterinarians in private small animal exclusive or predominant practice and proficiency expected of new veterinary school graduates. *J. Am. Vet. Med. Assoc.* **2004**, *224*, 1780–1787. [CrossRef]
11. Dentistry Now Required Part of Veterinary Curriculum. Available online: https://www.avma.org/javma-news/2020-11-01/dentistry-now-required-part-veterinary-curriculum (accessed on 24 June 2023).
12. Niemiec, B.; Gawor, J.; Nemec, A.; Clarke, D.; McLeod, K.; Tutt, C.; Gioso, M.; Steagall, P.V.; Chandler, M.; Morgenegg, G.; et al. World Small Animal Veterinary Association Global Dental Guidelines. *J. Small Anim. Pract.* **2020**, *61*, 395–403. [CrossRef]
13. Hunt, J.A.; Schmidt, P.; Perkins, J.; Newton, G.; Anderson, S.L. Comparison of Three Canine Models for Teaching Veterinary Dental Cleaning. *J. Vet. Med. Educ.* **2021**, *48*, 573–583. [CrossRef]
14. Perry, S.; Bridges, S.M.; Burrow, M.F. A review of the use of simulation in dental education. *Simul. Healthc.* **2015**, *10*, 31–37. [CrossRef] [PubMed]
15. Richter, M.; Peter, T.; Ruttermann, S.; Sader, R.; Seifert, L.B. 3D printed versus commercial models in undergraduate conservative dentistry training. *Eur. J. Dent. Educ.* **2022**, *26*, 643–651. [CrossRef]
16. Mahrous, A.; Elgreatly, A.; Qian, F.; Schneider, G.B. A comparison of pre-clinical instructional technologies: Natural teeth, 3D models, 3D printing, and augmented reality. *J. Dent. Educ.* **2021**, *85*, 1795–1801. [CrossRef] [PubMed]
17. Imran, E.; Adanir, N.; Khurshid, Z. Significance of Haptic and Virtual Reality Simulation (VRS) in the Dental Education: A Review of Literature. *Appl. Sci.* **2021**, *11*, 10196. [CrossRef]
18. Li, Y.; Ye, H.; Ye, F.; Liu, Y.; Lv, L.; Zhang, P.; Zhang, X.; Zhou, Y. The Current Situation and Future Prospects of Simulators in Dental Education. *J. Med. Internet Res.* **2021**, *23*, e23635. [CrossRef]
19. Plessas, A. Computerized Virtual Reality Simulation in Preclinical Dentistry: Can a Computerized Simulator Replace the Conventional Phantom Heads and Human Instruction? *Simul. Healthc.* **2017**, *12*, 332–338. [CrossRef]

20. Lumbis, R.H.; Gregory, S.P.; Baillie, S. Evaluation of a dental model for training veterinary students. *J. Vet. Med. Educ.* **2012**, *39*, 128–135. [CrossRef]
21. Goldschmidt, S.L.; Root Kustritz, M.V. Pilot Study Evaluating the Use of Typodonts (Dental Models) for Teaching Veterinary Dentistry as Part of the Core Veterinary Curriculum. *J. Vet. Med. Educ.* **2022**, *49*, 340–345. [CrossRef]
22. Hunt, J.A.; Simons, M.C.; Anderson, S.L. If you build it, they will learn: A review of models in veterinary surgical education. *Vet. Surg.* **2022**, *51*, 52–61. [CrossRef]
23. Read, E.K.; Vallevand, A.; Farrell, R.M. Evaluation of Veterinary Student Surgical Skills Preparation for Ovariohysterectomy Using Simulators: A Pilot Study. *J. Vet. Med. Educ.* **2016**, *43*, 190–213. [CrossRef]
24. McAlpin, E.; Levine, M.; Brenner, C.; Opazo, C.; Bathini, S.; Choi, S.J.V.; Louisville, M.; Grandhi, U. Evaluating the effectiveness of a virtual reality simulation for preclinical local anaesthesia dental education. *Eur. J. Dent. Educ.* **2022**. [CrossRef]
25. Abd-Shukor, S.N.; Yahaya, N.; Tamil, A.M.; Botelho, M.G.; Ho, T.K. Effectiveness of enhanced video-based learning on removable partial denture module. *Eur. J. Dent. Educ.* **2021**, *25*, 744–752. [CrossRef]
26. Fayaz, A.; Mazahery, A.; Hosseinzadeh, M.; Yazdanpanah, S. Video-based Learning Versus Traditional Method for Preclinical Course of Complete Denture Fabrication. *J. Dent.* **2015**, *16* (Suppl. S1), 21–28.
27. Jang, H.W.; Kim, K.-J. Use of online clinical videos for clinical skills training for medical students: Benefits and challenges. *BMC Med. Educ.* **2014**, *14*, 56. [CrossRef] [PubMed]
28. Roshier, A.L.; Foster, N.; Jones, M.A. Veterinary students' usage and perception of video teaching resources. *BMC Med. Educ.* **2011**, *11*, 1. [CrossRef] [PubMed]
29. Thilakumara, I.P.; Jayasinghe, R.M.; Rasnayaka, S.K.; Jayasinghe, V.P.; Abeysundara, S. Effectiveness of Procedural Video Versus Live Demonstrations in Teaching Laboratory Techniques to Dental Students. *J. Dent. Educ.* **2018**, *82*, 898–904. [CrossRef]
30. Higgins, D.; Hayes, M.J.; Taylor, J.A.; Wallace, J.P. How do we teach simulation-based dental education? Time for an evidence-based, best-practice framework. *Eur. J. Dent. Educ.* **2020**, *24*, 815–821. [CrossRef]
31. McGaghie, W.C.; Issenberg, S.B.; Cohen, E.R.; Barsuk, J.H.; Wayne, D.B. Does simulation-based medical education with deliberate practice yield better results than traditional clinical education? A meta-analytic comparative review of the evidence. *Acad. Med.* **2011**, *86*, 706–711. [CrossRef]
32. Scalese, R.J.; Issenberg, S.B. Effective use of simulations for the teaching and acquisition of veterinary professional and clinical skills. *J. Vet. Med. Educ.* **2005**, *32*, 461–467. [CrossRef]
33. Muca, E.; Cavallini, D.; Raspa, F.; Bordin, C.; Valle, E. Integrating new learning methods into equine nutrition classrooms: The importance of students' perceptions. *J. Equine Vet. Sci.* **2023**, *126*, 104537. [CrossRef]
34. Botelho, M.; Gao, X.; Bhuyan, S.Y. Mixed-methods analysis of videoed expert-student dialogue supporting clinical competence assessments. *Eur. J. Dent. Educ.* **2020**, *24*, 398–406. [CrossRef] [PubMed]
35. Guo, P.J.; Kim, J.; Rubin, R. (Eds.) How video production affects student engagement: An empirical study of MOOC videos. In Proceedings of the First ACM Conference on Learning@ Scale Conference, Atlanta, GA, USA, 4–5 March 2014; pp. 41–50. [CrossRef]
36. Annandale, A.; Scheepers, E.; Fosgate, G.T. The Effect of an Ovariohysterectomy Model Practice on Surgical Times for Final-Year Veterinary Students' First Live-Animal Ovariohysterectomies. *J. Vet. Med. Educ.* **2020**, *47*, 44–55. [CrossRef] [PubMed]
37. Coyne, E.; Rands, H.; Frommolt, V.; Kain, V.; Plugge, M.; Mitchell, M. Investigation of blended learning video resources to teach health students clinical skills: An integrative review. *Nurse Educ. Today* **2018**, *63*, 101–107. [CrossRef] [PubMed]
38. Kelly, R.F.; Mihm-Carmichael, M.; Hammond, J.A. Students' Engagement in and Perceptions of Blended Learning in a Clinical Module in a Veterinary Degree Program. *J. Vet. Med. Educ.* **2021**, *48*, 181–195. [CrossRef]
39. Cook, D.A.; Hamstra, S.J.; Brydges, R.; Zendejas, B.; Szostek, J.H.; Wang, A.T.; Erwin, P.J.; Hatala, R. Comparative effectiveness of instructional design features in simulation-based education: Systematic review and meta-analysis. *Med. Teach.* **2013**, *35*, e867–e898. [CrossRef]
40. Issenberg, S.B.; McGaghie, W.C.; Petrusa, E.R.; Lee Gordon, D.; Scalese, R.J. Features and uses of high-fidelity medical simulations that lead to effective learning: A BEME systematic review. *Med. Teach.* **2005**, *27*, 10–28. [CrossRef]
41. Little, W.B.; Artemiou, E.; Conan, A.; Sparks, C. Computer Assisted Learning: Assessment of the Veterinary Virtual Anatomy Education Software IVALA. *Vet. Sci.* **2018**, *5*, 58. [CrossRef]
42. Annandale, A.; Annandale, C.H.; Fosgate, G.T.; Holm, D.E. Training Method and Other Factors Affecting Student Accuracy in Bovine Pregnancy Diagnosis. *J. Vet. Med. Educ.* **2018**, *45*, 224–231. [CrossRef]
43. Agha, R.A.; Fowler, A.J. The role and validity of surgical simulation. *Int. Surg.* **2015**, *100*, 350–357. [CrossRef]
44. Maran, N.J.; Glavin, R.J. Low- to high-fidelity simulation-a continuum of medical education? *Med. Educ.* **2003**, *37* (Suppl. S1), 22–28. [CrossRef]
45. Homer, M.; Fuller, R.; Hallam, J.; Pell, G. Response to comments on: Shining a spotlight on scoring in the OSCE: Checklists and item weighting. *Med. Teach.* **2021**, *43*, 365–366. [CrossRef] [PubMed]
46. Daniels, V.J.; Pugh, D. Twelve tips for developing an OSCE that measures what you want. *Med. Teach.* **2018**, *40*, 1208–1213. [CrossRef] [PubMed]
47. Naeem, N.; van der Vleuten, C.; Alfaris, E.A. Faculty development on item writing substantially improves item quality. *Adv. Health Sci. Educ.* **2012**, *17*, 369–376. [CrossRef] [PubMed]

48. Yeates, P.; Moult, A.; Cope, N.; McCray, G.; Xilas, E.; Lovelock, T.; Vaughan, N.; Daw, D.; Fuller, R.M.; McKinley, R.K. Measuring the Effect of Examiner Variability in a Multiple-Circuit Objective Structured Clinical Examination (OSCE). *Acad. Med.* **2021**, *96*, 1189–1196. [CrossRef]
49. Royal, K.D.; Guskey, T.R. Does Mathematical Precision Ensure Valid Grades? What Every Veterinary Medical Educator Should Know. *J. Vet. Med. Educ.* **2015**, *42*, 242–244. [CrossRef] [PubMed]
50. Royal, K.D.; Hecker, K.G. Rater Errors in Clinical Performance Assessments. *J. Vet. Med. Educ.* **2016**, *43*, 5–8. [CrossRef]
51. Lin, C.-J.; Chang, J.Z.-C.; Hsu, T.-C.; Liu, Y.-J.; Yu, S.-H.; Tsai, S.S.-L.; Lai, E.H.-H.; Lin, C.-P. Correlation of rater training and reliability in performance assessment: Experience in a school of dentistry. *J. Dent. Sci.* **2013**, *8*, 256–260. [CrossRef]

Disclaimer/Publisher's Note: The statements, opinions and data contained in all publications are solely those of the individual author(s) and contributor(s) and not of MDPI and/or the editor(s). MDPI and/or the editor(s) disclaim responsibility for any injury to people or property resulting from any ideas, methods, instructions or products referred to in the content.

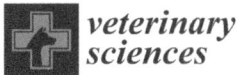

Review

Leadership Theories and the Veterinary Health Care System

Holger Fischer [1], Petra Heidler [2,3,4,*], Lisa Coco [1] and Valeria Albanese [1,*]

1. Tierärztliches Kompetenzzentrum für Pferde Großwallstadt Altano GmbH, 63868 Großwallstadt, Germany
2. Faculty of Health and Medicine, Department for Economy and Health, University for Continuing Education Krems, 3500 Krems, Austria
3. Department of Health Sciences, St. Pölten University of Applied Sciences, 3100 St. Pölten, Austria
4. Department of International Business and Export Management, IMC University of Applied Sciences Krems, 3500 Krems, Austria
* Correspondence: petra.heidler@donau-uni.ac.at (P.H.); vzalbanese@gmail.com (V.A.)

Simple Summary: Good leadership is necessary for the success of every company. The health care industry, including the veterinary sector, has been increasingly acknowledging the importance of an appropriate leadership, and the attention towards leadership theories in this field has steadily increased in the literature through the past one and a half decade. However, a consensus on what effective leadership is and on how it can contribute to the veterinary health sector is still lacking. This review aims to describe the most prominent leadership theories as well as leadership styles, as they may apply to the veterinary health care sector and to discuss transformational leadership in routine and crisis situation in the human and veterinary health care industry.

Abstract: This descriptive review aims to illustrate the different leadership theories as they may apply to the veterinary health care sector, and specifically, to the affection and sports animal subsectors. The increasing and ever-changing challenges veterinary health care operators and investors operating in these subsectors face are briefly described, as well as the most known leadership theories and styles, each with its possible advantages and disadvantages specific to its application to the veterinary health care system. The different theories are illustrated in their key aspects and their historical evolution. Finally, the discussion focuses on transformational leadership as it is seen as the most progressive and promising leadership style to hold up to said challenges in the veterinary health care system.

Keywords: leadership theory; leadership; transformational leadership; veterinary

Citation: Fischer, H.; Heidler, P.; Coco, L.; Albanese, V. Leadership Theories and the Veterinary Health Care System. *Vet. Sci.* **2022**, *9*, 538. https://doi.org/10.3390/vetsci9100538

Academic Editors: Simona Sacchini and Ayoze Castro-Alonso

Received: 11 August 2022
Accepted: 22 September 2022
Published: 29 September 2022

Publisher's Note: MDPI stays neutral with regard to jurisdictional claims in published maps and institutional affiliations.

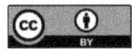

Copyright: © 2022 by the authors. Licensee MDPI, Basel, Switzerland. This article is an open access article distributed under the terms and conditions of the Creative Commons Attribution (CC BY) license (https://creativecommons.org/licenses/by/4.0/).

1. Introduction

Regardless of their business area and regardless of their size, companies benefit of good leaders to express their full potential and to thrive.

In particular, the health care sector is dynamic and complex. It experiences its own peculiar problems and challenges as well as those of organizations in other sectors [1–3]. Examples are the increasing expectations for transparency, the increasing threats of liability, the increasing influence of political groups and social media, and the shortage of young professionals willing and capable of replacing their aging counterparts, just to name a few [4–6]. External factors, such as government policies, globalization, changing population demographics, economic factors, progressing, and advancing medical technologies also have a substantial and increasing influence on the health care system [7–9]. The health care sector in these historical times is experiencing change at a pace that was not seen before. This change is a product of both internal and external factors that are largely outside the area of expertise of most health professionals. The health care industry is, therefore, calling for changes and reforms to meet the increasing expectations of patients and clients, the most important of which are safety, transparency, accountability, efficiency, and quality [10]. Cutting edge leadership is essential in establishing a vision for health care businesses and organizations, and in implementing necessary reforms and changes. Indeed, the topics "leadership" and "management" have received an unprecedented attention in the medical field in multiple countries since the turn of the century [3,11–24].

The primary goal of this review is to raise awareness on the topic of leadership in veterinary medicine.

Secondly, the authors aimed to review the major leadership theories and discuss, based on their experience, how they could apply to the veterinary health care sector.

Third and most importantly, the authors try to advise the readers on how the establishment of a conscious leadership culture could be helpful in facing the present and upcoming challenges of the veterinary profession, in daily practice management as well as in crisis management.

A very important aspect that is being investigated in the field of health care leadership is that of the skills and characteristics that the ideal leader should possess to be successful and to make their company thrive. Identifying these traits could help in the recruiting of potential leaders and also, perhaps more importantly, in the education and training of leaders-to-be, aimed at improving the team and organization performance in the medium to long run [22].

2. Literature Review

What is a leader and what does a leader do? What is expected from a successful leader in the health care sector, and especially in the veterinary health care system?

The Oxford dictionary defines a leader first as *A person in control of a group, a country or a situation*. This definition is tautological and not exhaustive, it does not explain in which sense a leader "ontrols", what tools they use to exert their control and why are they in such a position.

The same source continues: *A person who manages or controls other people, especially because of his or her ability or position*. This definition is more complete and starts to shine a light on what we will see as one of the most interesting aspects of this field of research: their *ability*. So, it appears that a leader is not only someone who sits on the leader chair, but someone who, in order to sit on said chair, needs to have something that others do not have [25].

Several leadership theories have been developed and researched through the years. Some of them have fallen out of favor, some new ones are developed continuously. A leadership theory is a slightly different concept than that of a leadership style.

"Theory provides the overarching sense-making frame for experience. Without a theoretical framework to connect and integrate experiences there is no sense-making, and thus there can be no learning" [26]. Leadership theories answer the questions of why and how some people become leaders and some do not.

Leadership theories tend to focus either on the traits or on the actions and demeanor that people should or should not display in order to be good leaders.

Over the years, the subject has been looked at from many different perspectives, and four prominent groups of theories can be identified. Newer leadership theories do not replace or discard the old ones, but rather they enrich and further on elaborate them, and look at them in a different way. Therefore, much of the information provided in this classification might appear redundant.

There are dozens of leadership theories, the most famous of which can be classified in four main groups: trait theories, functional theories, behavioral and style theories, and contemporary theories (Table 1).

Table 1. Leadership theories and their key points.

THEORY	KEY POINT
TRAIT THEORY	Leader's innate characteristics
FUNCTIONAL THEORY	Leader's functions
BEHAVIORAL THEORY	Leader's styles
	Authoritarian
	Democratic
	Permissive
	Bureaucratic
CONTINGENCY THEORY	Leader's ability to adapt to situations
MANAGEMENT THEORY	Rewards and punishments system
PARTICIPATIVE THEORY	Participations of the whole team to leadership
POWER THEORY	Power of the leader over his team
CONNECTIVE THEORY	Ability of the leader to connect people
TRANSFORMATIONAL THEORY	Leader's vision

2.1. Trait Theory

The trait theory, also known as the Great Man Theory, sustains that good leaders are born, not made. These people are destined and deserve to be good leaders thanks to their inborn special characteristics, special talents, and special capabilities, that cannot be taught or learned. Kohs and Irle [27], Bernard [28], Bingham [29], Tead [30], and Kilbourne [31] all explained leadership in definition of traits of character and personality [32]. By the 1950s, hundreds of studies had already been conducted exploring these traits [33]. Later on, these theories evolved to contemplate the possibility that such characteristics can be developed in others who were showing an innate disposition to them, and if not exactly taught or learned, at a minimum, they could be enhanced and further implemented.

Based on several research studies, Bass [32] developed a profile of traits that are evident in successful leaders. These are categorized into three areas:
1. Intelligence, including judgement, decisiveness, knowledge, and fluency.
2. Personality, including adaptability, alertness, integrity, and nonconformity.
3. Ability, including cooperativeness, popularity, and tact.

A spin-off of the Great Man Theory identifies the leader based on their charisma. Suasiveness, convincingness, personal appeal, seductiveness, aplomb, and whit are the main features of charismatic leaders. The leader's personality leverages loyalty and commitment, first to the person of the leader themselves, and second to the aims and goals of the organization that they represent. It is important to note that charismatic leadership is attributed based on what people *perceive and interpret* of the leader's behavior, and not by an objective set of characteristics and traits. Furthermore, one "charismatic" trait is not sufficient to identify a leader as charismatic, rather, there must be a constellation of traits and/or behaviors in order to entitle them to this attribute. Charisma, therefore, remains a concept that may seem easy to grasp but is very difficult to precisely define [34].

2.2. Functional Theory

Subsequent to trait theories of leadership, the functional theory of leadership was developed. This theory underscores the functions of the leader (and not their traits) and bypasses the dilemma between appointed vs. naturally emerging leader. It indicates that, in either case, the leader can and should learn to elicit the right functions at the right time. Kotter [35] suggests that, by focusing on the functions of the leader, their performance can be improved by training and, thereby, their leadership skills can further develop and be perfected. The same author also indicates that organizations should not wait for leaders to come along, but instead they should grow and train their own, by identifying employees with leadership potential and enabling them to develop those skills. This approach, therefore, also supports the idea that several members of a professional group can strive to develop their leadership potential. As an example, one widely accepted functional theory is Adair's action-centered leadership, according to which the leader has to take into account and consider three sets of needs of the organization: the technical needs or the tasks that need to be conducted, the needs of each single team member or individual needs, and the team needs or what needs to be performed to keep the group together efficiently. How successful the leader is, is decided by how effectively and harmonically they can take care of these three areas. Too much attention or effort in one over the others can cause imbalance and can interfere with the productiveness and effectiveness of the group. This could consequently affect the spirit of the group, and therefore, the quality of its performance and the overall outcome and achievements [36].

2.3. Behavioral Theory

The third group of leadership theories focuses on several possible styles of leadership. A leadership style is the way in which the leader carries out their functions, that is, the way in which the leader is perceived as typically behaving towards their followers (hence the definition of behavioral theory) [37]. Such leaders develop their styles through education, training, and life experiences. Therefore „style" refers to how, as leaders, we behave on a day-to-day basis, because we know or have learnt from previous experience that the way we do things works. The behavioral leadership theory is based on the assumption that these operating standards are repeatable and other leaders can duplicate them. Behind this theory is the concept that no inborn trait makes a leader successful, but rather a set of behaviors that can be replicated, taught, and learnt. The core point of leadership according to this theory is how the leader acts and not what their qualities or talents per se are. Actions are, therefore, the best predictors for success. Patterns of behavior are investigated and grouped into categories defined as "leadership styles".

In the perspective of behavioral theory, the potential leader gets to prospectively and somehow freely determine and plan their leadership style and act accordingly, which can be attractive. Nevertheless, leadership styles are fluid and flexible and can be adapted by changing patterns of behavior according to the circumstances. Furthermore, according to this theory, a leader does not necessarily possess innate traits that make them special, instead they become leader based on their actions, which in turn means that virtually anybody can become a leader, provided they behave as such. Of course, there is not a handbook that suggests a specific leadership style for every possible circumstance and every possible challenging situation in each and all possible industry, and it should not be expected that there is one. There are dozens of leadership styles that stem from the behavioral theory, but there is not a right one for every circumstance. The traditional classification of leadership styles within the behavioral theory is the following: authoritarian, democratic, permissive, and bureaucratic.

An authoritarian leader focuses on power and authority, exercises control and directive behavior, makes decisions alone and expects obedience of instructions, and uses coercion.

A democratic leader seeks, at least formally, the views of all relevant parties. They consult and work together with individuals and teams, engage in two-way communication, and encourage collaborative teamwork.

A permissive leader uses few established rules and policies. They monitor performance from a distance, which may make them seem detached, and permits individuals and teams to work autonomously.

A bureaucratic leader follows established policies and rules to the letter. Their rules are fixed and inflexible, and their communication is impersonal. Despite the approving and disapproving overtones of each of these styles of leadership, there are merits and weaknesses to each, depending on the situation, and especially in the health care setting.

Another way of classifying leaders based on the behavioral theory is task-oriented vs. people-oriented leader. The first type of leader will address problems always starting from within the workflow. The second type of leader, instead, will address problems starting from the individuals first. A leader who is too focused on people may be popular but not so productive, whereas a leader who is too focused on tasks may get a lot of work done, however the employees may be unhappy [37].

2.4. Contingency Theory

The contingency leadership theories, sometimes called situational theories, focus on the context of a leader. In the perspective of situational leadership theories, the efficacy of a leader has little to do with their personality, but it is rather a product of the circumstances the leader operates under. According to situational theories, changes in leadership styles dictated by the context are necessary for an effective leadership. In the interest of the further development of a company, these theories advise that there is a right leader for most specific circumstances, and that person should take over when the previous leader is no longer adapting to the present needs. Examples of contingency theories are the Hershey and Blanchard's Situational Theory [38], the Evans and House Path-Goal Theory [39], and Fiedler's Contingency Theory [40,41].

The contingency theories can be very inspiring. A very positive side to their perspective is that there would be an effective leadership for virtually any—no matter how challenging—context and situation. However, as it is often the case, there is not any very detailed source or handbook that one can consult to learn more details of specific situations and the challenges that it may present. Furthermore, contingency theories tend to focus on the context and the situation and to underscore them as they may be presented from factors outside the company itself, and in turn they may not give enough importance to the psychology of the employees and their wellbeing or to other types of inside factors. Moreover, these theories can appear somehow shallow as they fail to recognize that leadership evolves, also, because the person of the leader self-changes and grows and evolves in their role, independently from the circumstances. A leader is indeed influenced by a number of internal and external factors such as the type of company and what industry it is part of, how big the team is, how cohesive the team is, what type of person the leader is, and how they take success and failure are examples of internal factors that influence leadership. Economy, political events, social media influence, and customer reviews are examples of external factors that impact leadership [42].

2.5. Contemporary Theories

2.5.1. Management Theory

The transactional leadership theory or management theory is very common in the educational system, in the corporate world and to some extent, also, in the health care system. Its focus lies ultimately on the final performance of the group, and how to achieve success through organization and effective supervision. Transactional leadership consists of a system of benefits and penalties; when employees do right, they get rewarded. When they fail, they get warned and eventually punished. This theory is based on the principle that employees can only be motivated by rewards, and only dissuaded by penalties all directed to them personally. This theory discards the idea that people can behave a certain way because it is inherently right, or avoid doing something because it is inherently wrong [43].

Leading with punishments and rewards can be incredibly effective. Employees tend to appreciate and respond readily to positive reinforcement as they feel motivated and encouraged to succeed. However, strictly transactional leadership is seen critically because of how demoralizing punishments can feel to motivated employees who may feel treated unfairly and condescended upon. It can also be seen as a simplified and childish way of leading which does not live up to the standards and challenges of the modern world.

2.5.2. Participative Theory

Participative leadership or democratic leadership is not as represented as transactional leadership in the corporate world, but it is very common in the public health care system. Employees led in a democratic fashion are directly involved in the decision-making process of the organization they are part of, and the role of the leader is that of enabling and facilitating the communication, filtering the various suggestions and advice. The ultimate decision is still taken by the leader, but after the members of the team have had the chance of expressing themselves on the topic [44].

Intuitively employees will feel much more motivated when directly involved in decision-making, which is a clear advantage of this theory. However, detractors of this theory suggest that it may be an unnecessary, inefficient, and weak way of leading. Furthermore, leaders who lead this way may lose the focus on what the company as such actually needs, because they are too distracted by considering what everybody thinks and wishes and wants. Lastly, considering everyone's opinion is time consuming.

Bill Gates is a famous example of democratic or participative leader: participative leaders find a way to ask the team how they would manage a given situation. Employees in these organizations are encouraged to openly share and discuss their opinions. These leaders' strength is that they are capable of effectively take all the suggestions, process them, discuss them, and summarize them, ultimately considering them in their final decision. Employees, especially if educated, usually like this type of leaders; this is very important to consider, because democratically led organizations may, in the long run, attract more qualified and educated employees than organizations led in a less participative fashion. In the veterinary health care system, where most leaders and employees share the same education and have the same academic background, this theory is particularly appreciated, although it becomes less and less effective as the size of the company increases.

2.5.3. Power Theory

At the root of the power leadership theory is how the leader uses their power and their position to achieve their goals and those of the company they lead. An example of this is the French and Raven's Five Forms of Power [45], which describes how the power stemming from their person and from their position influences the conduct of the leaders and what outcomes they have.

Intuitively, in the short run, leaders with great power can be convincing and under this type of leadership things generally get conducted fast and reasonably well. So, it is easy to think this leadership theory describes one of the most efficient approaches to the topic. Once again though we cannot forget that employees are a dynamic factor, and leadership will influence the type of employees a company attracts. Educated employees tend to not like power leadership. The employees most companies aim to recruit (educated, accountable, and responsible) want a leader who does not enforce power over them, but works with them, encourages them, and helps them grow. A power leader instead makes employees feel dominated and controlled [46].

This leadership approach can be successful in very structured settings where hierarchy and promotion are underscored, such as in the military world, or in situations where the workforce is not educated at all and benefits of a stronger approach. In medical field organizations, employees in power led companies often see that their only chance to gain a place in the sun is to gain power of their own at all costs. This can have tremendously negative consequences such as low morale and inhospitable atmosphere [46]; especially when the health of the patients is at stake, the attention of the team may in the process get diverted from the mission of the organization.

2.5.4. Connective Theory

The focus of the connective leader lies on their interpersonal relationships and connections. The connective leadership theory underscores the fostering role of the leader in establishing collaborations within the organization to help achieve the goals of the organization itself. These leaders can exquisitely mentor their employees, allotting large slots of their time to this mission. These leaders believe in making work enjoyable for their team and employees and they are committed to creating and maintaining a conducive, virtuous working environment. Many educated and self-motivated employees can thrive under this type of leadership.

Charns and Tewksbury [47], who are key advocates of connective leadership, explained that the leader, in order to wire connections and to promote integration of mentees, needs to take the following steps:

- Scouting human resources to find collaborators.
- Creating and communicating a shared vision.
- Finding a role for their collaborators that enhances their value and adds value to the team.
- Facilitating communication.
- Building and maintaining social interactions and comfort.
- Defining positions and tasks.
- Documenting contributions and rewarding them properly.
- Structuring contributions and contributors formally when appropriate.

When led this way, employees trust and confide in their leaders. This kind of leadership also inspires workers to follow the leader's example and step up to a leadership role as well. Employees with growth prospects thrive under this leadership type and retention times tend to be long. Criticism to this leadership is mainly that being appropriately connected with similar other experts or individuals with similar interests through networking is already a recognized attribute of most effective leaders and it would not be enough per se to endorse a leading role. Other critics come from the thought that this type of leader would be so focused on interpersonal relationships that they would refrain from addressing problems with the employees in the fear of losing them or losing their appeal on them. However, it is generally agreed upon that connective leaders are, actually, quite effective overall.

2.5.5. Transformational Theory

Transformational leadership refers to the "ability of leaders to influence others by transforming their behavior without necessarily being in a position of authority" [48]. A systematic review of transformational leadership conducted by Holly and Igwee [49] identifies it as comprising intellectual stimulation by incentivizing new ideas, considering all employees individually, motivating and inspiring them, stimulating their creativity, conveying optimism and meaning for the mission of the organization, guiding the team in a coherent direction, acting exemplarily, and fostering a sense of belonging and motivation. Kouzes and Posner [50] identify the key attributes of ideal transformational leaders:

1. Leading by example.
2. Inspiring a shared vision.
3. Challenging the process.
4. Enabling the others to act.
5. Encouraging the heart.

Transformational leadership is, as in any other leadership model, not free from criticism. It may be seen as quite manipulative to have employees feel like they are part of something, that they belong to something bigger, although they, actually, rarely have a say on the major strategic or financial plans of the company, and they mostly do not own any stakes of it. Furthermore, transformational leaders are often criticized for focusing on small groups of people they consider worth their efforts, to further develop them. Lastly, the influence transformational leaders may exert on their employees can be detrimental if they are ill-minded or if their intentions are evil. In other words, if the leader has bad plans, followers might be deceived and be lured to go with whatever decisions the leader makes.

3. Discussion

The human medical profession has changed dramatically in the last century: medical care has changed, the education required to become medical doctors has changed, professional duties and offered services are different than they were, medical institutes are larger, more structured, and more organized, and the lifestyle of medical doctors has changed. In contrast to this, the veterinary profession has remained, until 10 years ago, relatively static: reading James Herriot's books we realize that not so long ago solo practitioners had comparable lifestyles, comparable duties, and comparable working hours to what they used to have almost a hundred years ago. In over 50 years of combined working experience in small and large animal practice in five countries, the authors have observed that many veterinarians, although thankfully not all of them, are quite reluctant to change and to innovate. The statement "we have always done it this way" backs up a variety of procedures who lack evidence base, both medically and from a managerial standpoint. Focusing on the latter, which is the core topic of this review, the authors have observed that the expectations on young workforce in terms of working hours, minimum salary, professional duties, and military acceptance of directions are unique and are also often justified by the thought that "we have always done it this way". Moreover, often veterinary practices lack an official emergency duty roster, an official distribution of the working load and a clear definition of the roles that the participants are called to fulfill, possibly generating confusion, frustration, and conflicts.

Nevertheless, clients are increasingly more informed, they are more educated, and they want the best for their animals, who are in part family members, in part valuable athletes, and in part an economical asset.

To accommodate the increasing expectations of the clientele, and to constantly improve the service provided to the animals, the clients, and the employees, the veterinary profession needs to accept innovation. Part of it is recognizing that a leadership culture is needed and must be established.

The abovementioned theories have advantages and disadvantages that make them more or less applicable to what the modern veterinary health care system needs to be.

The Great Man Theory has per se both proponents and critics. The main critic is that in its core, pure interpretation it fails to give credit to any learning process, work, or effort needed to become a leader. The Great Man Theory negates the modern concept that "you can if you want". Moreover, the traits are difficult to define clearly, and it is questionable whether a single individual could possess all traits identified in the various studies. Furthermore, most personality features considered to be associated with good leadership skills are masculine, which is also seen critically, and do not really match the actual description of countless leaders who have been successful [51].

Proponents of this theory cite giants as Abraham Lincoln or Alexander the Great or Queen Elizabeth as their examples, as these people utilized their inherited skills, their *traits* indeed, to lead armies and countries. Furthermore, leaders are often very ambitious and determined, observation that appears to support this theory, nevertheless.

Kouzes and Posner [50] identified in a large-scale questionnaire the following characteristics associated with leaders perceived as effective: honest (89% of respondents), forward looking (71%), competent (69%), and inspiring (65%). A lesser number of respondents mentioned the following features: intelligent, broad-minded, fair-minded, dependable, supportive, straightforward, cooperative, and determined. An even lesser number mentioned: courageous, ambitious, caring, loyal, imaginative, mature, self-controlled, and independent. This variety of responses shows that there is no universal agreement on the nature of a leader or on the innate features that are necessary for a good leader, observation that challenges the trait theory. However, based on the authors' experience, in the health care system, and more so in veterinary medicine, there are dozens of examples of solo practitioners, armed almost exclusively with strength, will, and grit, who founded a small clinic that progressively grew, acquired more employees, and became successful—a "great veterinarian" theory.

The risk associated with this theory, as it is applied to the veterinary world, is that of creating a practice that is centered around its leader and that it cannot function in their absence, which becomes a problem when the leader needs to take a leave for any reason.

The functional theory of leadership was innovative as it was developed in contrast to the trait theory, meaning that it underscored the importance of what the leaders do as opposed to what their innate characteristics are. This point has been largely absorbed and expanded by more modern theories to the point that the functional theory per se seems insufficient for the challenges presented by the contemporary veterinary health care system. In the authors' opinion, nonetheless, two points of this theory remain valid: the necessity to identify employees with leadership potential, to grow them and to train them, and the leader's obligation to juggle the three sets of need of the organization (technical, task, and individual).

The four major leadership styles, described by the behavioral theory, remain important in that any leader behaves in a way that falls predominantly in one of those categories: authoritarian, democratic, permissive, and bureaucratic, regardless of what their vision is, i.e., if they are transformational leaders or transactional leaders, for example.

The authors would like to provide the example of a leader of a local branch of a small animal corporate practice. Said leader may have an authoritarian style and like to personally assign every appointment to the staff veterinarian they consider most appropriate for each case. The central administration may also have transactional policies in place, such as a commission on top of the base salary, which the branch leader will apply.

Another example would be that of an equine hospital whose leader has a permissive style and a transformational vision; the staff veterinarian on call will take in an emergency, based on the duty roster. The leader will not intervene in any of the decisions or communications of the staff veterinarian unless requested. The performance and outcome of the staff veterinarian on call will be monitored from a distance, without direct interference. The leader will constantly reassure the employee on their ability of facing the situation and will offer advice and technical support at all times. Constructive, enthusiastic, and personalized feedback will be given by the leader in what the staff veterinarians have done properly. Criticism, where necessary, should not be avoided but it should never be aimed at humiliating or demeaning the employee, rather, at inspiring them to elevate their performance.

The contingency theory has been largely absorbed by subsequent theories. Nevertheless, it is very relevant to remind veterinary leaders how necessary changes in leadership styles can be when the context also changes. For example, the current paucity of young workforce in veterinary medicine has forced many leaders to change their style and policies in order to become more appealing for potential employees.

As previously mentioned, the management theory is also present in the health care system, especially in corporate medicine. An example of this management style is offering commission on top of a base salary, a widely used salary system in the veterinary health care system. The management theory is straightforward to understand and apply and can be very effective with the right type of employee. In the authors' observation, less ambitious veterinary doctors, part-time employees, and employees who do not have major medical, managerial, or financial responsibilities (janitors, entry level receptionists, and entry level nurses) are more likely to perform well under transactional leaders. However, eager veterinarians who want to grow professionally, higher level administrative personnel, and, in general, more ambitious individuals are unlikely to express their full potential under this type of leadership.

The participative theory of leadership offers advantages to the veterinary health care system especially at small to medium sized organizations. Staff veterinarians of any experience and age will obviously feel much more motivated when directly involved in decision-making. The leader must be careful to gauge the allotted freedom according to the experience of the individual on staff. The risks are that of making young veterinarians feel overwhelmed and insecure, and that of making more experienced staff members feel condescended upon. A certain degree of participation is, based on the authors' experience and observations, always appreciated, and received positively by all employees, veterinarians, nurses, administrative personnel, and barn crew.

Power leadership offers little advantage in the veterinary health care setting, as stated before, and therefore it will not be further discussed.

Working on establishing and maintaining connections, and using them at the right time, as advocated by the homonymous theory, has become increasingly important for veterinarians and veterinary leaders. Within a medium to large organization, it is important to choose the right people for the right tasks, and it is vital for the good outcome of the cases that communications between those people flow seamlessly. An example is that of a horse admitted after hours to a large equine referral practice for acute abdominal pain. The emergency service treats the horse conservatively based on the workup performed on admission. In the morning the horse's clinical picture worsens and it gets transferred from the emergency service to the day surgery service for celiotomy. The anesthesia service also must be called to anesthetize the patient and assist until recovery is completed. Three services (emergency, surgery, and anesthesia) must communicate openly and efficiently for the sake of the horse's life and wellbeing. This is much easier if the connections between those services are solid, friendly, established, and oiled, as it happens under an efficient connective leadership.

Transformational leadership is understood in terms of the leader's influence on followers [49], and is currently a widely advocated leadership approach especially for the health care sector. The positive impact of transformational leadership on the quality of health care provided is substantial, as stated by Fischer [52], as it is associated with a better performance of the team and with improved patient care, although the mechanisms by which this happens are not entirely clear.

Transformational leaders are visionary, balanced, self-aware, and confident [53]. They generate commitment of the employees to the vision and ideal of the organization, encouraging them to exercise leadership and achieve exceptional results. The transformational leader discourages dependence by stimulating growth and development. The term "transformational" implies being visionary, thus, having ideas and aspirations on how things could be different and better, and then implementing these visions. As a consequence, transformational leadership is widely advocated especially for health care and social settings. It is to be noted, however, that transformational leaders display substantially more energy and enthusiasm than those around them, and therefore could be seen as pushy by their followers.

Research on transformational leadership [49,54] for health care setting suggests that this is the most useful theory for healthcare professionals, because transformational leaders are seen to encourage followers to go beyond goals related to self-interest and toward goals of the organization [49]. Transformational leaders build capacity by role modelling the core values of the organization, and they build a unifying purpose which the staff feels a part of. Where there is transformational leadership, staff are more engaged and more productive, and organizational goals are met more consistently [54]. In the authors' opinion based on their experience and observations, this is also true in the veterinary health care sector.

Another aspect of what health care professionals face is crisis in health care, which poses a different set of leadership challenges compared to routine personal and public health care. Examples of crisis in public health care are the latest COVID-19 pandemic (2019 to present, still ongoing) or, in veterinary medicine, the Equine Herpesvirus epidemic (2021, 2022). The leadership skills required in these unique settings have been first examined by Deitchman [55] in their review and commentary.

A crisis is defined as a substantial threat to a social system and to the way it is structured, to its values, to its laws and regulations, threat that needs to be addressed quickly despite the uncertainty of times, through critical decisions [56]. A good leader in a time of crisis must withstand the enormous stress; must recognize that the crisis exists; must be able to make decisions, even unpopular ones, quickly and effectively and even in the absence of all necessary information; must be able to effectively and timely communicate; must be able to delegate without losing control.

Professionals employed in the public health sector are expected to lead responses to emergencies such as infectious diseases clusters, zoonotic diseases outbreaks, disease outbreaks in food animal impacting the food chain, or outbreaks of foodborne sicknesses. In this type of crises, however, the normal emergency measures are not effective in restoring the status quo [57]. Such crises can surge spontaneously or be initiated by hurricanes, tsunamis, draughts, extreme temperatures, and other natural causes; naturally occurring or laboratory-induced pandemics; biological terrorism; chemical spills; nuclear or radiological accidents. The authors have not been able to find in the literature any articles addressing the topic of health care leadership in critical circumstances and Deitchman was not either, according to their review's citations. Deitchman, therefore, branched out and reviewed the crisis response in the following groups: flight captains, military leaders in extremis (meaning in a situation where the leader's life and those of the team are perceived to be in danger), incident management team leaders such as firefighters or police officers, nuclear IMT commanders, and survivors of underground fires in mines. They observed that the surveyed disciplines display different requirements, challenges, training, working hours, work setting, and team size. A firefighting brigade on an accident scene may be composed by over 100 people, whereas a flight crew may be composed by as little as three. Firefighters and policemen are formally trained in the specifics of incident and crisis leadership. Military leaders and commanders of first response organizations receive formal training in incident leadership, but they may or may not have led a team in a real emergency situation before. Nonetheless it was noticed that effective crisis leaders seem to consistently display across the diverse settings some specific features, in that they have to be competent, decisive, self-confident, they need to be fast in receiving and processing external inputs, they have to communicate effectively, and they have to inspire trust in their team. Deitchman proposed therefore, based on the commonality displayed across the disciplines, a series of traits for the health care leader in times of crisis, which are: competence, decisiveness, situational awareness, acceptance of the inherited bidirectional communication responsibility towards both superiors and subordinates, coordination, inspiration of trust and self-confidence, and responsibility for the welfare of the team [55].

The crises the world experienced in the recent past in the global health system have challenged the existing training of health officers and leaders, and have demonstrated its inadequacy to withstand global emergencies such as the latest pandemic. In other words, it has become obvious that the traditional mix of basic management skills and medical knowledge is insufficient. Indeed, the large majority of the leadership has been taken by political forces and very little was left in the hands of health officers. As previously said, the public health environment benefits in normal times of a democratic, participative, and inclusive leadership which, however, may not be indicated for times of crisis, when the need arises of making decisions quickly despite the lack of complete information.

Because of this, some authors have advised for a more authoritarian decision-making process in terms of crisis, that should replace the conventional model in place in regular times [58]. Care should be taken, however, in promoting authoritarianism: these leaders in fact risk overlooking important contributions coming from the team, especially when team members have diverse, complementary areas of interest and expertise.

The truth is found probably somewhere in between the extremes of rigid mastery and never-ending search for general consensus. A leadership strategy that encourages open communication even in the face of crises seems to be more effective and safer [59]. The importance of open communication and approachability is exemplified by the experience of Captain Al Haynes in 1989. Captain Haynes and his crew managed to land a DC-10 despite the loss of its hydraulic controls. He gave credit to his team for using the so called CLR, crew leadership resource training. He admitted he would not have known better than any other crew member on that plane what to do, and therefore listening to the crew's opinions was very important for a successful outcome [60].

Team performance in the health care sector during crises has not been thoroughly investigated and researched. However, it is logical to think that it would follow the same trend and be better when the leadership allows and encourages team contributions, as it is the case with transformational leadership. Health care leaders in times of crisis have to juggle between authoritarianism and democracy, as they wear multiple hats soliciting opinions, reviewing data and statistics, receiving expert opinions, and, finally, making and executing decisions even if not all pieces of the puzzle are present or coincide [55].

In summary, transformational leadership is about a joint vision, about prospective, about common values and direction, and inspiration for the future. Transformational leaders look beyond the daily tasks and goals and rather establish a direction and a path for the organization to accomplish its goals and objectives. Transformational leaders are people who not only do things right, they strive to do the right thing. The difference is that the focus of these leaders is on their vision and judgment rather than on mastering daily technical tasks. Therefore, these leaders are not focused on being efficient, but rather on being effective. Our impression is that transformational leadership is the only theory that is visionary and flexible enough to apply to the contemporary veterinary health care system and its never-ending set of challenges and changes, as it enhances the skills of every team member, it promotes their involvement and encourages them to go the extra mile. We feel that transformational leadership fosters the sense of belonging, it promotes necessary change following a broad-minded vision, and it prepares the individuals and teams for responsiveness in crisis situation, ultimately improving and enhancing the experience for employers, employees, clients, and patients (Figure 1).

In order to collect evidence to prove or to challenge our impressions, basic research is needed amongst human resources in the veterinary health care system, to investigate their needs, their fears, their goals, and their vison. This research has already begun in the small animal sector of the system [61], traditionally more advanced and more inclined to follow the progresses of the human medical world. The more traditional large animal sector is, on the other hand, still to be explored.

A first important step would be to administer human resources employed in large animal hospitals questionnaires modeled after the small animal works [61], to examine their conduct and retention time in relation to the type of practice they are employed in, and to investigate what variables influence them.

Motivated, competent, and professionally satisfied personnel should perform better and be retained longer, in turn ensuring better and more continuous patient care, as well as better outcomes for the patients and the sector they are part of. This speculation should be proven by prospective research that examines how different leadership strategies results in several objective and subjective parameters referred to all parties involved (personnel, patients, owners, industrial, and/or commercial partners).

Human resources are ultimately the most valuable asset of the veterinary business, and only an established leadership culture that considers every team member as valuable will withstand the challenges that the future of the large animal veterinary industry will bring.

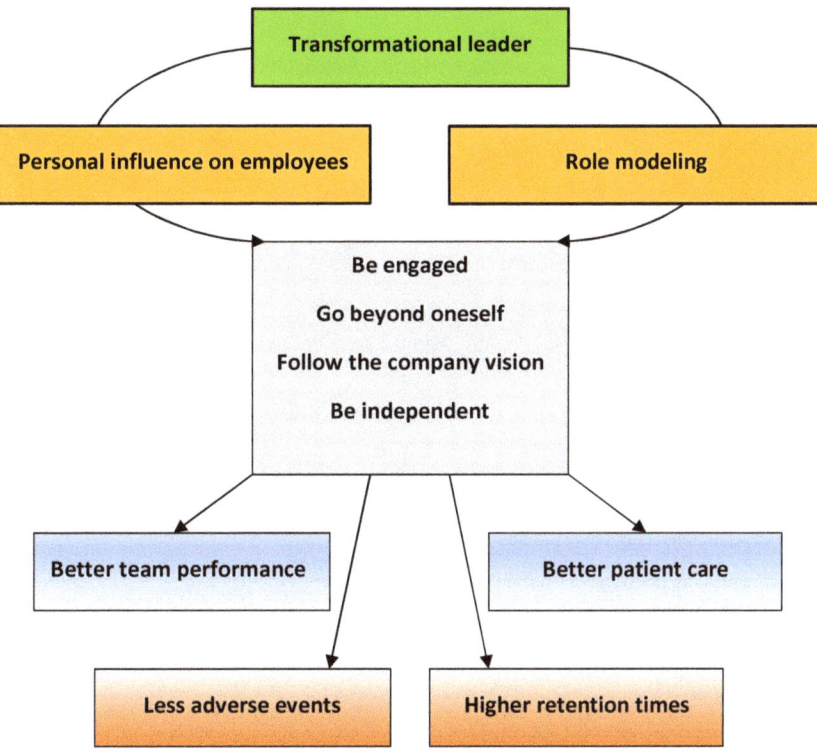

Figure 1. Potential effects of transformational leadership in health care.

Author Contributions: All Authors (H.F., L.C., P.H., V.A.) contributed equally. All authors have read and agreed to the published version of the manuscript.

Funding: This research received no external funding.

Institutional Review Board Statement: Not applicable.

Informed Consent Statement: Not applicable.

Data Availability Statement: Not applicable.

Conflicts of Interest: The authors declare no conflict of interest.

References

1. Counte, M.A.; Newman, J.F. Competency-based health services management education: Contemporary issues and emerging challenges. *J. Health Adm. Educ.* **2002**, *20*, 113–122.
2. Garman, A.; Scribner, L. Leading for quality in healthcare: Development and validation of a competency model. *J. Healthc. Manag.* **2011**, *56*, 373–384. [CrossRef]
3. Liang, Z.; Howard, P.F. Competencies required by senior health executives in new South Wales, 1990–1999. *Aust. Health Rev.* **2010**, *34*, 52–58. [CrossRef]
4. Liang, Z.; Short, S.D.; Brown, C.R. Senior health managers in the new era: Changing roles and competencies in the 1990s and early 21st century. *J. Health Adm. Educ.* **2006**, *23*, 281–301.
5. Stefl, M. Common competencies for all healthcare managers: The healthcare leadership alliance model. *J. Healthc. Manag.* **2008**, *53*, 360–373. [CrossRef]
6. Wallick, W.G.; Stager, K.J. Healthcare managers' roles, competencies, and outputs in organizational performance improvement/practitioner response. *J. Healthc. Manag.* **2002**, *47*, 390–401.
7. Leggat, S.G. Teaching and learning teamwork: Competency requirements for healthcare managers. *J. Health Adm. Educ.* **2007**, *24*, 135–149.

8. Guo, K.L.; Anderson, D. The new health care paradigm: Roles and competencies of leaders in the service line management approach. *Leadersh. Health Serv.* **2005**, *18*, 12–20. [CrossRef]
9. Gertner, E.J.; Sabino, J.N.; Mahady, E.; Deitrick, L.M.; Patton, J.R.; Grim, M.K.; Geiger, J.F.; Salas-Lopez, D. Developing a culturally competent health network: A planning framework and guide/practitioner application. *J. Healthc. Manag.* **2010**, *55*, 190–204.
10. Ayeleke, R.O.; Dunham, A.; North, N.; Wallis, K. The concept of leadership in the health care sector. In *Leadership*; Davut Göker, S., Ed.; IntechOpen: London, UK, 2018; pp. 83–95.
11. Liang, Z.; Leggat, S.G.; Howard, P.F.; Koh, L. What makes a hospital manager competent at the middle and senior levels? *Aust. Health Rev.* **2013**, *37*, 566–573. [CrossRef]
12. Liang, Z.; Howard, P.F.; Koh, L.C.; Leggat, S. Competency requirements for middle and senior managers in community health services. *Aust. J. Prim. Health* **2013**, *19*, 256–263. [CrossRef] [PubMed]
13. Lockhart, W.; Backman, A. Health care management competencies: Identifying the GAPs. *Health Manag. Forum* **2009**, *22*, 30–37. [CrossRef]
14. MacKinnon, N.J.; Chow, C.; Kennedy, P.L.; Persaud, D.D.; Metge, C.J.; Sketris, I. Management competencies for Canadian health executives: Views from the field. *Healthc. Manag. Forum* **2004**, *17*, 15–20. [CrossRef]
15. McCarthy, G.; Fitzpatrick, J.J. Development of a competency framework for nurse managers in Ireland. *J. Contin. Educ. Nurs.* **2009**, *40*, 346–350. [CrossRef]
16. Díaz-Monsalve, S.J. The impact of health-management training programs in Latin America on job performance. *Cad. Saúde Pública* **2004**, *20*, 1110–1120. [CrossRef]
17. North, N.; Park, E. Potential for a web-based tool to confirm and update health management and leadership competencies. Experiences of a pilot survey in New Zealand 2012. *Asia Pac. J. Health Manag.* **2014**, *9*, 13–20.
18. Pillay, R. Defining competencies for hospital management: A comparative analysis of the public and private sectors. *Leadersh. Health Serv.* **2008**, *21*, 99–110. [CrossRef]
19. Pillay, R. The skills gap in hospital management: A comparative analysis of hospital managers in the public and private sectors in South Africa. *Health Serv. Manag. Res.* **2010**, *23*, 30–36. [CrossRef] [PubMed]
20. Pillay, R. The skills gap in nursing management in the south African public health sector. *Public Health Nurs.* **2011**, *28*, 176–185. [CrossRef]
21. Robbins, C.J.; Bradley, E.H.; Spicer, M.; Mecklenburg, G.A. Developing leadership in healthcare administration: A competency assessment tool/practitioner application. *J. Healthc. Manag.* **2001**, *46*, 188–202.
22. Calhoun, J.G.; Dollett, L.; Sinioris, M.E.; Wainio, J.A.; Butler, P.W.; Griffith, J.R.; Warden, G.L. Development of an interprofessional competency model for healthcare leadership. *J. Healthc. Manag.* **2008**, *53*, 375–390. [CrossRef]
23. Landry, A.Y.; Stowe, M.; Haefner, J. Competency assessment and development among health-care leaders: Results of a cross-sectional survey. *Health Serv. Manag. Res.* **2012**, *25*, 78–86. [CrossRef]
24. Reischl, T.M.; Buss, A.N. Responsive evaluation of competency-based public health preparedness training programs. *J. Public Health Manag. Pract.* **2005**, *11*, 100–105. [CrossRef]
25. Leader. Oxford Online Dictionary. 2021. Available online: https://en.oxforddictionaries.com/definition/leader (accessed on 13 January 2022).
26. Day, D.; Harrison, M.; Halpin, S. Leader development through learning from experience. In *An Integrative Approach to Leader Development*; Routledge: New York, NY, USA, 2009; pp. 111–137.
27. Kohs, S.C.; Irle, K.W. Prophesying army promotion. *J. Appl. Psychol.* **1920**, *4*, 73–87. [CrossRef]
28. Bernard, L.L. The quality of leaders. In *An Introduction to Social Psychology*; Henry Holt and Co.: New York, NY, USA, 1926; pp. 528–540.
29. Bingham, W.V. *Leadership/The Psychological Foundations of Management*; New York, NY, USA, 1927.
30. Tead, O. *The Art of Leadership*; McGraw-Hill, Co.: New York, NY, USA, 1935.
31. Kilbourne, C.E. The elements of leadership. *J. Coast Artill.* **1935**, *78*, 437.
32. Bass, B.M. *Bass and Stogdills Handbook of Leadership: Theory, Research and Managerial Applications*, 3rd ed.; Free Press: New York, NY, USA, 1990.
33. Handy, C. *Understanding Organizations*, 4th ed.; Penguin Books Ltd.: London, UK, 2007.
34. Conger, J. Charismatic Leadership. In *Wiley Encyclopedia of Management*; John Wiley and Sons: Hoboken, NJ, USA, 2015; Volume 11. [CrossRef]
35. Kotter, J. What leaders really do. In *Discovering Leadership*; Billsberry, J., Ed.; Palgrave Macmillan: Basingstoke, UK, 2009.
36. Adair, J.E. *How to Grow Leaders: The Seven Key Principles of Effective Leadership Development*; Kogan Page Publishers: London, UK, 2005.
37. Gopee, N.; Galloway, J. *Leadership and Management in Health Care*, 3rd ed.; Sage: London, UK, 2017.
38. Hersey, P.; Blanchard, K.H. Life Cycle Theory of Leadership. *Train. Dev. J.* **1969**, *23*, 26–34.
39. Evans, M.G. Path-goal theory of leadership. In *Leadership*; Neider, L.L., Schriesheim, C.A., Eds.; Information Age Publishing: Greenwich, CT, USA, 2002; Volume 2, pp. 115–138.
40. Fiedler, F.E. Validation and extension of the contingency model of leadership effectiveness: A review of empirical findings. *Psychol. Bull.* **1971**, *76*, 128–148. [CrossRef]
41. Fiedler, F.E. The contingency model and the dynamics of the leadership process. *Adv. Exp. Soc. Psychol.* **1978**, *11*, 59–112.

42. Ogbonna, E.; Harris, L.C. Leadership style, organizational culture and performance: Empirical evidence from UK companies. *Int. J. Hum. Resour. Manag.* **2000**, *11*, 766–788. [CrossRef]
43. Bass, B.M.; Riggio, R.E. *Transformational Leadership*, 2nd ed.; Psychology Press: New York, NY, USA, 2006; pp. 1–18. [CrossRef]
44. Gastil, J. A definition and illustration of democratic leadership. *Hum. Relat.* **1994**, *47*, 953–975. [CrossRef]
45. French, J.R.; Raven, B.; Cartwright, D. The bases of social power. *Class. Organ. Theory* **1959**, *7*, 311–318.
46. Wood, J. Fight the power: Comparing and evaluating two measures of French and Raven's bases of social power. *Curr. Res. Soc. Psychol.* **2014**, *21*, 37–49.
47. Charns, M.P.; Tewksbury, L.S. *Collaborative Management in Health Care: Implementing the Integrative Organization*; Jossey-Bass: San Francisco, CA, USA, 1993.
48. Morgan, C. Growing your own- a model for encouraging and nurturing aspiring leaders. *Nurs. Manag.* **2005**, *11*, 27.
49. Holly, C.; Igwee, G. A systematic review of the influence of transformational leadership style on nursing staff in acute care hospitals. *Int. J. Evid.-Based Health Care* **2011**, *9*, 301. [CrossRef]
50. Kouzes, J.M.; Posner, B.Z. *The Leadership Challenge*, 5th ed.; Jossey-Bass: San Francisco, CA, USA, 2012.
51. McGregor, D.M. *The Human Side of Enterprise*; McGraw-Hill: New York, NY, USA, 2006; pp. 243–258.
52. Fischer, S.A. Transformational leadership in nursing: A concept analysis. *J. Adv. Nurs.* **2016**, *72*, 2644–2653. [CrossRef]
53. Murphy, L. Transformational Leadership: A cascading chain reaction. *J. Nurs. Manag.* **2005**, *13*, 128–136. [CrossRef]
54. Lipley, N. Two-Year Funding to train more leaders. *Nurs. Manag.* **2004**, *11*, 4–5. [CrossRef]
55. Deitchman, S. Enhancing Crisis Leadership in Public Health Emergencies. *Disaster Med. Public Health Prep.* **2013**, *7*, 534–540. [CrossRef]
56. Rosenthal, U.; Charles, M.T.; Hart, P.T. *Coping with Crises: The Management of Disasters, RIOTS and Terrorism*; Charles C Thomas: Springfield, IL, USA, 1989.
57. Lagadec, P. *Preventing Chaos in a Crisis: Strategies for Prevention, Control and Damage Limitation*; McGraw Hill: New York, NY, USA, 1993.
58. Kizer, K.W. Lessons learned in public health emergency management: Personal reflections. *Prehospital Disaster Med.* **2000**, *15*, 83–88. [CrossRef]
59. Driskell, J.E.; Adams, R.J. *Crew Resource Management: An Introductory Handbook*; Department of Transportation, Federal Aviation Administration: Washington, DC, USA, 1992; pp. 8–11.
60. Haynes, A. The Crash of United Flight 232. Edwards, California: NASA Ames Research Center, Dryden Flight Research Facility. 24 May 1991. Available online: http://clear-prop.org/aviation/haynes.html (accessed on 28 November 2011).
61. D'Souza, E.; Barraclough, R.; Fishwick, D.; Curran, A. Management of occupational health risks in small-animal veterinary practices. *Occup. Med.* **2009**, *59*, 316–322. [CrossRef]

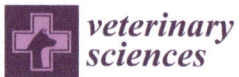 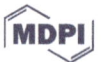

Review

Current Perspectives on the Challenges of Implementing Assistance Dogs in Human Mental Health Care

Sandra Foltin [1,*] and Lisa Maria Glenk

[1] Department of Biology, University of Duisburg-Essen, 45141 Essen, Germany
[2] Comparative Medicine, The Interuniversity Messerli Research Institute of the University of Veterinary Medicine Vienna, 1210 Vienna, Austria
* Correspondence: sfoltin@web.de

Citation: Foltin, S.; Glenk, L.M. Current Perspectives on the Challenges of Implementing Assistance Dogs in Human Mental Health Care. *Vet. Sci.* **2023**, *10*, 62. https://doi.org/10.3390/vetsci10010062

Academic Editors: Ayoze Castro-Alonso and Simona Sacchini

Received: 30 November 2022
Revised: 7 January 2023
Accepted: 11 January 2023
Published: 15 January 2023

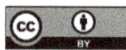

Copyright: © 2023 by the authors. Licensee MDPI, Basel, Switzerland. This article is an open access article distributed under the terms and conditions of the Creative Commons Attribution (CC BY) license (https://creativecommons.org/licenses/by/4.0/).

Simple Summary: Accounting for the global rise in mental health disorders, sustainable therapeutic strategies are urgently needed. However, despite the increasing interest in dogs that support their owners with a mental illness such as post-traumatic stress disorder, depression or autism, some issues including inconsistent use of terminology and the variability or lack of certification procedures across countries have remained unresolved. Moreover, to date, only few studies have addressed the tasks these dogs accomplish and there is only little information available on the canine welfare status related to the performance in human mental health support. This scoping review stresses the need for stringent procedures in legislation, certification, training of desired tasks and animal welfare management practices. Considering the challenges associated with a mental health diagnosis, collaborations of dog provider organizations and health care professionals would be desirable to continuously assess the efficiency of the human-dog dyad regarding their overall compatibility, general satisfaction and mutual well-being.

Abstract: The prevalence of mental health disorders, driven by current global crises, is notably high. During the past decades, the popularity of dogs assisting humans with a wide spectrum of mental health disorders has significantly increased. Notwithstanding these dogs' doubtless value, research on their legal status, certification processes, training and management practices, as well as their welfare status, has been scarce. This scoping review highlights that in contrast to other assistance dogs such as guide dogs, there exists no consistent terminology to mark dogs that assist humans with impaired mental health. Legal authorities monitoring the accreditation process, training and tracking of mental health supporting dogs are broadly lacking, with only few exceptions. This review emphasizes the need to address several topics in the promotion of progress in legal and welfare issues related to assistance dogs as well as emotional support dogs for humans with a mental health disorder. The current body of knowledge was assessed in three different areas of focus: (1) the legal dimension including definitions and certification processes; (2) the dimension of performed tasks; and (3) the dog welfare dimension including aspects of the relationship with the handler and risks associated with children recipients. Considering the challenges associated with a mental health diagnosis, collaborations of dog provider organizations and health care professionals would be desirable to continuously assess the efficiency of the human-dog dyad regarding their overall compatibility, general satisfaction and mutual well-being.

Keywords: mental health; service dog; assistance dog; emotional support animal; psychiatric dog; PTSD service dog; autism spectrum disorder; post-traumatic stress disorder

1. Introduction

The current global crises have cumulative effects and resulted in a significant rise in mental health diseases in recent years [1,2]. Accounting for this emerging trend, appropriate interventions are needed to address the specific needs of mentally vulnerable populations.

Assistance or service dogs' duties have diversified to aid and support people with physical, mental and/or emotional challenges. In the widest sense, they are a versatile group of working dogs that are trained or proficient to assist humans with different types of impairment [3]. The past decade has been characterized by a significant increase in both dogs serving humans with a mental illness [4] and studies that sought to measure the effects on human health outcomes [5]. Notwithstanding these dogs' doubtless value, research on their legal status including terminology, definition, authorization as well as their repertoire of trained behaviors and overall welfare has been scarce [3]. Apart from assistance dogs, similarly, emotional support dogs (ESDs) seek to positively affect human mental health, although these animals do not receive any training or preparation to fulfil their assigned role [6]. These aspects have contributed to inconsistencies and confusion regarding legal, public and social privileges for the human-dog dyads.

The aim of this scoping review was to address recent advances and challenges of implementing assistance dogs in human mental health care by analyzing and discussing the state of knowledge on three dimensions: The legal dimension, the dimension of performed tasks and the welfare dimension. Moreover, we sought to elucidate the differences between assistance dogs and ESDs on the respective domains.

Inclusion criteria for literature were the publication in a peer-reviewed scientific journal, book publications or book chapters, legal documents or statements, position papers or guidelines. Exclusion criteria included duplicate publication, publication as a monograph or academic thesis and language other than English or German.

Scientific databases (including ScienceDirect, SCOPUS and PubMed), Google and Google Scholar were screened for the following terms: psychiatric assistance dog, psychiatric service dog, emotional support animal or dog, legal status, trained tasks or behavior, performed tasks or behavior, animal or dog welfare. The available literature was screened for relevant information covering the three main areas of interest: the legal dimension, the dimension of performed tasks and the welfare dimension.

2. The Legal Dimension

Despite the rapidly increasing numbers of assistance dogs accomplishing various roles, terminology and definition lack clarity and thus impact the question of legal protections given to the owner or handler as well as the dogs. The situation has been complicated in that some jurisdictions afford legal protections also to emotional support animals similar to assistance animals, even though former lack all training requirements [6].

2.1. Assistance Dog: Terminology, Definition, Numbers, Legal Status

A panel of experts recently addressed the issue of flawed terminology (i.e., assistance or service dog versus emotional support dog) across countries, laws and organizations and provided some recommendations to facilitate working dog classification. Thereby, Howell and colleagues suggest promoting the term assistance dog instead of service dog when referring to a dog that has been trained to perform defined tasks [7]. However, past usage has established the inclusive term service dog [8] in the United States (U.S.), whereas, internationally, "assistance dog" is the most common term [9,10]. Therefore, in this paper, either term, service or assistance dog, are used interchangeably. Terms and definitions are depicted in Table 1.

Walther et al. [4] researched placement (2013-2014) with persons with disabilities (including mobility, autism spectrum disorder (ASD), psychiatric diseases, diabetes, seizures) on the statistics and varieties of dogs of U.S. and Canadian non-profit organizations of Assistance Dogs International (ADI) and the International Guide Dog Federation (IGDF) besides non-accredited U.S. assistance dog organizations. U.S. and Canadian replying accredited organizations (55 of 96: 57%) assigned 2374 dogs; non-accredited U.S. organizations (22 of 133: 16.5%) consigned 797 dogs. Autism service dogs were the third-highest group allocated by accredited organizations for these two years in the U.S. and Canada (n = 205 dogs) as well as for U.S. non-accredited organizations (n = 72 dogs). The assignment of autism service dogs rose by 16% from 2013 to 2014 in the U.S and Canada for accredited organizations [4]. Autism service dogs particularly support children who were diagnosed with ASD and their caregivers. Psychiatric service dogs were fourth-most common in accredited assignments (n = 119) and accounted for most allocations (n = 526) in non-accredited organizations. The accreditation status of the assistance dog organization was significantly connected with the categories of dogs they assigned. Non-accredited facilities allocated primarily psychiatric service and seizure alert dogs. Accredited organizations often bred their own dogs or used other breeders, but did not utilize clients' pets or shelter dogs. Non-accredited facilities on the other hand frequently made use of the clients' own pets or dogs from shelters and did not breed their own dogs. A majority of both facilities train and prepare dogs contingent on the requirements of recipients [4]. A comparable pattern was reported in Europe, but is not represented on an international level, where organizations tend to typically place dogs of only one category [4]. Accordingly, the fastest growing groups (both by accredited and non-accredited organizations) were dogs that assist with autism and psychiatric disabilities.

ADI [11], an organization linking not-for-profit programs that train and assign assistance dogs, estimates that currently there are 16,766 assistance dogs in the U.S. This number, however, does not take account of assistance dogs trained by their disabled owners. Therefore, it is challenging to establish a precise number of assistance dogs in the U.S. For instance, ShareAmerica.com [12] estimates that there are all in all approximately 500,000 service dogs at work in the U.S., where all states have laws regarding assistance dogs, but individual states differ in their definitions [4]. All breeds and body sizes of dogs are being utilized in assisting roles. In fact, a study of dogs that were registered in California as assistance dogs included equal numbers of large and small dogs, and a lesser number of medium sized dogs [13]. Under the Fair Housing Act (FHA) [14], the law obliges homeowners and housing providers not to discriminate and to make available reasonable accommodation for service dogs. Under the Air Carrier Access Act (ACAA) [15], airline operators in the U.S. are required to accept service dogs as passengers and transport them on flights to, within, and from the U.S. This is exclusive to service dogs and does not apply to emotional support animals and other animal species. The Americans with Disabilities Act (ADA) [16] provides service dogs the right to enter public areas and facilities. Allergies or cynophobia (fear of dogs) are not considered as legitimate reasons for a service dog team to be denied access. The laws safeguard the assistance dog teams, not the assistance dog alone. If the assistance dog is being handled by a secondary handler (such as a parent or caretaker), or (in some states) by a professional trainer, the assistance dog loses the right to be in public places. Legislation and regulations in the U.S. guarantee persons with disabilities the right to have public access with their service dogs that execute tasks related to the recipients' disability [17]. Although it is mandatory that the dog is trained in these tasks, the method and source of the training are unspecified and no certification process or special identification is obligatory for the dog or the handler [18].

The assistance dogs report published by the European Union Program PROGRESS postulates that comprehensive EU-wide laws are lacking [19]. This deficiency has negative consequences ranging from complications concerning the definition and recognition of the various types of service dogs (e.g., by government institutions) up to individual challenges in the dogs' and owners' everyday life, for instance, their freedom of movement in public areas and by using the train or airplane. National laws addressing the diverse types of service dogs are fragmented and vary across EU countries [20]. Currently, the European Standards Agency, TC/452, is attempting to establish an applicable assistance dog standard [7].

Regulations have been implemented by the European Parliament concerning the rights of humans with disabilities when travelling by plane specifying that service dogs may be transported in the cabin; however, it is subject to national regulations [21]. Furthermore, airlines have specific guidelines for the transportation of service dogs which may be at variance, sometimes requiring certification by certain assistance dog provider organizations. British Airways permits service dogs to accompany their owner in the airplane if the dog is certified by a member of ADI or of the International Guide Dog Federation (IGDF) [22]. Lufthansa, a German airline, on the other hand necessitates the dog to be a "recognized" service dog in order to travel with the handler in the cabin free of charge, without restricting the permission to service dogs certified from specific organizations [23].

Austria has implemented laws maintaining requirements and procedures for the official qualification and recognition of assistance dogs. The Messerli Research Institute [24], part of the University of Veterinary Medicine Vienna, was appointed in 2014 as the official coordinating authority for assistance dogs. Requirements and prerequisites to be officially qualified and recognized as an assistance dog in Austria encompass a health and behavioral suitability check as well as a two-step procedure working performance screening [25].

In Denmark, service dogs for adults with mental illnesses were first legally recognized in 2012, with emerging numbers of people who request a dog. A case study on the implementation of an assistance dog to relieve symptoms of post-traumatic stress disorder (PTSD) raised the question whether these dogs can be legally considered as helping aids to support daily activities of mentally ill people similarly as for the physically disabled [26].

Most countries lack centralized registration processes, thus not requiring any specific accreditation procedure to verify the training and authorization of the dogs and even permitting owners to train their individual assistance dogs. Exceptions are Japan [27], Taiwan [28] Austria [29] and Queensland, Australia [30], where a centralized authority for certifying and tracking assistance dogs exists. In Japan, the Act on Assistance Dogs for Physically Disabled Persons was established in 2002 [31] with the aim to facilitate the quality of assistance dogs and the use of public facilities for people with physical disabilities. It guarantees patient and dog open access as facilities cannot deny access to certified guide, service and hearing dogs. In Japan, the term "assistance dogs" refers to guide dogs, mobility service dogs and hearing dogs certified in accordance with the Act [31]. All other dogs are categorized as "pets". The Act specifies the rights and duties of assistance dogs training organizations, certifying organizations, and eligible assistance dog partners. In 2019, Japan had 26 training organizations for service dogs [32] and seven organizations certifying service dogs. Sixty-six service dogs were registered in 2019 [33]. In Japan, service dogs are solely used for people with physical and not emotional or psychological disorders. The service dogs are lent to the handler by a training organization gratuitously. The handler is responsible for the health and well-being of the dog, which may become challenging depending on his or her medical condition [32]. Once the dog has completed its training and passed the examination, it becomes an official and registered service dog. The training organization remains responsible for continuing training and assistance and is obligated to provide re-training in the event of changing circumstances [34].

2.2. Emotional Support Dog (ESD): Terminology, Definition, Numbers, Legal Status

According to Service Dog Certifications (SDC) [35], an ESD is a pet dog to offer a health benefit and/or support for those that suffer from an emotional or mental disability (see Table 1). ESDs are used for an extensive range of mental illnesses such as Attention Deficit Disorder; Learning Disorders; ASD; General Anxiety Disorder; Gender Identity; Bipolar; Cognitive disorders; Depression; Severe anxiety and/or PTSD. The Americans with Disabilities Act (ADA) does not necessitate an ESD registration [14]. The number of ESDs has similarly increased significantly within the last years [36]. ESDs in the widest sense are dogs that offer some type of companionship or support that will aid alleviate at least one aspect of their owner's disability [7]. The U.S. Centers for Disease Control and Prevention estimate that in 2019, there were nearly 200.000 emotional support animals (ESA) in the U.S. [37].

At present, a valid letter signed by a qualified, licensed healthcare provider is prerequisite to have a dog legally designated as an ESD for the purpose of housing accommodations [8]. The ESD designation does not however grant public access in any other contexts. The dog must be of importance to assist in a person's daily functioning. No special training or suitability screening is obligatory [6,38].

The lack of standards, procedures and certifications regarding ESDs has resulted in much confusion [7,39], fostering a market for falsely "certifying" pets. This led to a bill in in the state of Michigan that will penalize people who sell online certificates [40]. The American Disabilities Act and Department of Justice do not recognize any form of certificate or identification card as a proof of an animal's designation as a service animal or an ESD [41]. A "registration" or "certification" does not constitute appropriate documentation of any kind of helper animal [40].

Table 1. Assistance Dogs and Emotional Support Dogs (ESD): Terminology, definitions, recipient.

	Assistance Dog/Service Dog [7,14]	Emotional Support Dog (ESD) [7,16]
Definition	"An animal living with and highly trained to mitigate the impacts of the owner's disability, and with legal protections" ([7], p.3) The ADA defines service dogs as "dogs that are individually trained to do work or perform tasks for people with disabilities" [14] The U.S. Department of Justice uses the following definition: "Service animals are defined as dogs that are individually trained to do work or perform tasks for people with disabilities. Service animals are working animals, not pets. The work or task a dog has been trained to provide must be directly related to the person's disability. Dogs whose sole function is to provide comfort or emotional support do not qualify as service animals under the ADA" [15]. "an animal who performs at least one identifiable task or behavior (not including any form of protection, comfort, or personal defense) to help a person with a disability to mitigate the impacts of that disability, and who is trained to a high standard of behavior and hygiene appropriate to access public spaces that are prohibited to most animals" ([7], p.6)	An emotional support animal (ESA) may be an animal of any species (domestic, rare or exotic) that provides some emotional or therapeutic support to an individual with a mental health condition or emotional disorder [20]. "an animal who lives with and provides emotional benefit and/or support for the person, as confirmed by an appropriate qualified health care professional." ([7], p.7)
Recipient	Individuals with a physical or psychological disability as defined by the Americans with Disabilities Act (ADA).	Any individual whose need is expressed in a request by a qualified physician, psychiatrist, or other mental health professional based upon a disability-related need.

2.3. Organizations and Health Care Providers

Ethical principles and codes of conduct state that mental health clinicians provide only services within the realm of their competency. When offering novel services, clinicians have to take on pertinent education, training or study. The American Psychological Association (APA) Ethics Code 2.01b states that "psychologists have or obtain the training, experience, consultation, or supervision necessary to ensure the competence of their services, or they make appropriate referrals ... (c) Psychologists planning to provide services, teach or conduct research involving populations, areas, ... new to them undertake relevant education, training, supervised experience, consultation, or study" (American Psychological Association, 2017, paras. 2–3). The American Counseling Association (ACA), 2014, p. 8 states: "While developing skills in new specialty areas, counselors take steps to ensure the competence of their work and protect others from possible harm" [42].

Mental health providers should consequently have comprehensive knowledge on the subject of therapeutic human-dog interactions, canine behavior, and a thorough understanding of the policies surrounding ESDs at the local, state and federal level. Without this knowledge, clinicians, regardless of discipline, risk practicing outside their scope of competence. Regarding ESD prescription, mental health providers should consult or cooperate with dog trainers, behaviorists, veterinarians and/or providers of animal-assisted interventions. Given the absence of accrediting organizations and of federal or state mandates, the mental health provider has to ensure ethical practices43]. The mental health professional must conduct a thorough assessment of a person applying for an ESD to define disability-related need [43]. Prior to endorsing an ESD, the mental health provider has to make reasonable efforts to ensure that the client can provide adequate food, water, housing and veterinary care and fulfill the emotional requirements of the dog, despite their disability. Illness, undue stress from being handled by a person or persons without specialized training in animal welfare, or injury from interactions with the public have to be discussed and minimized.

It is critical that organizations and health care providers have extensive expertise and knowledge regarding a future dog handler's specific disability, cognitive ability, the types of prescribed medication and consumption of addictive substances as well as the effect of comorbid conditions prior to dog adoption. Expectations of first-time handlers regarding the dog must be evaluated. Unrealistic expectations should be minimized as they negatively impact perceived success and satisfaction with the dog. Organizations and health care providers must delineate resources required for successful integration of a dog into the recipient's life. This involves several aspects. Does the handler receive extensive ongoing support? Do the providers maintain contact with handlers with multifaceted disabilities? Do organizations and health care providers have the resources to attend to complex cases? Are alternative placement models an option, such as offering initial training prior to dog adoption, particularly for individuals with complex disabilities and cognitive impairment and/or additional support throughout the assignment duration, perhaps for the entire lifetime of the dog?

2.4. Outlook

Future legislation should aim at addressing fundamental aspects such as providing internationally consistent definitions of the various types of service dogs or ESD for people with mental health disorders; the implementation of qualification procedures for these individuals; and the establishment of an official registration system to provide transparency for government institutions with regard to dog and human data (number of dogs, distribution, age, breed, assessment results, etc.). This database could moreover offer the option to track individual dogs, to assess their welfare state, and to provide dog owners with the opportunity to regularly participate in educational initiatives in order to improve their individual knowledge about dog training and welfare maintenance.

3. The Dimension of Performed Tasks

3.1. Psychiatric Assistance Dog

As indicated in Table 2, psychiatric assistance dogs (PAD) are trained to provide disability-specific support to one person (i.e., the recipient) [44,45]. The tasks these dogs are proficient to perform typically include physical chores [46], and emotional, social and psychological benefits [47] to increase the recipient's well-being [48] and quality of life [49]. According to findings by Lloyd et al. [50], psychiatric conditions in Australian PAD handlers most commonly included depression (84%), anxiety (social 61%; generalized 60%), PTSD (62%) and panic attacks (57%), while fewer study respondents suffered from Obsessive-Compulsive Disorder, ASD and eating disorders.

Table 2. Assistance Dogs and Emotional Support Dogs (ESD): Performed tasks and training.

	Assistance Dog/ Service Dog [7,14]	Emotional Support Dog (ESD) [7,14]
Performed tasks	Dogs perform at least one specific assistive task for individuals with a physical or psychological disability as defined by the Americans with Disabilities Act (ADA). Disability-mitigating tasks include the following: Opening and closing doors; turning light switches off and on; barking to indicate that help is needed; providing deep pressure; pulling a wheelchair; alerting to a medical crisis; providing assistance in a medical crisis; grounding their handler during a flashback; guiding their handler home during a dissociative episode; initiating tactile intervention when a handler experiences sensory overload; alleviating symptoms of hypervigilance.	ESD provide companionship, affection and support to people diagnosed with mental and emotional disabilities, autism, anxiety and panic attacks, depression and various phobias. They provide comfort or emotional support by their mere presence [6].
Training	Service dogs are usually professionally trained but may also be trained by their owner. A service animal must be under the control of its handler. Under the ADA, service animals must be harnessed, leashed or tethered, unless the individual's disability prevents using these devices or these devices interfere with the service animal's safe, effective performance of tasks. In that case, the individual must maintain control of the animal through voice, signal, or other effective controls [13].	ESDs do not require specific training, licensing, registration, or certification and do not have to be trained for any particular task [7,14].

The most common associated tasks performed by the assistance dogs were anxiety reduction through tactile stimulation (94%); nudging or pawing to disrupt dissociative states (71%); interrupting an undesirable behavioral state (51%); maintaining constant body contact (50%); deep pressure stimulation (45%); and blocking contact from other people (42%) [50]. Other performed tasks reported by Lloyd et al. [50] included alerting the recipient to leave the bed or house; reminding the recipient to take medications; providing safety; sensing recipient's emotions and behaviors; and providing a "reality check" from anxiety or dissociation/hallucination. While no statistically significant associations emerged between the recipients' mental health diagnoses and the tasks the dog performed, reductions in the consumption of mental health care services were caused by fewer suicide attempts, less hospitalizations and less medical requirements. However, in 54% of the study participants, having a PAD was not linked to a lesser need for seeking psychiatric or mental health care.

According to Tseng [51], assistance dogs may help to alert and/or interrupt potentially problematic repetitive or self-stimulating behaviors in children with ASD. In addition, dogs can apply pressure stimulation to the children that resembles patterns of touch therapy that are commonly practiced by occupational therapists with the aim of alleviating arousal and anxiety [51,52]. Dogs may provide a calming presence and decrease the numbers of disruptive behaviors including tantrums [53,54]. In addition, parents with an assistance dog perceived the public to react more responsibly and respectfully towards their children [54]. Moreover, reductions of child salivary cortisol levels have been related to the presence of an autism assistance dog [55]. A recent assessment of chronic cortisol in hair or nail specimen points at reduction in cortisol levels for both parents and children. Reduced chronic cortisol concentrations were further paralleled by reductions in stress levels as perceived by the parents [51].

To prevent an autistic child from elopement, a special belt connecting the child to the dog's vest has been previously used. While a parent or adult may hold the dog's lead, the performed behavior of the dog is to passively resist with its body weight or lay down if the child attempts to escape, thereby securing it in public spaces or near roads [52–55].

3.2. PTSD Service Dog for Veterans

Up to 23% of the United States military personnel deployed to Iraq and Afghanistan returned with diagnosed symptoms of PTSD [56]. PTSD has been defined by the APA by avoidance, re-experiencing traumatic events, impaired cognition and mood as well as agitation [57]. Symptom alleviations in terms of behavioral adjustments are anticipated from the support of the PTSD service dog. PTSD service dogs for veterans are supposed to alert to and interrupt anxiety and panic attacks and are frequently trained for positional commands such as standing behind the veteran in public and "watching their back", thereby providing a sense of safety [58].

The demand for PTSD service dogs is immense and it may take months or years to acquire a dog [4,59]. One reason for the extraordinary demand may be that PTSD service dogs are not as publicly stigmatized in contrast to other mental health treatment options [60]. Empirical assessments of the specifically trained tasks the dog is supposed to perform for military veterans with PTSD, such as the therapeutic components of the intervention, remain mostly undefined. Several proposed criterions for PTSD service dog training propose that the dogs must be able to lessen the veteran's PTSD symptoms [61]. These trained assignments, however, vary widely across service dog providers, are not specified and have to be applied to a veteran's individual requirements [62]. Accordingly, no assessments exist on how significant untrained versus trained behaviors are for decreasing PTSD symptoms.

Rodriguez et al. [63] assessed the relevance of trained and untrained behaviors of PTSD service dogs regarding their relevance, frequency of use and PTSD-symptom specificity for post-9/11 veterans. Research findings suggest that calming and interrupting anxiety were considered as the most important and most frequently used trained tasks to mitigate symptoms of PTSD. Veterans who had an intense relationship with their dog relied on trained tasks more often and veterans who had their service dogs longer less frequently required trained tasks. Cover and interrupt/alert to anxiety were considered as the second- and third-most important behaviors [63]. Other symptoms helped by the service dog were decreasing intrusive memories of a traumatic event, feeling distressed and having intense bodily responses (e.g., palpitations and sweating). Veterans on the waitlist had higher expectations compared to veterans with a service dog. The most relevant untrained behavior for relieving PTSD-related symptoms was to express love for the dog and to feel loved in return, while the least important task was to provide social help in public [63].

Other studies similarly propose that anxiety-reducing behaviors displayed by service dogs are the most essential and key mechanistic components to veterans for reducing hyperarousal and dealing with re-experiencing events [58,59,64–66]. The cover task was the second-most frequently used and is thought to replicate aspects of military comradeship by "watch my back" missions in which soldiers will guard each other during combat. Veterans described that their service dogs, similarly to themselves, are constantly on alert or aware of approaching people [58]. When performing "wake up from nightmare" task, the dog responds to stress indicators at night and interrupts the troubled sleep episode of the veteran. The dogs were to reduce the symptoms of intrusive memories or flashbacks as well as internal and physical distress by the trained tasks of "calm/comfort to anxiety" [59]. Williamson et al. [67] integrated the multifaceted support provided by a PTSD service dog into the four principal components of the Zooeyia model, thus labeling the service dog as a builder of social capital, agent of harm reduction, motivator for health-related behavior adaption and active participant in healthcare.

3.3. Emotional Support Dog (ESD)

Given that ESDs do not require any training, only few data exist on the tasks they perform. As shown in Table 2, ESDs provide emotional support, thereby alleviating specific symptoms or disability by their mere presence [68]. To this end, ESDs primarily provide companionship, relieve loneliness, and sometimes contribute to improve symptoms of depression, anxiety, and certain phobias. ESD are used in various heterogeneous environments for emotional support, including rides on airplanes, being taken to educational or working settings [69] or assisting during daily activities such as shopping without having had any prior training.

Brooks et al. [70] reviewed 17 studies regarding ESAs. Of the 17 studies, eight were conducted in the USA, four in the UK, two in Canada, one in the Netherlands, one in Australia and one in Sweden. Fifteen reported positive features of dog ownership for individuals suffering mental health problems whereas nine described negative elements. In military veterans with PTSD, positive effects were centered on decreasing feelings of loneliness, depression, worry and irritability, and, moreover, having a source of comfort and affection [71]. Owner described that their dogs provided a source of physical warmth and companionship, opportunities for communication, reducing feelings of isolation, provided a safe environment and "their dogs allowed them to express their feelings and clarify their thoughts without the concern that they will interrupt, offer criticism or advice or betray confidence" [72]. The studies further indicated that the dogs provided unconditional love and affection fostering self-acceptance and congruence, supporting emotional stability, aiding in stress management and coping with challenging life events [73]. For people living alone, dogs were a source of "connectedness" [74], reassurance, and normalcy [75]. The dogs contributed to their owner's feelings of security by distracting from particular symptoms such as hearing voices or panic attacks and through decreasing symptoms of their mental health disorder [70,71,75,76].

However, a recent survey study failed to expose any model for evaluating individuals reporting need for an ESA [77], outlining the general deficiency of awareness regarding the ESA policy of many mental health professionals and the absence of reliable assessment standards.

3.4. Training Methods

Employing exclusively reward-based (positive reinforcement) training methods is more effective than aversive, compulsive, punishment-based (e.g., shock collars) or mixed methods [78,79]. Solely utilizing positive reinforcement was linked to more optimistic dogs, who learn faster and exhibit more consistent behavioral responses, less pain and suffering as well as lower incidences of negative affect, aggression and problematic behaviors (e.g., unwanted barking) [79,80]. In many instances, the working equipment, such as collars, leads and harnesses, is outdated [81]. Preliminary research considering the trained behaviors of service dogs has mainly focused on assessments to advance the selection and performance to enhance program success rates, which are estimated approximately 50% across different working dog populations [82]. Assessments of behavioral characteristics should be measured regarding their prognostic value linked to working suitability [83]; the genetics of service dog behavior [84]; maternal care in service dog breeding programs [85]; and development and testing of cognitive skills [86]. Terminology used to designate behavior however differs extensively between and across industry sectors, potentially producing irritations for researchers, dog trainers and dog handlers/recipients alike [82]. Further research is essential to debate the difference and value of untrained versus trained behaviors of the service dog as they may dually contribute to the therapeutic efficacy.

4. The Welfare Dimension

Animal welfare refers to the quality of life experienced by the animal, positive or negative, with respect to the domains of nutrition, environment, physical health, behavioral interactions and mental health state of the animal [87]. The Five Domains Model encourages the requirement to provide opportunities within each domain that lead to positive affective states [87]. Modern animal management practices are critical to industries reliant on animal use, including working dogs [88]. Risk assessment to safeguard the welfare of assistance dogs at the operational level recognizes a widespread lack of transparency, stakeholder commitment and partaking of best practice and standards [82]. Acknowledgment that dogs are sentient animals, having intrinsic value beyond their consideration as properties, equipment or working aid has been somewhat mirrored in advances to legislation and politics globally (e.g., Australia, European Union, New Zealand, Canada, United States and United Kingdom) [89–91]. Service or assistance dogs are permanently housed with individuals with disabilities to aid in their day-to-day life [5] and their welfare must be a principal consideration moving toward a greater degree of concern [92,93]. Concerns such as absence of a day-to-day routine, lack of sufficient "time off", being overweight, and (un)intentional harm and mishandling of the dog by recipients/owners must be addressed. To this end, provider organizations necessitate transparent, long-term procedures and processes for animal welfare [94,95].

Cultural difference clearly exists with respect to the perception of assistance dogs. An Australian study [96] researched the Australian public's opinion toward both assistance and companion dogs. There was an equal interest in both groups of dogs. Assistance dogs were rated as happier than companion dogs by the study respondents. The survey revealed some ethical concerns regarding the use of animals for human benefit. These included conditions in which the dogs might not profit from their role as working animals and the prevalence of inappropriate behaviors from strangers in public environments such as touching the dog while working. There was only little disapproval of the intensity of training imposed on the dogs as well as the straining and restrictive nature of assistance dog work. It emerged that some study respondents expressed some concern about the ability of recipients with disability to appropriately take care for their dogs, while others stated that assistance dogs may even be better cared for because of the recipients' dependency on them and the greater amount of time spent together [96]. The past decade has been associated with some advancement in considering the welfare of assistance dogs [82,87,97]. Numerous researchers in animal welfare science have stressed that professionals working with service or therapy dogs (and other animals) must consider welfare issues [92,97,98]. It is vital to understand that if the working experiences repeatedly cause discomfort, pain or fear the dog is inevitably subject to distress which has severe consequence for both its physical and mental health [97].

The "ethics of care" approach endeavors to respect all parties participating by emphasizing sustainable relationships and establishing a human-dog bond [99]. Within this model, the dog should be provided with an optimal rather than a sufficient quality of life [82]. The "rights approach" concentrates on protecting and respecting the rights of all individuals involved and furthermore contemplates the advantages and disadvantages from the dog's perspective. According to the "utilitarian approach", a cost benefit analysis must determine what should be acted upon subsequently, founded on all the morally relevant consequences (typically harms and benefits for sentient individuals) [100].

4.1. Relationship and Attachment

After adoption, guide dogs were broadly considered as family members by their owners [101] and similarly, service or assistance dogs frequently have multiple handlers. Dogs perform differently for respective handlers [102] based on the interplay of canine and human personalities, the strength and style of attachment [103] and recipient beliefs [104]. A majority of recipients experience mental health challenges which may influence their concentration, fatigue, stress, motivation and determination. Some recipients may have extended hospital admissions, not being able to care for their dog during that time span. Recipients with an intellectual disability or a lack of maturity may experience more challenges related to memory and consistency in handling the dog and, thus, impacting its welfare.

Therapy dogs are most commonly visiting dogs that are temporarily brought to a setting to support individuals diagnosed with a mental health illness or to interact with people with other diagnoses, for recreation purposes or social facilitation. They are usually accompanied by their owner or a closely familiar person who acts as the responsible person to safeguard the dog's welfare at any time [105]. In contrast, mental health service dogs are constantly paired with their owners who themselves frequently have trouble to regulate their inner tension and mental states. Individuals with impaired mental health may experience extended periods of dissociation, where they do not at all respond to their social environment. However, similar to a child, a dog requires attention, social interaction, food, water and needs to be taken outside irrespective of the current constitution of the handler. And the question that instantly emerges is whether people who struggle to maintain their own well-being can be the responsible person to safeguard their dog's welfare and provide a safe haven in case the dog needs emotional support.

Measurements of cortisol as a strategy to monitor the adrenocortical activity in response to stress have been broadly applied in canine welfare science [105]. In comparison to saliva, in which cortisol typically rises in response to an acute stressor, analyses of hair may represent the long-term cortisol status [106]. Research by Sundman et al. [107] demonstrated significant interspecies associations in long-term stress when dog hair cortisol levels were correlated with human hair cortisol concentrations. This is particularly interesting since cortisol in hair of PTSD service dogs for veterans did not differ from concentrations of regular pet dogs, suggesting no profound effect of their working task on their long-term stress profile [108,109]. In line with these findings, van Houtert et al. [109] also stated that salivary cortisol, a representative of acute arousal, appeared to be lower in PTSD dogs for veterans during training sequences than concentrations measured upon arrival at the training site or after an episode of free play. According to these recent studies on adrenocortical activity related to supporting veterans with PTSD, the data do not raise any concern about compromised animal welfare. Although the two recent studies have not found any evidence of altered stress levels, both acute and long-term, in PTSD service dogs for veterans [108,109] it would be essential to run long-term research including regular, continuous physiological and psychological follow-ups. As we have mentioned before in therapy dogs [97], studies would benefit from adding measurements of the recipients' emotional competence, attitude and empathy towards their dog.

Yarborough et al. [60] described difficulties in coping with the additional stressors of sustaining the dog's training, integrating the dog into the family, and receiving unwanted attention in public which may cause added stress, anxiety and fatigue. Additionally, findings from a recent exploratory study by Williamson et al. [67] point at difficulties such as establishing a sustainable emotional and working relationship with the service dog as well as integrating it into the family (including socialization with preexisting pets). In case of unsuccessful matches, dogs may need to be rehomed or reassigned to another veteran. Furthermore, preexistent pet dogs may not necessarily be ideal candidates for PTSD service due to challenges of coping with the newly assigned tasks, as Williamson et al. revealed [69].

According to Glintborg and Hansen [26] people with PTSD can benefit from their service dog through ventriloquizing (i.e., talking about the nonverbal animal by implicitly referring to oneself) which may facilitate social interactions and psychotherapeutic processes. However, the fact that people with a mental health disorder may regularly have their service dog accompany them to psychotherapy, especially in group sessions, necessitates attention from an animal welfare point of view due to interindividual emotional contagion of behavior and physiology [110] that may negatively impact the dog [111].

4.2. Children Recipients

Dog assistance may benefit children affected by neuro-developmental disorders such as ASD [112–114]. However, families may have unrealistic expectations of the recipient/owner-dog relationship [115], and insufficient information regarding the impact on the dog and the basic welfare guidelines to protect the animal [116].

Living in close proximity with children may negatively affect dog well-being and quality of life [117,118], conceivably augmenting the risk of child-directed aggression. The majority of dog bite accidents (about 75%) occur in the household environment [119] indicating a great necessity to intensify parent sentience about contexts and child activities that may trigger a dog bite [120]. Dogs do not necessarily enjoy being physically close to and tactile with a child [121]. Studies suggest that dogs may well find close interactions such as kissing or petting stressful, as evidenced by increases in cortisol [122] and behavioral indices [123,124].

A number of studies provide data on the impact of child-dog interactions for dog quality of life [125–127], with one considering the quality of life of pet dogs around children [127]. Oher studies referred to therapy dogs [128,129], other animal-assisted intervention dogs [126] and autism service dogs [53].

Four papers specified possible sources of stress (for service dogs, therapy dogs and pet dogs), either as identified through the parent/handler [53,127] or through researcher observations [53,129].

Hall et al. [127] as well as Burrows et al. [53] reported that child meltdowns and tantrums were particularly stressful for pet dogs [127] or assistance dogs [53]. Stress indicators observed were barking, jumping up and shaking. Both papers indicated that the dog was being at risk from potentially aggressive behaviors from the child, either because the dog was the closest target for the child or because the parent had encouraged the dog to interrupt the display of aggression to calm the child. At times, Hall et al. [127] observed that the dog spontaneously interjected in a meltdown by seeking physical proximity with the child, reflecting its efforts to appease a stressful situation and defuse a perceived conflict [130].

Not all negative attention directed to the dog was the consequence of meltdowns or tantrums, as it was reported that the child jumped, prodded and poked the dog aggressively and in a rough manner during various daily interactions [53,127].

Lack of predictable routines, uninterrupted resting times, children handling the dog on the lead [127], environmental instability, erratic unpredictable movements, such as those involving wheeled toys or the child bouncing around, as well as loud noises [53,127] and activities from child visitors [127] were considered as major sources of stress for dogs. Recreational activities, in particular sleep and off-duty time, were seen as vital to ensure physical and psychological health [53]. Children's toys and games had a negative effect on some dog's well-being as indicated by a proliferation in stress behaviors associated with avoidance (e.g., pet dogs hiding and running away [127]). Interestingly, parents believed that the dog enjoyed being "dressed-up" by the child [127]; however, other studies indicated more stress when children put a bandana on the dog [129]. Behaviors displayed by the dog during child-dog interactions included paw chewing, lip-licking, grooming, yawning and panting [53,127–129], running away, shaking, urinating and defecating [53,127], safety seeking behaviors (hiding, going to their safe place or seeking the parent/handler), all of which may be indicators of heightened stress levels [131]. Dogs living full time with children displayed a spectrum of physical health conditions associated with chronic stress due to impaired immunity [119], such as ear, eye and skin infections [53,127]. Social effects exhibited by the dog were displaying distress when left alone with the child shown by whining, scratching, seeking behavior, particularly if the dog had to sleep in the same room as the child [53], or if the child created stressful situations for the dog [127], with the dog also withdrawing from the child [127].

Arousal-reducing interactions that comfort the child (e.g., tactile stimulation from the dog lying on the child, fiddling with the dog's ears and medallion, and being able to rub the feet on their dog) as reported by Appleby et al. [52] may cause considerable discomfort in the dog, especially if performed for extended periods of time. For appropriate supervision of children and dogs, parents must be aware of the dog's communication and signaling as reaction to their own or their children's interactions.

Parents of neuro-typically developing children and children with neuro-developmental disorders identified various behaviors that pose a risk to the dog. Parent surveys also indicated that children were often not sufficiently supervised around their dogs. Even though dog-child interactions did not differ much between families, study findings revealed that neuro-typically developing children displayed fewer outbursts of anger, crying, meltdowns and tantrums compared to children with a neuro-developmental disorder [127]. The shorter the time the dog had lived with the child, the greater the score on canine excitability in meltdowns and with child visitors. Scores on fearfulness were significantly higher when the child-dog interaction included physical interactions with the dog, such as rough contact, meltdowns and grooming/bathing. Moreover, smaller dogs, older dogs and younger children were linked with increased levels of fearfulness.

Displays of acute and chronic stress [132] include, e.g., chewing, lip-licking, yawning and panting, cowering, shaking, running away and aggressive behaviors. Another point of concern is that children and adults had difficulty recognizing signs of stress in their dog [121,133,134]. Hall et al. [127] found that the main caregivers tended to report lower signs of fearfulness-related behavior of the dog either indicating desensitization with repeat exposure, or reduced observation of the behavior because they did not recognize relevant behaviors and/or they were unwilling to report them.

If the dog lives full time with the child, the duration of child-dog contact time and the nature of exposure the dog experiences have been considered critical [53,127]. Thus, increased precautions must be taken when an assistance dog or ESD is first placed into a family to support a child diagnosed with ASD.

4.3. Physical and Mental Health

The physical health of a service dog must be considered from the time of birth or recruitment, throughout the dog's working life and into retirement [95], requiring standards for breeding, rearing and/or recruitment of the dogs; housing, transportation; training techniques and equipment; trainer and owner/handler education; enrichment, maintenance of a good welfare state, as well as animal agency [135]. Older dogs naturally become less resilient, need more time to recover from stress, and thus, may not be as adept at managing social situations [136,137]. However, there are no data available about the ideal age for a dog to start working or when to retire [97].

Preventive veterinary care is critical to maintain service dog health and an example of minimum requirements are described in the AAHA (American Animal Hospital Association) recommendations [138]. Physical fitness is an essential welfare consideration [87]. Research and rethinking of the importance of veterinarians in detecting and reporting animal abuse and cruelty in the context of service or assistance as well as emotional support dogs is needed. Optimal rest and sleep are critical for all but especially for working dogs. Sleep is connected with emotional states and essential for learning, immune function, performance and recovery [139,140]. It is furthermore critical that service dogs' social and emotional needs are met by providing them social, environmental and mental enrichment [141] and by allowing dogs to engage freely with their environment under their own motivation. This is referred to as agency [142] and promotes behavioral variety and welfare [143]. Supporting regular occasions for service dogs to exercise agency in environmental and social contexts is vital.

One activity shown to induce positive judgement bias in dogs is nosework [144]. Allowing dogs to engage in olfactory-based sniffing activities resulted in them exercising autonomy and increased optimism [144]. Behavioral problems are a key contributing factor to the extraordinary failure rates in service dog programs [145]. Improved assessment and personalized maintenance for dogs ensure welfare benefits [83]. Community stances and media debate have encouraged modifications in some segments that historically euthanized working dogs as an end point to their training or working life [e.g., Royal Australian Air Force Wilson: [146]; US Military: Alger and Alger [147,148]]. The identification of behavioral displays of affective state and welfare regarding training, operational environments, kennel facilities and home settings should be focused on in-depth [149].

A One Health framework [117,150] for the spectrum of dogs supporting human mental health, outlining under which circumstances no tradeoff of human benefits against animal health and well-being may be found, is essential. Assistance dogs must no longer be perceived as objects other than pet dogs being instrumentalized to fulfill a plethora of tasks. As dogs do not share equal privilege, right or power as the recipient, it is questionable whether dogs may give any form of free and informed consent to fulfill the numerous tasks assigned to them [97]. Current perspectives on animal status denote that latter should not be seen as "less than" or "tools" but as individuals with likes, dislikes and limitations [151]. If we maintain the concept of animals as sentient beings whose rights and dignity may be inseparable from our own, then the ethical principles of autonomy, beneficence, nonmaleficence and justice ought to be applied [152].

5. Conclusions and Future Directions

During the past decades, the popularity of dogs assisting humans with various mental health disorders has significantly increased. This article highlights that in contrast to other assistance dogs such as guide dogs, there exists no consistent terminology to mark dogs that assist humans with impaired mental health. Legal authorities monitoring the accreditation process, training and tracking of mental health supporting dogs are broadly lacking, with only few exceptions. To advance the field of working dogs in mental health, stringent procedures in safeguarding dog welfare need to be established. Considering the challenges associated with a mental health diagnosis, collaborations of dog provider organizations and health care professionals would be desirable to continuously assess the efficiency of the human-dog dyad regarding their overall compatibility, general satisfaction and mutual well-being.

A limitation of this scoping review is the relatively narrow focus on specific topics rather than a holistic synthesis of the literature and internet-based content. One facet that has merely received scarce attention is the efficiency and appropriateness of training and management practices. Future research is challenged to raise methodological rigor and uniformity in terminology and definitions. Dog selection processes and the definition of desired traits and performed tasks need to be transparent, allowing a comprehensive evaluation of research. This refers to both assistance dogs and ESDs that are paired with people who suffer from a mental health disorder. Future studies must also determine appropriate and individualized parameters and feasible methods to investigate the ideal life phase for dog retirement and to prepare the recipient for such. Accounting for the variations in which dogs are working within the assistance or emotional support context, comprehensive, long-term studies using objective and multiple measures of welfare are warranted. Methods to measure the relative resilience of dogs to stressful events and the development of optimal protocols to enhance such resilience are certainly needed.

Author Contributions: Conceptualization, S.F. and L.M.G.; investigation, S.F. and L.M.G.; writing—original draft preparation, S.F. and L.M.G.; writing—review and editing, S.F. and L.M.G. All authors have read and agreed to the published version of the manuscript.

Funding: This research received no external funding.

Institutional Review Board Statement: Not applicable.

Informed Consent Statement: Not applicable.

Data Availability Statement: Not applicable.

Conflicts of Interest: The authors declare no conflict of interest.

References

1. Nochaiwong, S.; Ruengorn, C.; Thavorn, K.; Hutton, B.; Awiphan, R.; Phosuya, C.; Ruanta, Y.; Wongpakaran, N. Global prevalence of mental health issues among the general population during the coronavirus disease-2019 pandemic: A systematic review and meta-analysis. *Sci. Rep.* **2019**, *11*, 1–18. [CrossRef] [PubMed]
2. Riad, A.; Drobov, A.; Krobot, M.; Antalová, N.; Alkasaby, M.A.; Peřina, A.; Koščík, M. Mental Health Burden of the Russian–Ukrainian War 2022 (RUW-22): Anxiety and Depression Levels among Young Adults in Central Europe. *Int. J. Environ. Res. Public Health* **2022**, *19*, 8418. [CrossRef] [PubMed]
3. Bremhorst, A.; Mongillo, P.; Howell, T.; Marinelli, L. Spotlight on Assistance Dogs-Legislation, Welfare and Research. *Animals* **2018**, *7*, 129. [CrossRef]

4. Walther, S.; Yamamoto, M.; Thigpen, A.P.; Willits, N.H.; Hart, L.A. Geographic Availability of Assistance Dogs: Dogs Placed in 2013–2014 by ADI- or IGDF-Accredited or Candidate Facilities in the United States and Canada, and Non-accredited U.S. Facilities. *Front. Vet. Sci.* **2019**, *6*, 349. [CrossRef]
5. Leighton, S.C.; Nieforth, L.O.; O'Haire, M.E. Assistance dogs for military veterans with PTSD: A systematic review, meta-analysis, and meta-synthesis. *PLoS ONE* **2022**, *9*, e0274960. [CrossRef] [PubMed]
6. Schoenfeld-Tacher, R.; Hellyer, P.; Cheung, L.; Kogan, L. Public Perceptions of Service Dogs, Emotional Support Dogs, and Therapy Dogs. *Int. J. Environ. Res. Public Health* **2017**, *14*, 642. [CrossRef] [PubMed]
7. Howell, T.J.; Nieforth, L.; Thomas-Pino, C.; Samet, L.; Agbonika, S.; Cuevas-Pavincich, F.; Fry, N.E.; Hill, K.; Jegatheesan, B.; Kakinuma, M.; et al. Defining terms used for animals working in support roles for people with support needs. *Animals* **2022**, *12*, 1975. [CrossRef]
8. U.S. Department of Justice, Civil Rights Division, Disability Rights Section. Available online: https://www.justice.gov/crt/disability-rights-section (accessed on 25 October 2022).
9. Australian Human Rights Commission. Assistance Animals and the Disability Discrimination Act 1992 (Cth). 2016. Available online: https://humanrights.gov.au/our-work/disability-rights/projects/assistance-animals-and-disability-discriminationact-1992-cth (accessed on 17 December 2022).
10. Equality and Human Rights Commission. *Assistance Dogs: A Guide for All Businesses*; Equality and Human Rights Commission: Manchester, UK, 2017.
11. Assistance Dog International. Available online: https://assistancedogsinternational.org/ (accessed on 1 October 2022).
12. Share America. Available online: https://shareamerica.com/ (accessed on 3 October 2022).
13. Yamamoto, M.; Lopez, M.T.; Hart, L.A. Registrations of assistance dogs in California for identification tags: 1999–2012. *PLoS ONE* **2015**, *10*, e0132820. [CrossRef]
14. Fair Housing Act. Available online: https://www.hud.gov/program_offices/fair_housing_equal_opp/fair_housing_act_overview (accessed on 28 July 2022).
15. Air Carrier Access Act. Available online: https://www.accessibility.com/air-carrier-access-act (accessed on 3 October 2022).
16. Americans with Disabilities Act. Available online: https://www.dol.gov/general/topic/disability/ada (accessed on 28 July 2022).
17. U.S. Department of Justice. Available online: https://adata.org/service-animal-resource-hub/differences (accessed on 28 July 2022).
18. U.S. Department of Justice (DOJ). ADA 2010 Revised Requirements. Service Animals. 2011. Available online: https://www.ada.gov/service_animals_2010.htm (accessed on 27 July 2022).
19. PROGRESS–European Commission–DG Justice Unknown Label (europa.eu). Available online: https://eur-lex.europa.eu/eli/reg/2006/1107/oj (accessed on 27 July 2022).
20. European Guide Dog Federation. European Standard for Assistance Dogs-Progress Report. 2019. Available online: https://www.egdfed.org/news-information/reports/report-of-2019-conference-in-tallin-estonia/european-standard-for-assistance-dogs-progress-report/ (accessed on 17 December 2022).
21. Service dog Training School Interantion. Available online: https://www.servicedogtrainingschool.org/service-dog-legalities (accessed on 12 January 2023).
22. British Airways. British Airways Service Animal Policies–Dogs on Planes. Available online: https://www.britishairways.com/en-gb/information/disability-assistance/travelling-with-your-assistance-dog (accessed on 3 October 2022).
23. Lufthansa Airlines. Available online: https://www.lufthansa.com/de/de/assistenzhunde (accessed on 3 October 2022).
24. Messerli Research Institute, Vienna. Available online: https://www.vetmeduni.ac.at/assistenzhunde/richtlinien (accessed on 27 July 2022).
25. The Austrian Law Addressing Assistance Dogs Was Amended on 1 January 2015, and Integrated into the Austrian Federal Law for Disabled People [Bundesbehindertengesetz]. Article 39a of the Bundesbehindertengesetz Defines the Characteristics and Requirements to Officially Qualify and Acknowledge a Dog as an Assistance Dog. An Additional Directive on Assistance Dogs [Richtlinie Assistenzhunde] Further Details the Practical Implementation of this Law. Available online: https://www.jusline.at/gesetz/bbg (accessed on 3 October 2022).
26. Glintborg, C.; Hansen, T. How Are Service Dogs for Adults with Post Traumatic Stress Disorder Integrated with Rehabilitation in Denmark? A Case Study. *Animals* **2017**, *7*, 33. [CrossRef]
27. Ministry of Health, Labour and Welfare. Act on Assistance Dogs for Physically Disabled Persons. 2002. Available online: http://elaws.e-gov.go.jp/search/elawsSearch/elaws_search/lsg0500/detail?lawId=414AC1000000049 (accessed on 2 October 2022).
28. Taiwan Guide Dog Association. Available online: http://www.guidedog.org.tw/aboutguidedog/about-2.html (accessed on 2 October 2022). (In Chinese).
29. Republic of Austria. Protection Federal Ministry of Labour Social Affairs and Consumer. Directive on Assistance Dogs [Richtlinie Assistenzhunde]. Available online: https://www.sozialministerium.at/cms/site/attachments/1/5/6/CH3434/CMS1450709884090/richtlinien_assistenzhunde.pdf (accessed on 2 September 2022).
30. Queensland Guide, Hearing and Assistance Dogs Act 2009. 2013. Available online: https://www.legislation.qld.gov.au/view/pdf/inforce/2013-12-06/act-2009-004 (accessed on 12 July 2022).
31. Ministry of Health, Labour and Welfare. A List of Training Facilities of Service Dogs and Hearing Dogs. 2019. Available online: https://www.mhlw.go.jp/content/000468562.pdf (accessed on 18 December 2022).
32. Ministry of Health, Labour and Welfare. Number of Working Assistance Dogs (2019). Available online: https://www.mhlw.go.jp/stf/seisakunitsuite/bunya/0000165273.html (accessed on 18 December 2022).

33. Matsunaka, K.; Koda, N. Acceptance of dog guides and daily stress levels of dog guide users and nonusers. *J. Vis. Impair. Blind.* **2008**, *102*, 295–304. [CrossRef]
34. Takayanagi, T.; Yamamoto, M. The Use of Service Dogs for People with Physical Disabilities in Japan in Accordance with the Act on Assistance Dogs for Physically Disabled Persons. *Front. Vet. Sci.* **2019**, *21*, 198. [CrossRef]
35. Service Dog Certifications. Available online: https://www.servicedogcertifications.org/emotional-support-animal-id/ (accessed on 3 October 2022).
36. National Service Animal Registration. Available online: https://www.nsarco.com/ (accessed on 1 October 2022).
37. U.S. Centers for Disease Control and Prevention. Available online: https://www.cdc.gov/ncbddd/disabilityandhealth/ (accessed on 22 October 2022).
38. Kogan, L.; Schoenfeld-Tacher, R.; Hellyer, P.; Rishniw, M. US Veterinarians' Knowledge, Experience, and Perception Regarding the Use of Cannabidiol for Canine Medical Conditions. *Front. Vet. Sci.* **2019**, *5*, 338. [CrossRef]
39. Enders-Slegers, M.J.; Hediger, K.; Beetz, A.; Jegatheesan, B.; Turner, D. Animal-assisted interventions with in an international perspective: Trends, research, and practices. In *Handbook on Animal-Assisted Therapy: Foundations and Guidelines for Animal-Assisted Interventions*; Fine, A., Ed.; Elsevier: Amsterdam, The Netherlands, 2019; pp. 465–477.
40. Michigan State Legislation. Available online: https://eu.detroitnews.com/story/news/local/michigan/2022/10/16/influx-of-emotional-support-animals-fake-certificates-prompts-michigan-legislation/69565194007/ (accessed on 3 November 2022).
41. U.S. Department of Justice (DOJ). Part 35. Nondiscrimination on the Basis of Disability in State and Local Government Services (as Amended by the Final Rule Published on September 15, 2010). Available online: http://www.ada.gov/regs2010/titleII_2010/titleII_2010_withbold.htm (accessed on 22 October 2022).
42. State Board of Licensed Professional Counselor Examiners v. Stanford Sutherland. 2016. Available online: https://www.dora.state.co.us/pls/real/ddms_public.display_document?p_section=DPO&p_source=ELIC_PUBLIC&p_doc_id=473699&p_doc_key=C9581B58DF08B56A95AF03C3B36FB50C (accessed on 9 September 2022).
43. Younggren, J.N.; Boness, C.L.; Bryant, L.M.; Koocher, G.P. Emotional Support Animal Assessments: Toward a Standard and Comprehensive Model for Mental Health Professionals. *Prof. Psychol. Res. Pr.* **2020**, *4*, 156–162. [CrossRef] [PubMed]
44. Spence, H.R. How Feasible Is It to Compare Effects of Companion Dogs and Service Dogs on Quality of Life in People with Movement Disorders? Ph.D. Thesis, University of Auckland, Auckland, New Zealand, 2015.
45. Camp, M.M. The use of service dogs as an adaptive strategy: A qualitative study. *Am. J. Occup. Ther.* **2001**, *55*, 509–517. [CrossRef]
46. Fairman, S.K.; Huebner, R.A. Service dogs: A compensatory resource to improve function. *Occup. Ther. Health Care* **2001**, *13*, 41–52. [CrossRef]
47. Valentine, D.; Kiddoo, M.; LaFleur, B. Psychosocial implications of service dog ownership for people who have mobility or hearing impairments. *Soc. Work Health Care* **1993**, *19*, 109–125. [CrossRef]
48. Plowman, S.; Bowan, P.; Williams, D. "Okay girl, it's up to you" a case study of the use of a seizure alert dog to improve the wellbeing of a student with epilepsy. *J. Stud. Wellbeing.* **2009**, *3*, 40–51. [CrossRef]
49. Shintani, M.; Senda, M.; Takayanagi, T.; Katayama, Y.; Furusawa, K.; Okutani, T.; Kataoka, M.; Ozaki, T. The effect of service dogs on the improvement of health-related quality of life. *Acta Med. Okayama.* **2010**, *64*, 109–113. [PubMed]
50. Lloyd, J.; Johnston, L.; Lewis, J. Psychiatric Assistance Dog Use for People Living with Mental Health Disorders. *Front. Vet. Sci.* **2019**, *6*, 166. [CrossRef]
51. Tseng, A. Brief Report: Above and Beyond Safety: Psychosocial and Biobehavioral Impact of Autism-Assistance Dogs on Autistic Children and their Families. *J. Autism. Dev. Disor.* **2022**, *1*, 1–16. [CrossRef]
52. Appleby, R.; Wright, S.; Williams, L.; Stanley, M. Australian parents' experiences of owning an autism assistance dog. *Health Soc. Care Comm.* **2022**, *10*, e4113–e4121. [CrossRef] [PubMed]
53. Burrows, K.E.; Adams, C.L.; Spiers, J. Sentinels of safety: Service dogs ensure safety and enhance freedom and well-being for families with autistic children. *Qual. Health Res.* **2008**, *18*, 1642–1649. [CrossRef] [PubMed]
54. Burgoyne, L.; Dowling, L.; Fitzgerald, A.; Connolly, M.; Browne, J.P.; Perry, I.J. Parents' perspectives on the value of assistance dogs for children with autism spectrum disorder: A crosssectional study. *Brit. Med. J. Op.* **2014**, *4*, e004786. [CrossRef] [PubMed]
55. Wojtaś, J.; Karpiński, M.; Czyżowski, P. Salivary Cortisol Interactions in Search and Rescue Dogs and their Handlers. *Animals* **2020**, *4*, 595. [CrossRef]
56. Fulton, J.J.; Calhoun, P.S.; Wagner, H.R.; Schry, A.R.; Hair, L.P.; Feeling, N.; Elbogen, E.; Beckham, J.C. The prevalence of posttraumatic stress disorder in Operation Enduring Freedom/Operation Iraqi Freedom (OEF/OIF) Veterans: A meta-analysis. *J. Anxiety Disord.* **2015**, *31*, 98–107. [CrossRef]
57. American Psychiatric Association. *Diagnostic and Statistical Manual of Mental Disorders: DSM-V*; American Psychiatric Association: Washington, DC, USA, 2013.
58. Krause-Parello, C.A.; Morales, K.A. Military veterans and service dogs: A qualitative inquiry using interpretive phenomenological analysis. *Anthrozoös* **2018**, *31*, 61–75. [CrossRef]
59. Walther, S.; Yamamoto, M.; Thigpen, A.P.; Garcia, A.; Willits, N.H.; Hart, L.A. Assistance dogs: Historic patterns and roles of dogs placed by aDior igDF accredited facilities and by non-accredited US facilities. *Front. Vet. Sci.* **2017**, *4*, 1. [CrossRef]
60. Yarborough, B.J.H.; Stumbo, S.P.; Yarborough, M.T.; Owen-Smith, A.; Green, C.A. Benefits and challenges of using service dogs for veterans with posttraumatic stress disorder. *Psychiatr. Rehabil. J.* **2018**, *41*, 118–124. [CrossRef]

61. Assistance Dogs International. Assistance Dogs International's Guide to Assistance Dog Laws. Available online: http://www.assistancedogsinternational.org/wp-content/uploads/2012/01/ADI20062ndprint.pdf (accessed on 22 October 2022).
62. Futeran, N.; Mackenzie, L.; Wilkes-Gillan, S.; Dickson, C. Understanding the participation outcomes for persons with disability when partnered with assistance dogs: A scoping review. *Aust. Occup. Ther. J.* **2022**, *8*, 475–492. [CrossRef]
63. Rodriguez, K.E.; LaFollette, M.R.; Hediger, K.; Ogata, N.; O'Haire, M.E. Defining the PTSD service dog intervention: Perceived importance, usage, and symptom specificity of psychiatric service dogs for military veterans. *Front. Psychol.* **2020**, *11*, 1638. [CrossRef]
64. Vincent, C.; Belleville, G.; Gagnon, D.H.; Auger, É.; Lavoie, V.; Besemann, M.; Dumont, F. A logic model as the sequence of needs and experience that lead PTSD patients to seek a service dog and concerns related to it: A stakeholders' perspective. *Int. J. Neurorehabil.* **2017**, *4*, 268. [CrossRef]
65. Bergen-Cico, D.; Smith, Y.; Wolford, K.; Gooley, C.; Hannon, K.; Woodruff, R.; Spicer, M.; Gump, B. Dog ownership and training reduces post-traumatic stress symptoms and increases self-compassion among veterans: Results of a longitudinal control Study. *J. Alternat. Complement Med.* **2018**, *24*, 1166–1175. [CrossRef]
66. Crowe, T.K.; Sanchez, V.; Howard, A.; Western, B.; Barger, S. Veterans transitioning from isolation to integration: A look at veteran/service dog partnerships. *Disabil. Rehabi.* **2018**, *40*, 2953–2961. [CrossRef] [PubMed]
67. Williamson, L.; Dell, C.; Chalmers, D.; Cruz, M.; De Groot, P. Strengthening Zooeyia: Understanding the Human-Animal Bond between Veterans Living with Comorbid Substance Use and Posttraumatic Stress Disorder and their Service Dogs. *Human-Anim. Interact Bull.* **2022**, *10*, 20–47. [CrossRef]
68. Ligatti, C. *No Training Required: The Availability of Emotional Support Animals as a Component of Equal Access for the Psychiatrically Disabled under the Fair Housing Act*; U.S. Department of Housing and Urban Development: Washington, DC, USA, 2012.
69. Notman, N. Let the Dog in: How Institutions and Colleagues Can Help Scientists Who Require Support Animals. *Nature* **2021**, *589*, 627–630. Available online: https://www.nature.com/articles/d41586-021-00190 (accessed on 11 November 2022). [CrossRef] [PubMed]
70. Brooks, H.L.; Rushton, K.; Lovell, K.; Bee, P.; Walker, L.; Grant, L.; Rogers, A. The power of support from companion animals for people living with mental health problems: A systematic review and narrative synthesis of the evidence. *BMC Psychiat.* **2018**, *2*, 31. [CrossRef]
71. Stern, S.L.; Donahue, D.A.; Allison, S.; Hatch, J.P.; Lancaster, C.L.; Benson, T.A.; Johnson, A.L.; Jeffreys, M.D.; Pride, D.; Moreno, C.; et al. Potential benefits of canine companionship for military veterans with posttraumatic stress disorder (PTSD). *Soc. Anim.* **2013**, *21*, 568–581. [CrossRef]
72. Wells, D.L. Associations between pet ownership and self-reported health status in people suffering from chronic fatigue syndrome. *J. Altern. Complement Med.* **2009**, *15*, 407–413. [CrossRef]
73. Bystrom, K.M.; Persson, C.A. The meaning of companion animals for children and adolescents with autism: The parents' perspective. *Anthrozoös* **2015**, *28*, 263–275. [CrossRef]
74. Hunt, M.G.; Stein, C.H. Who let the dogs in? A pets policy for a supported housing organization. *Am. J. Psychiatr. Rehabil.* **2007**, *10*, 163–183. [CrossRef]
75. Pehle, M.A. *Healing Relationships with Companion Dogs in the Therapeutic Process: An exploratory Qualitative Study*; California Institute of Integral Studies: San Francisco, CA, USA, 2010; p. 3365.
76. Zimolag, U.; Krupa, T. The occupation of pet ownership as an enabler of community integration in serious mental illness: A single exploratory case study. *Occup. Ther. Ment. Health* **2010**, *26*, 176–196. [CrossRef]
77. Boness, C.L.; Younggren, J.N.; Frumkin, I.B. The certification of emotional support animals: Differences between clinical and forensic mental health practitioners. *Prof. Psychol. Res. Pract.* **2017**, *48*, 216–223. [CrossRef]
78. Arhant, C.; Bubna-Littitz, H.; Bartels, A.; Futschik, A.; Troxler, J. Behaviour of smaller and larger dogs: Effects of training methods, inconsistency of owner behaviour and level of engagement in activities with the dog. *Appl. Anim. Behav. Sci.* **2010**, *123*, 131–142. [CrossRef]
79. Hiby, E.F.; Rooney, N.J.; Bradshaw, J.W.S. Dog training methods: Their use, effectiveness and interaction with behaviour and welfare. *Anim. Welf.* **2004**, *13*, 63–70. [CrossRef]
80. Rooney, N.; Gaines, S.; Hiby, E.F. A practitioner's guide to working dog welfare. *J. Vet. Behav. Clin. Appl. Res.* **2009**, *4*, 127–134. [CrossRef]
81. Webber, S.; Cobb, M.L.; Coe, J. Welfare Through Competence: A Framework for Animal-Centric Technology Design. *Front. Vet. Sci.* **2022**, *6*, 885973. [CrossRef]
82. Cobb, M.L.; Otto, C.M.; Fine, A.H. The Animal Welfare Science of Working Dogs: Current Perspectives on Recent Advances and Future Directions. *Front. Vet. Sci.* **2021**, *8*, 666898. [CrossRef]
83. Bray, E.E.; Otto, C.M.; Udell, M.A.; Hall, N.J.; Johnston, A.M.; MacLean, E.L. Enhancing the selection and performance of working dogs. *Front. Vet. Sci.* **2021**, *8*, 430. [CrossRef]
84. Kwon, Y.-J.; Choi, B.-H.; Eo, J.; Kim, C.; Jung, Y.-D.; Lee, J.-R.; Choi, Y.; Gim, J.-A.; Lee, D.-H.; Ha, J.-H.; et al. Genetic structure and variability of the working dog inferred from microsatellite marker analysis. *Genes Genom.* **2014**, *36*, 197–203. [CrossRef]
85. Bray, E.E.; Sammel, M.D.; Cheney, D.; Serpell, J.A.; Seyfarth, R.M. Effects of maternal investment, temperament, and cognition on guide dog success. *Proc. Natl. Acad. Sci. USA* **2017**, *114*, 9128–9133. [CrossRef]
86. Hare, B.; Ferrans, M. Is cognition the secret to working dog success? *Anim. Cogn.* **2021**, *24*, 1–7. [CrossRef]

87. Mellor, D.J.; Beausoleil, N.J.; Littlewood, K.E.; McLean, A.N.; McGreevy, P.D.; Jones, B.; Wilkins, C. The 2020 five domains model: Including human–animal interactions in assessments of animal welfare. *Animals* **2020**, *10*, 1870. [CrossRef]
88. Cobb, M.; Branson, N.; McGreevy, P.; Lill, A.; Bennett, P. The advent of canine performance science: Offering a sustainable future for working dogs. *Behav. Process.* **2015**, *110*, 96–104. [CrossRef]
89. Cruse, S.D. Military working dogs: Classification and treatment in the US Armed Forces. *Anim. Law.* **2014**, *21*, 249.
90. Leon, K.C. The legislative history of the treatment of military working dogs in the United States. *Univ. Detroit. Mercy Law Rev.* **2019**, *97*, 1.
91. Chaney, P.; Rees-Jones, I.; Fevre, R. Exploring the substantive representation of non-humans in UK parliamentary business: A legislative functions perspective of animal welfare petitions, 2010–2019. *Parliam. Aff.* **2021**, *75*, 1–29. [CrossRef]
92. Serpell, J.A.; Coppinger, R.; Fine, A.H.; Peralta, J.M. Welfare Considerations in Therapy and Assistance Animals. In *Animal Assisted Therapy*, 3rd ed.; Fine, A.H., Ed.; Elsevier: San Diego, CA, USA, 2010; pp. 481–583. [CrossRef]
93. Lane, D.; McNicholas, J.; Collis, G.M. Dogs for the disabled: Benefits to recipients and welfare of the dog. *Appl. Anim. Behav. Sci.* **1998**, *59*, 49–60. [CrossRef]
94. Howell, T.; Bennett, P.; Shiell, T. *A Reviewing Assistance Animal Effectiveness: Literature Review, Provider Survey, Assistance Animal Owner Interviews, Health Economics Analysis and Recommendations*; La Trobe University: Bendigo, VIC, Australia, 2016. Available online: https://www.ndis.gov.au/medias/documents/hf5/hc0/8799673090078/Assistance-Animals-PDF-1-MB-.pdf (accessed on 1 October 2022).
95. Winkle, M.; Johnson, A.; Mills, D. Dog welfare, well-being and behavior: Considerations for selection, evaluation and suitability for animal-assisted therapy. *Animals* **2020**, *10*, 2188. [CrossRef]
96. Gibson, P.E.; Oliva, J.E. Public Perceptions of Australian Assistance Dogs: Happier and Better Used Than Companion Dogs. *J. Appl. Anim. Welf. Sci.* **2022**, *25*, 18–30. [CrossRef]
97. Glenk, L.M.; Foltin, S. Therapy Dog Welfare Revisited: A Review of the Literature. *Vet. Sci.* **2021**, *12*, 226. [CrossRef]
98. Zamir, T. The moral basis of animal-assisted therapy. *Soc. Anim.* **2006**, *14*, 179–199. [CrossRef]
99. Peralta, J.M.; Fine, A.H. (Eds.) The welfarist and the psychologist: Finding common ground in our interactions with therapy animals. In *The Welfare of Animals in Animal Assisted Interventions*; Springer Veterinary Medicine: Heidelberg, Germany, 2021; pp. 265–284.
100. Francione, G.L. Animal rights theory and utilitarianism: Relative normative guidance. *Between Species* **2003**, *13*, 5. [CrossRef]
101. Glenk, L.M.; Přibylová, L.; Stetina, B.U.; Demirel, S.; Weissenbacher, K. Perceptions on Health Benefits of Guide Dog Ownership in an Austrian Population of Blind People with and without a Guide Dog. *Animals* **2019**, *9*, 428. [CrossRef]
102. Jamieson, L.T.J.; Baxter, G.S.; Murray, P.J. You are not my handler! Impact of changing handlers on dogs' behaviours and detection performance. *Animals* **2018**, *8*, 176. [CrossRef]
103. Lockyer, J.M.; Oliva, J.L. Better to have loved and lost? Human avoidant attachment style towards dogs predicts group membership as 'Forever Owner'or 'Foster Carer'. *Animals* **2020**, *10*, 1679. [CrossRef]
104. Lit, L.; Schweitzer, J.B.; Oberbauer, A.M. Handler beliefs affect scent detection dog outcomes. *Anim Cogn.* **2011**, *14*, 387–394. [CrossRef] [PubMed]
105. Glenk, L.M. Current Perspectives on Therapy Dog Welfare in Animal-Assisted Interventions. *Animals* **2017**, *7*, 7. [CrossRef] [PubMed]
106. Heimbürge, S.; Kanitz, E.; Otten, W. The use of hair cortisol for the assessment of stress in animals. *Gen. Comp. Endocrinol.* **2019**, *1*, 10–17. [CrossRef] [PubMed]
107. Sundman, A.-S.; Van Poucke, E.; Holm, A.-C.S.; Faresjö, Å.; Theodorsson, E.; Jensen, P. Long-term stress levels are synchronized in dogs and their owners. *Sci. Rep.* **2019**, *9*, 7391. [CrossRef]
108. van Houtert, E.A.E.; Endenburg, N.; Vermetten, E.; Rodenburg, T.B. Hair Cortisol in Service Dogs for Veterans with Post-traumatic Stress Disorder Compared to Companion Dogs (CanisFamiliaris). *J. Appl. Anim. Welf. Sci.* **2022**, *17*, 1–11. [CrossRef]
109. van Houtert, E.A.E.; Endenburg, N.; Rodenburg, T.B.; Vermetten, E. Do Service Dogs for Veterans with PTSD Mount a Cortisol Response in Response toTraining? *Animals* **2021**, *11*, 50. [CrossRef]
110. Herrando, C.; Constantinides, E. Emotional Contagion: A Brief Overview and Future Directions. *Front. Psychol.* **2021**, *12*, 712606. [CrossRef]
111. Katayama, M.; Kubo, T.; Yamakawa, T.; Fujiwara, K.; Nomoto, K.; Ikeda, K.; Mogi, K.; Nagasawa, M.; Kikusui, T. Emotional Contagion from Humans to Dogs Is Facilitated by Duration of Ownership. *Front. Psychol.* **2019**, *10*, 1678. [CrossRef]
112. Purewal, R.; Christley, R.; Kordas, K.; Joinson, C.; Meints, K.; Gee, N.; Westgarth, C. Companion animals and child/adolescent development: A systematic review of the evidence. *Int. J. Environ. Res. Public Health* **2017**, *14*, 234. [CrossRef]
113. Hall, S.S.; Wright, H.F.; Mills, D.S. What factors are associated with positive effects of dog ownership in families with children with autism spectrum disorder? The development of the Lincoln autism pet dog impact scale. *PLoS ONE* **2016**, *11*, e0149736. [CrossRef]
114. Carlisle, G.K. The social skills and attachment to dogs of children with autism spectrum disorder. *J. Autism Dev. Disord.* **2015**, *45*, 1137–1145. [CrossRef]
115. Powell, L.; Chia, D.; McGreevy, P.; Podberscek, A.L.; Edwards, K.M.; Neilly, B.; Guastella, A.J.; Lee, V.; Stamatakis, E. Expectations for dog ownership: Perceived physical, mental and psychosocial health consequences among prospective adopters. *PLoS ONE* **2018**, *13*, e0200276. [CrossRef]

116. Rendle, M.; Jones, B. One Health. BSAVA Manual of Practical Veterinary Welfare. Edited by Matthew Rendle and Jo Hinde-Megarity. 2022. Available online: https://www.bsavalibrary.com/content/chapter/10.22233/9781910443798.chap9 (accessed on 18 December 2022).
117. Diesel, G.; Brodbelt, D.; Pfeiffer, D.U. Characteristics of relinquished dogs and their owners at 14 rehoming centers in the United Kingdom. *J. Appl. Anim. Welf. Sci.* **2010**, *13*, 15–30. [CrossRef]
118. Mills, D.; Karagiannis, C.; Zulch, H. Stress–Its effects on health and behavior: A guide for practitioners. *Vet Clin Small Anim Pract.* **2014**, *44*, 525–541. [CrossRef]
119. Schalamon, J.; Ainoedhofer, H.; Singer, G.; Petnehazy, T.; Mayr, J.; Kiss, K.; Höllwarth, M.E. Analysis of dog bites in children who are younger than 17 years. *Pediatrics* **2006**, *117*, e374–e379. [CrossRef] [PubMed]
120. Meints, K.; De Keuster, T. Brief report: Don't kiss a sleeping dog: The first assessment of "the blue dog" bite prevention program. *J. Pediatr. Psychol.* **2009**, *34*, 10. [CrossRef]
121. Melson, G.F.; Kahn, P.H.; Beck, A.; Friedman, B.; Roberts, T.; Garrett, E.; Gill, B.T. Children's behavior toward and understanding of robotic and living dogs. *J. Appl. Dev. Psychol.* **2009**, *30*, 92–102. [CrossRef]
122. Handlin, L.; Hydbring-Sandberg, E.; Nilsson, A.; Ejdebäck, M.; Jansson, A.; Uvnäs-Moberg, K. Short-term interaction between dogs and their owners: Effects on oxytocin, cortisol, insulin and heart rate–An exploratory study. *Anthrozoös* **2011**, *24*, 301–315. [CrossRef]
123. Petersson, M.; Uvnäs-Moberg, K.; Nilsson, A.; Gustafson, L.L.; Hydbring-Sandberg, E.; Handlin, L. Oxytocin and cortisol levels in dog owners and their dogs are associated with behavioral patterns: An exploratory study. *Front. Psychol.* **2017**, *8*, 1796. [CrossRef]
124. Reisner, I.R.; Nance, M.L.; Zeller, J.S.; Houseknecht, E.M.; Kassam-Adams, N.; Wiebe, D.J. Behavioural characteristics associated with dog bites to children presenting to an urban trauma centre. *Inj. Prev.* **2011**, *17*, 348–353. [CrossRef] [PubMed]
125. Burrows, K.E.; Adams, C.L.; Millman, S.T. Factors affecting behavior and welfare of service dogs for children with autism spectrum disorder. *J. Appl. Anim. Welfare Sci.* **2008**, *11*, 42–62. [CrossRef] [PubMed]
126. Marinelli, L.; Normando, S.; Siliprandi, C.; Salvadoretti, M.; Mongillo, P. Dog assisted interventions in a specialized centre and potential concerns for animal welfare. *Vet. Res. Commun.* **2009**, *33*, 93–95. [CrossRef]
127. Hall, S.S.; Wright, H.F.; Mills, D.S. Parent perceptions of the quality of life of pet dogs living with neuro-typically developing and neuro-atypically developing children: An exploratory study. *PLoS ONE* **2017**, *12*, e0185300. [CrossRef]
128. Palestrini, C.; Calcaterra, V.; Cannas, S.; Talamonti, Z.; Papotti, F.; Buttram, D.; Pelizzo, G. Stress level evaluation in a dog during animal-assisted therapy in pediatric surgery. *J. Vet. Behav. Clin. Appl. Res.* **2017**, *17*, 221–222. [CrossRef]
129. McCullough, A.; Jenkins, M.A.; Ruehrdanz, A.; Gilmer, M.J.; Olson, J.; Pawar, A.; Holley, L.; Sierra-Rivera, S.; Linder, D.E.; Pichette, D.; et al. Physiological and behavioral effects of animal-assisted interventions on therapy dogs in pediatric oncology settings. *Appl. Anim. Behav. Sci.* **2018**, *200*, 86–95. [CrossRef]
130. Custance, D.; Mayer, J. Empathic-like responding by domestic dogs (*Canis familiaris*) to distress in humans: An exploratory study. *Anim. Cog.* **2012**, *15*, 851–859. [CrossRef]
131. Beerda, B.; Schilder, M.B.; Van Hooff, J.A.; De Vries, H.W.; Mol, J.A. Behavioural, saliva cortisol and heart rate responses to different types of stimuli in dogs. *Appl. Anim. Behav. Sci.* **1998**, *58*, 365–381. [CrossRef]
132. Mills, D.; Westgarth, C. *Dog Bites: A Multidisciplinary Perspective*; 5M Publishing: Sheffield, UK, 2017.
133. Mariti, C.; Gazzano, A.; Moore, J.L.; Baragli, P.; Chelli, L.; Sigheri, C. Perception of dogs' stress by their owners. *J. Vet. Behav.* **2012**, *7*, 213–219. [CrossRef]
134. Lakestani, N.N.; Donaldson, M.L.; Waran, N. Interpretation of dog behavior by children and young adults. *Anthrozoös* **2014**, *27*, 65–80. [CrossRef]
135. Ng, Z.; Fine, A. Paving the path toward retirement for assistance animals: Transitioning lives. *Front. Vet. Sci.* **2019**, *6*, 39. [CrossRef]
136. Roth, L.S.V.; Jensen, P. Assessing companion dog behavior in a social setting. *J. Vet. Behav.* **2015**, *10*, 315–323. [CrossRef]
137. Mongillo, P.; Pitteri, E.; Adamelli, S.; Bonichini, S.; Farina, L.; Marinelli, L. Validation of a selection protocol of dogs involved in Animal Assisted Intervention. *J. Vet. Behav.* **2015**, *10*, 103–110. [CrossRef]
138. American Animal Hospital Association; American Veterinary Medical Association. AAHA-AVMA Canine Preventive Healthcare Guidelines. 2011. Available online: https://www.aaha.org/globalassets/02-guidelines/preventive-healthcare/caninepreventiveguidelines_ppph.pdf (accessed on 1 July 2022).
139. Kis, A.; Szakadát, S.; Gácsi, M.; Kovács, E.; Simor, P.; Török, C.; Gombos, F.; Bódizs, R.; Topál, J. The interrelated effect of sleep and learning in dogs (*Canis familiaris*); an EEG and behavioural study. *Sci. Rep.* **2017**, *7*, 1–6. [CrossRef]
140. Mondino, A.; Delucchi, L.; Moeser, A.; Cerdá-González, S.; Vanini, G. Sleep disorders in dogs: A pathophysiological and clinical review. *Top Compan. Anim. Med.* **2021**, *43*, 100516. [CrossRef]
141. Rooney, N.J.; Clark, C.C.; Casey, R.A. Minimizing fear and anxiety in working dogs: A review. *J. Vet. Behav.* **2016**, *16*, 53–64. [CrossRef]
142. Špinka, M. Animal agency, animal awareness and animal welfare. *Anim. Welf.* **2019**, *28*, 11–20. [CrossRef]
143. Miller, L.J.; Vicino, G.A.; Sheftel, J.; Lauderdale, L.K. Behavioral diversity as a potential indicator of positive animal welfare. *Animals* **2020**, *10*, 1211. [CrossRef]
144. Duranton, C.; Horowitz, A. Let me sniff! Nosework induces positive judgment bias in pet dogs. *Appl. Anim. Behav. Sci.* **2019**, *211*, 61–66. [CrossRef]

145. Leighton, E.A.; Hare, E.; Thomas, S.; Waggoner, L.P.; Otto, C.M. A solution for the shortage of detection dogs: A detector dog center of excellence and a cooperative breeding program. *Front. Vet. Sci.* **2018**, *5*, 284. [CrossRef]
146. Wilson, C. Royal Australian Air Force Military Working Dogs Considered for Retirement. ABC News (Australia) (28 October 2013). Available online: https://www.abc.net.au/news/2013-10-28/retirement-program-formilitary-working-dogs-at-amberley-airbase/5046626?nw=0 (accessed on 1 July 2022).
147. Alger, J.M.; Alger, S.F. Canine soldiers, mascots, and stray dogs in US wars: Ethical considerations. In *Animals and War*; Hediger, R., Ed.; Brill: Boston, MA, USA, 2013.
148. Landa, M. From war dogs to service dogs: The retirement and adoption of military working dogs. *Anim. L.* **2018**, *24*, 39.
149. Starling, M.; Spurrett, A.; McGreevy, P. A pilot study of methods for evaluating the effects of arousal and emotional valence on performance of racing greyhounds. *Animals* **2020**, *10*, 1037. [CrossRef]
150. Menna, L.F.; Santaniello, A.; Todisco, M.; Amato, A.; Borrelli, L.; Scandurra, C.; Fioretti, A. The Human-Animal Relationship as the Focus of Animal-Assisted Interventions: A One Health Approach. *Int. J. Environ. Res. Public Health* **2019**, *16*, 3660. [CrossRef]
151. International Association of Human-Animal Interaction Organizations. IAHAIO White Paper. 2018. Available online: http://iahaio.org/wp/wpcontent/uploads/2018/04/iahaio_wp_updated-2018-final.pdf (accessed on 12 October 2022).
152. Beauchamp, T.L.; Childress, J.F. *Principles of Biomedical Ethics*; Oxford University Press: Oxford, UK, 2009.

Disclaimer/Publisher's Note: The statements, opinions and data contained in all publications are solely those of the individual author(s) and contributor(s) and not of MDPI and/or the editor(s). MDPI and/or the editor(s) disclaim responsibility for any injury to people or property resulting from any ideas, methods, instructions or products referred to in the content.

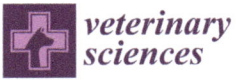

Article

Veterinary Education and Training on Non-Traditional Companion Animals, Exotic, Zoo, and Wild Animals: Concepts Review and Challenging Perspective on Zoological Medicine

Jaime Espinosa García-San Román [1,*], Óscar Quesada-Canales [2], Manuel Arbelo Hernández [2], Soraya Déniz Suárez [3] and Ayoze Castro-Alonso [2,*]

[1] Department of Animal Pathology, Veterinary School, University of Las Palmas de Gran Canaria (ULPGC), 35413 Arucas, Spain
[2] Veterinary Histology and Pathology, Institute of Animal Health and Food Safety (IUSA), University of Las Palmas de Gran Canaria (ULPGC), 35413 Arucas, Spain; oscar.quesada@ulpgc.es (Ó.Q.-C.)
[3] Veterinary Infectious Diseases and Ichthyopathology, Veterinary School, University of Las Palmas de Gran Canaria (ULPGC), 35413 Arucas, Spain
* Correspondence: jaime.espinosa@ulpgc.es (J.E.G.-S.R.); ayoze.castro@ulpgc.es (A.C.-A.)

Citation: Espinosa García-San Román, J.; Quesada-Canales, Ó.; Arbelo Hernández, M.; Déniz Suárez, S.; Castro-Alonso, A. Veterinary Education and Training on Non-Traditional Companion Animals, Exotic, Zoo, and Wild Animals: Concepts Review and Challenging Perspective on Zoological Medicine. *Vet. Sci.* **2023**, *10*, 357. https://doi.org/10.3390/vetsci10050357

Academic Editor: Ihab Habib

Received: 31 March 2023
Revised: 27 April 2023
Accepted: 11 May 2023
Published: 17 May 2023

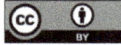

Copyright: © 2023 by the authors. Licensee MDPI, Basel, Switzerland. This article is an open access article distributed under the terms and conditions of the Creative Commons Attribution (CC BY) license (https://creativecommons.org/licenses/by/4.0/).

Simple Summary: In the recent past, the concepts of exotic animal medicine and zoological medicine have been used wrongly or interchangeably. The veterinary community should adopt zoological medicine as the appropriate term to cover the veterinary medicine of non-traditional companion animals, zoo animals, and wildlife animals. Furthermore, zoological medicine should be also integrated into the ecosystem health evaluation (environmental medicine) and the "One Health" approach. Beyond the terminology, zoological medicine has evolved and expanded its activities and action fields from its historical roots to afford new and challenging scenarios. In this context, the practice of zoological medicine includes its exercise in private veterinary clinics and hospitals, zoos and bioparks, and directly on wildlife. Several studies and international organisations have stressed the importance of high-quality veterinary training in this discipline, at the beginning and continuously during the professional practice. This fact is consistent with an increased societal demand for skilled and trained veterinarians concerning a broader species target and a wider scientific and technical scope including fields including eco-biology, environmental management, public health, welfare, and conservation. These challenging scenarios can only be correctly met by implementing more related compulsory subjects in the veterinary curriculum and post-degree specialisation and accreditation.

Abstract: The role of veterinarians is becoming more significant and necessary to support the welfare and health not only of non-traditional companion animals and wildlife animals, but also of humans and the environment. The importance of the One Health/One World concept and its social impact is increasing significantly, accompanied by the notoriety of new emerging and reemerging zoonoses. This paper aims to review and anchor the main concepts and professional applications of zoological medicine, which has been extensively discussed and adapted in recent decades. In addition, we analyse the main social demands, training, and educational needs and the perception of veterinary professionals relating to this specialised veterinary discipline. Our final goal is to reinforce the use of the term zoological medicine and contribute to highlight the need to foster and underpin specific educational policies and programs on this matter in the veterinary curricula. Zoological medicine should be the appropriate and agreed-upon term in the academic language concerning the veterinary medicine of pets, wild, or zoo species, excluding traditional domestic animals, and integrating the principles of ecology and conservation, applied to both natural and artificial environments. This discipline has suffered an intense evolution covering applications in private clinics, zoos, bioparks, and wildlife. All this implies current and future challenges for the veterinary profession that can only be addressed with greater and better attention from multiple perspectives, especially the education and training of professionals to improve and specialise in their professional scope of services.

Keywords: zoological medicine; exotic animals; veterinary; One Health; education; NTCAs; companion animals

1. Introduction

Veterinary sciences have been concerned with animal health since ancient times (BAM 159 cuneiform tablet, Code of Hammurabi, Ugaritic text, Roman veterinary medicine). The focus has been established mostly on domestic animals, whether they are for production or companionship. In the last decades, the term "companion animals" has notably been extended from just traditional pets (cats, dogs, small birds, and rodents) to integrate new species such as exotic birds, rabbits, ferrets, snakes, lizards, and others which are legally covered to be kept in homes [1,2].

Human pressure on ecosystems and the continued loss of habitats and biodiversity have made necessary the implementation of important conservation and preservation measures where the role of veterinarians has progressively expanded and their contributions have increased in the last decades. Among these measures, it has been crucial to reorientate zoo policies from being menageries to becoming true centres of environmental education and ex situ conservation [3,4].

In addition, recent events, such as the SARS-CoV-2 pandemic or monkeypox, have highlighted the relevance of establishing robust health surveillance and monitoring programs for wild species populations and fostering the One Health/One World approach, that is, that human, animal, and environmental health are inextricably interconnected [5,6].

Veterinary science should no longer be focused exclusively on the maintenance of production or traditional domestic and companion animals. Instead, its scope of action is much broader, covering new species and scenarios [7]. These facts generate relevant challenges in adaptation and transformation in the veterinary profession, which needs to implement essential changes in educational and training programs to face these challenges and lead the job to a more open vision of health and welfare, not only animal, but also human and their environments.

This paper aims to review and anchor the main concepts and professional applications of zoological medicine, which has been extensively discussed and adapted in the last decades. In addition, we provide an analysis of main social demands, training, and educational needs and the perception of veterinary professionals relating to this specialised veterinary discipline. Our final goal is to reinforce the use of the term "zoological medicine" and contribute to highlight the need to foster and underpin specific educational policies and programs on this matter in the veterinary curricula.

2. Material and Methods

To produce this work, we have developed a scientific review, mainly at European and American scales, to consolidate past and current concepts of zoological medicine, to improve the understanding of the evolution of its scope and professional framework, and, finally, to contribute to update and define social demand and educational and training needs for this veterinary specialisation. In addition, to directly verify the implementation status of the clinical practice and professional perception of zoological medicine, a brief and anonymous survey has been conducted at the national level with the cooperation of regional veterinary professional associations in Spain.

To contribute to focusing on and clarifying the concept of zoological medicine, our analysis starts with the descriptions of the terms "one medicine" (1964) and "conservation medicine" (1996). We describe later the initial discussions of different authors at the beginning of the decade of 2000, mainly focused on the definition of the type of animals included under this concept, whether exotic or non-traditional companions animals. Finally, this review is expanded to the decades of 2010 and 2020, to integrate the importance of health applied to animals, humans, and the environment.

In this document, we understand that zoological medicine is a vast concept that encompasses different species and fields, including non-traditional companion animals, zoo animals, wildlife animals, aquatic animals, production and environmental medicines [1,7]. However, it could be really challenging to try to classify the professional application of zoological medicine based on the different species involved. Instead, our work affords this organisation based on the principal place to conduct veterinary services, including (i) private clinics, (ii) zoos and parks, and (iii) wildlife.

Lastly, this work analyses the social demands and educational needs of zoological medicine from the veterinary perspective. It includes reports based on direct studies and surveys to understand better the application of professional veterinary services to non-traditional companion animals and wild species in different parts of the world (Europe, Canada, USA, and South America). In addition, a brief national survey has been conducted among the professional veterinary associations in Spain (primarily private clinics) to reinforce and update these results. The survey was distributed on the internet and focused on obtaining data from veterinarians referring to their level of experience in zoological medicine, type of professional application, type of animals, main reasons for consultancy, their professional confidence, and training/educational needs. The participation in the survey was voluntary and anonymous and, before accessing the questions, all respondents agreed to and authorised the use of their answers for educational and research purposes. No personal data were collected, and all the information was aggregated for statistical purposes. This survey was outside of the scope of ethical concern and data protection law according to the EU General Data Protection Regulation (GDPR; Directive (EU) 2016/680).

3. Results and Discussion

3.1. Consolidating the Concepts and the Appropriate Terminology: Zoological Medicine and One Health

The terms "zoological medicine" and "exotic animal medicine" have often been used interchangeably, referring to animals other than those known as traditional domestic animals, i.e., dogs, cats, horses, or other farm animals [1,5]. However, these terms should be distinct. Zoological medicine has been defined as encompassing companion animal medicine (small mammals, birds, reptiles, amphibians, and fish), zoo animal medicine, aquatic animal medicine (marine mammals, display fish), production medicine (farmed/ranched wildlife, game birds, and aquaculture), and environmental medicine (free-ranging wildlife, conservation/preservation, and ecosystem health) [1,7].

In contrast, exotic animal medicine is commonly applied only to certain species of small mammals, reptiles, and birds kept as pets. The term "exotic" is defined in multiple veterinary dictionaries as relating to "an animal that is not indigenous to a location where it currently lives". In this sense, a European rabbit could be native to mainland Spain but exotic in the United Kingdom, Australia, or the United States. In addition, as a small-prey herbivore species, the rabbit would behave much more like a wild animal than a domesticated dog [1].

In the European continent, the British Small Animal Veterinary Association (BSAVA) prefers the term "non-traditional companion animal" (NTCA) over the term "exotic pet" as it considers that this better describes the species involved [2]. In addition, it would be a mistake to infer that the diagnostic and treatment techniques used are markedly different if the animal is kept in a pet, zoo, or wildlife situation. They have more things in common for their approach to the taxon than based on the degree of domestication or the place of maintenance. For these reasons, it would be preferable to use the term zoological medicine for everything that covers the medicine of pets, wild or zoo species of reptiles, birds, and mammals excluded from traditional domestic ones such as dogs, cats, horses, and farm animals [1,2,8].

In the USA, the confusion about these terms, which were used to refer to the veterinary responsibilities of non-domestic or non-traditional animals, was addressed in the year 2000 in an intensive workshop that took place in White Oak, convened by the ACZM

(American College of Zoological Medicine). As a result, there was a solid consensus to adopt a single consistently defined term to represent the wide range of activities related to non-domestic species. Eventually, the term "zoological medicine" was explicitly established by the White Oak Accords as the appropriate umbrella concept which integrates veterinary medicine and the principles of ecology and conservation applied in both natural and artificial environments [5].

Scaling up the framework of zoological medicine, there are other terms, even higher, which need clarification; these are One Medicine, conservation medicine, and the One Health concepts.

As early as 1964, Dr Schwabe coined the term "One Medicine" and proposed veterinary and human health professionals collaborate to combat zoonotic diseases [9]. Similarly, in 1996, Kock introduced the concept of conservation medicine in response to the growing concern about the adverse effects of anthropogenic environmental changes on humans, animals, and ecosystem health [10].

More recently, in the early 2000s, the One Health initiative emerged. The One Health approach (Figure 1) summarises a concept known for more than a century—that human, animal, and plant health are interdependent and bound to the health of the ecosystems in which they exist. The Food and Agriculture Organization of the United Nations (FAO), the World Organisation for Animal Health (OIE), the United Nations Environment Programme (UNEP), and the World Health Organization (WHO) have established a common advisory panel proposing the following definition: "One Health is an integrated, unifying approach that aims to sustainably balance and optimise the health of people, animals, and ecosystems. It recognises the health of humans, domestic and wild animals, plants, and the wider environment (including ecosystems) are closely linked and interdependent. The approach mobilises multiple sectors, disciplines, and communities at varying levels of society to work together to foster well-being and tackle threats to health and ecosystems while addressing the collective need for clean water, energy and air, safe and nutritious food, taking action on climate change, and contributing to sustainable development".

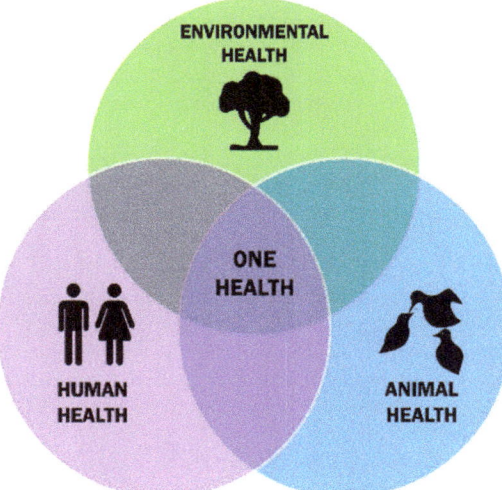

Figure 1. Graphical representation of One Health approach (licensed under the Creative Commons Attribution-Share Alike 4.0 International license (https://creativecommons.org/licenses/by-sa/4.0/deed.en, accessed on 26 April 2023)).

Based on this definition, it is evident that veterinarians play a key integral role in the One Health approach because animals both impact and are impacted by people and the environment. Nevertheless, even today, human, animal, and environmental science studies are largely conducted independently [11]. Furthermore, veterinarians, being experts in animal production, welfare, and food safety and its technology, and public health under the One Health concept, are scarcely informed in environmental aspects, which would help them to understand and face the consequences of climate change [12].

3.2. The Practice of Zoological Medicine: From the Historical Roots to the Current New Scenarios

The role of veterinarians in dealing with wild and exotic animals is continuously increasing and changing. Progress and evolution have been different according to diverse factors. This section reviews and summarises this evolution according to the main application sectors.

3.2.1. Zoological Medicine Applied to Non-Traditional Companion Animals (NTCAs) in Private Veterinary Clinics and Hospitals: From Just "Collecting Animals" to Responsible Ownership of Exotic and Non-Conventional Pets

The habit of collecting animals, particularly wild and exotic animals, is an ancient and common practice (Mesopotamia, Egypt, China, Greece, and Rome). The interest in owning wild animals was widespread among the European aristocracy between the 16th and 18th centuries because these possessions were considered prestigious and symbols of luxury and power of the nobility of those times [3,13,14].

Since these antique practices, the desire and interest in keeping wild animals in captivity have increased. During the last decades, this growth has been extended to other homes of other social classes, notably the increasing number of owners of exotic animals as new pets or non-traditional companion animals (NTCA). The European Pet Food Industry Federation (FEDIAF) estimates that NTCAs kept in captivity in European households are more than 48 million birds, more than 16 million fishes, 29 million small mammals, and 11 million reptiles and terrarium animals [15].

In the US, the same tendency has been reported. In this country, the notable increase must be highlighted, up to the highest registers in a decade, of new acquisition levels of pets other than dogs and cats, due to the motivation of COVID-19 pandemic lockdowns. Nowadays, 12.2% of US households own NTCAs as pets, up from 10.8% 4 years before, according to the 3rd edition of the Fish, Small Mammal, Herptile, and Bird Products: U.S. Market Trends and Opportunities Report [16].

Therefore, NTCAs are acquiring an increasingly important role as pets as the penetration rate into homes becomes more remarkable. Consequently, the demand for specialised veterinary care, specific knowledge, and competencies must be improved and increased in parallel. It should be remembered that the legal possession of unconventional pets is associated with attention to specialised requirements and their specific anatomical and physiological characteristics, which do not allow extrapolating procedures from the traditional medicine of dogs and cats [8].

This particularity of requirements has led different organisations, such as the Federation of Veterinarians of Europe (FVE), to request the creation of white lists of animals that can be kept in captivity as pets. That has been reinforced by the general knowledge that most emerging infectious diseases worldwide are zoonotic [17]. Some European countries that have already implemented white lists are Belgium, Croatia, Luxembourg, Greece, the Netherlands, and Norway. In addition, some states in USA and provinces in Canada have also established white lists [18].

The development of this kind of list can mean a decrease in the number of species kept in captivity and, therefore, in the number of individuals. On the other hand, it may mean a concentration of individuals in certain species which could generate greater specialisation from the point of view of veterinary care. Consequently, private veterinarians have an increasing role in supporting non-traditional pets' welfare and health, preventing zoonosis, and acting under the One Health approach.

3.2.2. Zoological Medicine Applied to Exotic and Wild Fauna in Captivity on Zoos and Parks: From "Menageries" to Bioparks

The practice of wild animal collecting, described above, depending on certain circumstances and due to various motivations, may contribute to explaining the beginnings of many zoos in different European countries [3,13].

Zoological parks have evolved from a merely exhibitionist perception to a more conservationist one. They were initially conceived as menageries [3,19,20] where wild and exotic animals were simply exposed to the public, without fulfilling any additional function than the mere entertainment and enjoyment of visitors. However, they have experienced a resounding change, and although there are still zoos with this archaic vision, many others have spent years developing education, research, conservation, and captive breeding to contribute to the survival of threatened species [8]. These zoos have become bioparks, rescue centres, or reserves that often allow visitors to see animals in more natural and less intrusive environments, replacing the barred cages with semi-open facilities based on the zoo or landscape immersion concept [3,21].

Nowadays, in most countries of the world, zoos and animal exhibitions are requested to be adapted not only to ethical but also to legal requirements to develop ex situ conservation programs, species survival programs, environmental education, and even directly, or indirectly, participation in in situ projects. Unfortunately, for some species, breeding programs and captivity maintenance are the only way to avoid extinction [22,23].

In all this, it is vital to highlight the work carried out by the veterinarians in this new concept of zoos for maintenance of fauna in captivity, not to be just a doctor dedicated to taking care of the health of captive specimens but to participate in notions of animal welfare, conservation, education, and research.

3.2.3. Zoological Medicine Applied to Wildlife: From Hunting Management to Eco-Pathology and Rehabilitation Centres

Wildlife management is a complex process that should not focus exclusively on the animal but must be understood as integral management considering biological, health, sociological, and economic aspects. Consequently, the involvement of veterinary sciences is crucial [24].

Hunting and fish management programs were scarce or even non-existent until very recently. However, such management requires measures to guarantee the rational exploitation of a limited natural resource. In the past, game management focused primarily on hunting pieces and the exploitation of natural resources, and veterinarians could be hired to perform tasks such as inspecting bushmeat to ensure its quality. Over time, game management has become more focused on the conservation and sustainable management of wildlife populations [24].

Wildlife rehabilitation centres are places often managed and under the responsibility of veterinarians. They provide medical attention and care to injured or sick wild animals to recover and return them to their natural habitat. The creation of the first wildlife rehabilitation centres dates to the 1970s [25]. Since then, these facilities have spread and evolved, with governmental, non-governmental, or individual support, covering the protection of a variety of terrestrial and aquatic species. Their initiatives and actions have also evolved from providing clinical and medical care to also acting as sentinel centres evaluating and reporting on the health status of wild populations, contributing to the detection and diagnosis of key environmental threats, affecting ecosystems, and supporting the essential role of environmental education [20].

The work of veterinarians in wildlife management and rehabilitation centres provides opportunities for biomonitoring and identification of anthropogenic sources of injuries and critical threats such as environmental pollutants and new diseases [24]. The veterinarian is the only professional who combines knowledge about genetics, reproduction, zootechnics, ethology, welfare, and animal health and those authorised to handle and apply anaesthetics and euthanasia [24].

3.3. Social Demand and Training Needs on Zoological Medicine

WOHA (formerly OIE) set out in its recommendations the minimum competencies expected of newly licensed veterinarians to ensure the quality of national veterinary services and highlighted their essential contribution to society in ensuring the health and welfare of animals, people, and ecosystems. Furthermore, WOHA stressed the importance of high-quality veterinary training, initially and continuously during the professional exercise. This fact is consistent with an increased societal demand for skilled and trained professionals concerning biology, management, health, and conservation of wild species.

In the last decades, the emergence of zoonotic diseases on production animals derived from wildlife populations (e.g., the recent cases of MERS and SARS, monkey virus, nipha virus, etc.) has increased global awareness of the importance of zoological medicine in protecting both production livestock and public health. In this demand, zoological medicine has expanded to a wider variety of subspecialties beyond clinical care to encompass conservation, research, nutrition, reproductive physiology, molecular genetics, and others.

Veterinarians work with a unique comparative approach to conduct zoonosis research. However, in most veterinary curricula, the prevalence of domestic animal studies and the need for a system from a population-scale and ecosystem perspective pose an obstacle and create a knowledge gap in veterinary careers. With increasing funding and interest in studying the ecology of emerging infectious diseases, both human and wildlife, there is likely to be dramatically greater demand for veterinarians, ecologists, and other professionals who understand these concepts in an integrated manner [25,26]. Furthermore, knowledge of the principles of ecology and ecosystems should be acquired during pre-veterinary studies or, at least, at the beginning of the veterinary curriculum. At the graduate level, master's degrees in preventive veterinary medicine, ecology, environmental health, or public health with an emphasis on infectious diseases should be offered to veterinarians seeking job opportunities in public health and wildlife management [27].

It is essential to take a multidisciplinary approach to deepen the study of the incidences of diseases in wild populations. Veterinary science plays a central role in this regard. Currently, the two disciplines that lead the studies of diseases in wild species are epidemiology on the side of medical sciences and ecology on the side of biology. However, given the complexity of the issue, it is necessary to promote the formation of multidisciplinary teams to address the health aspects of fauna, species conservation, animal production, ecosystem health, and public health [28].

Therefore, conservation medicine and zoological medicine face challenges in the academic field, where they must make their way into a space theoretically already occupied by different disciplines and subdisciplines. Ecosystem health and conservation medicine agree that an approach to health and treatment should be part of the basic training received by health sciences students in general and among veterinarians [29].

It is time for veterinarians to create formal mechanisms within academic institutions to promote and increase enthusiasm for wildlife and ecosystem health. This transdisciplinary view will encourage a more global, generational, and preventive approach to health care. Veterinary faculties have a unique opportunity to collaborate in teaching these complexities, as veterinary schools employ specialists working from the ecosystem and population levels to the environmental and molecular. Thus, progress has been made in expanding veterinary curricula to provide basic critical knowledge and skills needed to provide medical care to captive non-domestic or non-traditional species. Furthermore, most recent veterinary curriculum revisions have already been considered, including studying animal populations and their environmental interactions [30].

3.4. Educational Programs and Veterinary Perception of Professional Skill and Competence in Zoological Medicine

Europe has a long and distinguished history in veterinary science and education, and it was here that the first professional investigations of pathological conditions in zoo animals were carried out. However, despite the increasing number of veterinarians working with wildlife, education in zoological and wildlife medicine has only recently and partially been included as part of formal veterinary training at the undergraduate level.

Due to the large number and diversity of nation-states in Europe, current educational opportunities in zoological medicine vary widely across Europe, both in availability and composition and at both undergraduate and post-graduate levels. The need to establish agreed-upon standards in education across Europe and to encourage the mobility of students and teaching staff is reflected in international agreements such as the Bologna Process and the ERASMUS-Socrates program and is likely to help reduce these differences and have a positive effect on the role of zoo and wildlife medicine in veterinary education [31,32].

Different European studies have tried to assess the degree of competence, educational programs, and availability of specialised veterinarians in zoological medicine and exotic and non-traditional companion animals. As early as 1994, Zwart investigated undergraduate training in zoological medicine in 27 European veterinary faculties, revealing that although there was a growing interest in exotic animal medicine, exotic animal diseases were taught separately as electives [31].

During the spring–summer of 2005, Mazet and colleagues conducted a survey designed to identify the educational and training needs of people entering the fields of wildlife medicine and ecosystem health. Data revealed that only some wildlife veterinarians believed that the training they received in veterinary school adequately prepared them to acquire and succeed in their field. Instead, wildlife veterinarians and their employers rated mentorship with an experienced veterinarian, leadership and communication training, wildlife health courses and internships, and additional formal training beyond the veterinary degree as necessary in preparing for success. In addition, survey responses from employers, wildlife veterinarians, and job seekers demonstrate that understanding and maintaining ecosystem health is a crucial component of the wildlife veterinarian's job description, as it is critical to protecting animal health, including human health [30].

A survey conducted in Ireland in 2020 by Goins and colleagues revealed a third of respondents had an exotic pet, and 50% of them had requested a veterinary consultation in the previous year. Most of them found barriers to accessing veterinary services, highlighting the perception of a lack of species-specific competence in the provision of veterinary services [33].

In parallel, another survey conducted by the same authors showed that the prevalence of veterinary services for exotic pets in Ireland was present in 82% of small and mixed animal clinics. Furthermore, more than four out of five veterinary professionals in small or mixed animal practices surveyed were willing to treat exotic pets. This fact contradicts the views expressed by respondents in the other survey, which indicated a limited availability of veterinary services. This contradiction could be explained because veterinarians offer a first aid or primary care approach. At the same time, pet owners may seek veterinarians who specialise and have post-graduate training in their pet's species [15].

Ostovic and collaborators surveyed in the academic year 2019–2020 veterinary students from Zagreb (Croatia) from different courses related to the veterinary medicine of reptiles. The study also revealed the need to invest in efforts to update the veterinary curriculum to introduce additional education for future Croatian veterinarians in reptile medicine since, in addition to clinical practice, this problem has implications for the health and safety of humans and other animals, as well as for the protection of the environment [34].

Recently, a study by Roopnarine and collaborators aimed to explore the faculty perceptions in medical, veterinary, and public health programs on the need, opportunities, and challenges of developing the concept of One Health in curricula, revealing that faculty perceived education in One Health as crucial to preparing veterinary students for collaborative practice. Successful One Health development is vital to prepare students for future threats to global health and promote a culture of shared learning [35].

In North America, advances in zoological medicine education were notably facilitated by the deliberations and recommendations of the White Oak Accords of 2000. A group of veterinarians teaching at universities in the United States created a steering committee and organised a workshop under the auspices of the ACZM to study and implement improvements in North American veterinary curricula in birds, reptiles, small pet mammals, non-traditional companions, aquatic and zoos animals, wildlife medicine, and environmental health and conservation. The committee and the ACZM recognised that the most significant demand was in providing medical care to companion animals due to the large proportion of graduates who wished to pursue careers in small animal clinical practice. Five years after these agreements, a review of curricular opportunities at USA and Canadian veterinary schools showed that progress had been made in implementing those recommendations. However, there is still room for improvement [7].

A survey conducted in 2000 by Stoskopf et al. revealed that 21 of the 31 North American veterinary colleges included aspects of zoological medicine within the curriculum and all offered educational opportunities in zoological medicine. The same authors recommended to the AVMA (American Veterinary Medical Association) that all veterinary schools train students to work in small animal medicine by acquiring proficiency in birds, reptiles, small mammals, and fish and that, at a minimum, they should teach clinical skills, comparative anatomy, physiology, and behaviour.

Although specialisation in zoological medicine is well-established in the UK, USA, and Australia, the number of residency programs in zoological medicine currently needs to be increased to meet the needs of this field. Therefore, veterinary schools, zoos/aquariums, or alliances between these institutions must establish additional training opportunities for veterinarians in this discipline [1,31,35].

Other geographical contexts have also assessed the implementation of zoological medicine and the work with exotic animals and NTCAs. For instance, a study conducted in Guatemala in 2018 revealed the lack of confidence that most veterinarians surveyed have when they must work with wild and exotic animals; even though they indicated that 92.3% were directly attended to and treated, only 5.6% were referred to another clinic, and 2.1% were not attended [36].

In Turkey, a study was also carried out on the perception of the training received for the clinical practice of exotic animals at the Istanbul Faculty of Veterinary Medicine. A total of 90% of the veterinarians felt they needed additional training at the university. More than 65% thought they had adequate knowledge about managing, transmitting, preventing, diagnosing, and treating avian diseases but did not have that knowledge regarding turtles, other reptiles, and fish. The frequency of care of exotic pets significantly affected veterinarians' confidence in treating them. Knowledge and confidence in the diagnosis and treatment of exotic pets were considerably lower than for dogs and cats [37].

To contribute to and update these studies, we launched a survey to evaluate some key parameters of the implementation of zoological medicine in Spain. The survey was anonymous and distributed online among professional veterinary associations between December 2022 and January 2023. A number of 120 professionals answered it. The results showed that 89.3% of respondents work in the small animal practice, similar to the data reported by Goins and Lepe-Lopez in Ireland and Guatemala, respectively.

Among these veterinarians in Spain, 83.3% confirmed they receive non-traditional companion animals in their consultancies (Figure 2). Most of them (47.5%) said to provide first aid care as an essential service and readdress the case to a reference centre specialised in medical care for these animals. Only 6.7% declared to attend exclusively exotic or non-traditional animals and 32.5% to have a specific member of the staff who has the knowledge, competencies, and skills to attend non-traditional companion animals in their clinics (Figure 3).

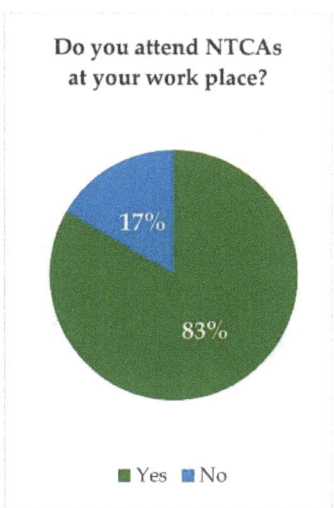

Figure 2. Spanish survey: percentage of veterinarians who attend NTCAs.

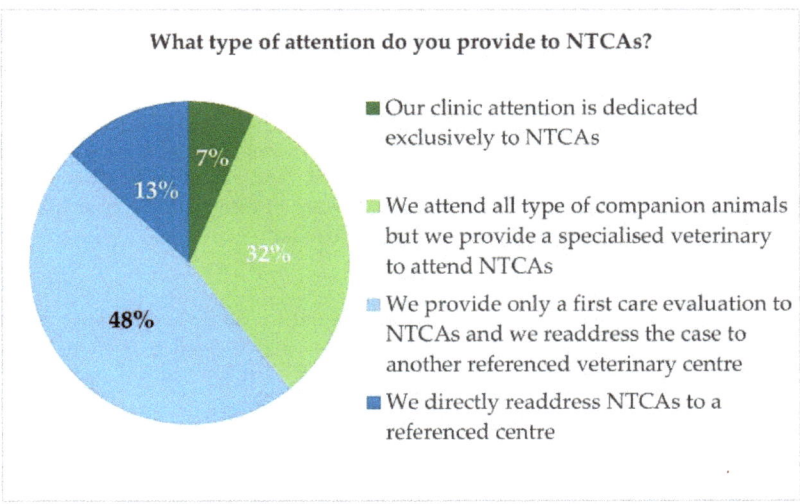

Figure 3. Spanish survey: type of attention applied to NTCAs.

The only taxa where respondents said they mostly felt confident were rabbits (68.3%) and small mammals (54.2%). They felt little or no confidence in dealing with other birds (57.5%), reptiles (72.5%), amphibians (91.7%), fish (95%), or other non-traditional companion animals (90%) (Figure 4).

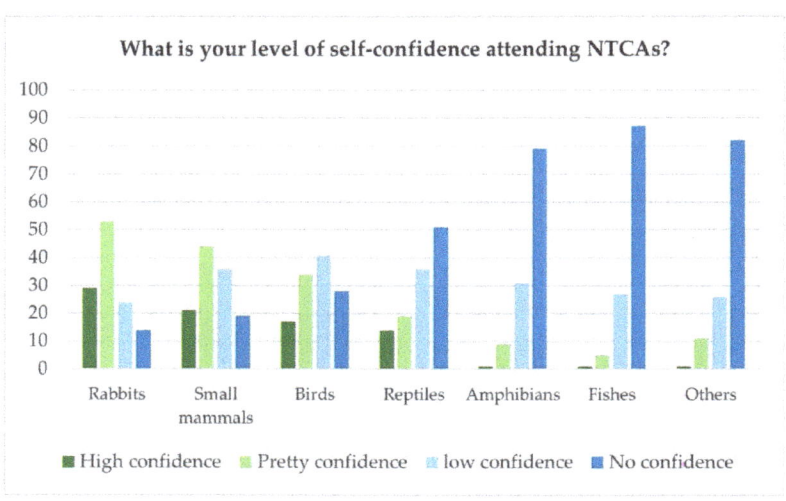

Figure 4. Spanish survey: level of self-confidence attending different NTCAs.

When they were asked if the education received at the university was enough, on a Likert scale from 1 to 5, 67.2% considered it as null (1), 31.9% medium (2–4), and only 1 person estimated it as enough (Figure 5). The average was established at 1.17. Further, 77.5% of the respondents declared the need to increase the number of specific subjects of zoological medicine and NTCAs in the Veterinary curricula (Figure 6). These results are in coincidence with those reported by Mazet et al., 2006, from veterinarians' answers in North America, Mexico, the Philippines, Australia, New Zealand, France, Brazil, South Africa, and Scotland (UK). All these surveys and studies imply the need for pre-and post-graduate veterinary education to support the veterinary community in providing services to NTCA pet owners and to wildlife care.

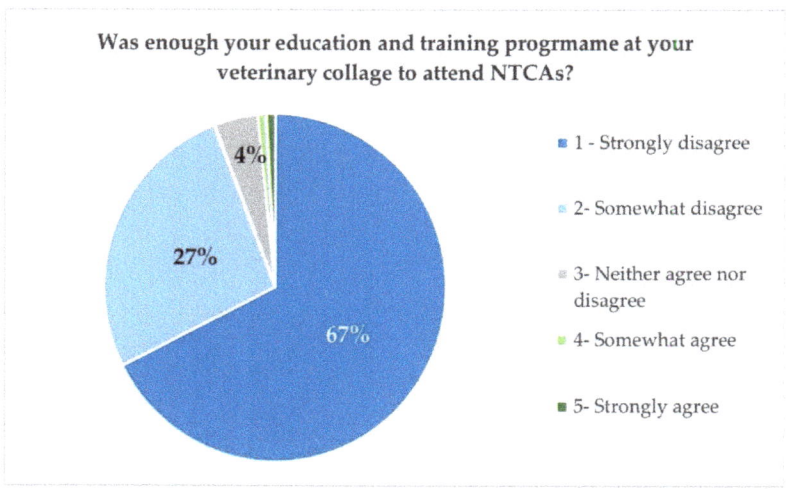

Figure 5. Spanish survey: level of specialised education received at the veterinary college.

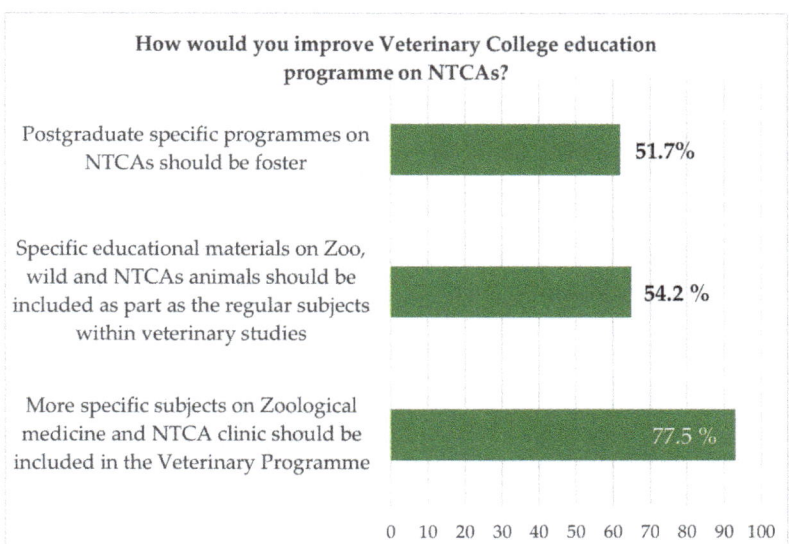

Figure 6. Spanish survey: suggested measures to improve NTAC specialised training. More than one option could be selected by respondents.

The curriculum should address the enormous diversity of wild animals, from amphibians to marine mammals and from insects to fish, seen in a zoo, aquarium, park, or veterinary practice, including an understanding of the local and global implications of emerging infectious diseases and preventive medicine in zoological collections. Training related to veterinary ethics and animal welfare science applied to zoos and wildlife should also be required [38].

4. Conclusions

Every day the role of veterinarians is more relevant and necessary in supporting the welfare and health of non-traditional companion animals and wildlife animals, and also human and environmental health. The importance of the One Health/One World concept and its social impact is increasing, especially accompanied by the notoriety of new emerging and reemerging zoonoses.

Within this framework, zoological medicine should be the appropriate and agreed-upon term in the academic language concerning the veterinary medicine of pets, wild, or zoo species, excluding traditional domestic animals, and integrating the principles of ecology and conservation, applied to both natural and artificial environments. Zoological medicine has evolved from its historical roots to the current new scenarios in a different way depending on the fields of work. These fields, even sharing focus and objectives, have their particularities and demand specific lines of action.

In this sense, private veterinarians' role in supporting non-traditional pets' welfare and health is increasing as these animals' penetration rate into homes becomes more notable. At the same time, veterinarians can contribute to the prevention of zoonosis under the One Health approach.

Zoological medicine applied to exotic and wild fauna in captivity in zoos and parks has evolved from the old conceptions of menageries to centres of conservation, education, and research, and the veterinarians working in these places should not focus only on the health of captive specimens. In the same way, the work of veterinarians in wildlife management and rehabilitation centres should contribute to recovering injured animals and identifying and monitoring environmental threats.

All this implies current and future challenges for the veterinary profession, at all international levels, that can only be addressed with greater and better attention from multiple perspectives, especially the education and training of professionals to improve and specialise in their professional scope of services.

The present work reinforces that new approaches are needed in training, both undergraduate and post-graduate, in all veterinary schools throughout the world and in Spain and the rest of Europe. This situation should be more comprehensive than including certain content in core subjects or elective courses, but instead, more compulsory courses and truly accredited training itineraries should be generated. Different studies and surveys across the world, including our survey, support this position.

Author Contributions: Conceptualization and methodology, J.E.G.-S.R. and A.C.-A.; Investigation, analysis and survey assessment, J.E.G.-S.R. and Ó.Q.-C.; Writing—original draft preparation, J.E.G.-S.R. and A.C.-A.; finally, writing—review and editing, M.A.H. and S.D.S. All authors have read and agreed to the published version of the manuscript.

Funding: This research received no external funding.

Institutional Review Board Statement: Ethics approval is not required for this research. Our Ethics Committee based its functions on the European Directive 2016/680—General Data Protection Regulation. The Regulation establishes clearly that if the research does not involve biological samples or personal data, especially those concerning sensible information about human health, and if it is anonymous, ethical considerations and Data protection are not necessary.

Informed Consent Statement: Informed consent was obtained from all subjects involved in the study.

Data Availability Statement: All data are available on request.

Acknowledgments: We would like to express our gratitude to the Spanish Official Colleges of Veterinarians which have provided their support distributing our survey among their associates. Many thanks to: Ilustre Colegio Oficial de Veterinarios de Las Palmas de Gran Canaria, de Santa Cruz de Tenerife, Sevilla, Asturias, Bizkaia, Gipuzkoa, Valencia, Salamanca, La Rioja, Navarra, Almería, Palencia, Zamora, Valladolid, and Ourense. In addition, we wish to thank to all respondents of our survey who dedicated time to complete it.

Conflicts of Interest: The authors declare no conflict of interest.

References

1. Redrobe, S. Redefining and developing exotic animal medicine. *J. Small Anim. Pract.* **2008**, *49*, 429–430. [CrossRef] [PubMed]
2. Chitty, J. Non-Traditional Companion Animals. 2022. Available online: https://www.bsava.com/position-statement/non-traditional-companion-animals/ (accessed on 29 March 2023).
3. Sampaio, M.B.; Schiel, N.; Souto, A.D.S. From exploitation to conservation: A historical analysis of zoos and their functions in human societies. *Ethnobiol. Conserv.* **2020**, *9*, 2. [CrossRef]
4. Rose, P.E.; Riley, L.M. Expanding the role of the future zoo: Wellbeing should become the fifth aim for modern zoos. *Front. Psychol.* **2022**, *13*, 1018722. [CrossRef]
5. Stoskopf, M.K. Current perspectives on curriculum needs in zoological medicine. *J. Vet. Med. Educ.* **2006**, *33*, 331–337. [CrossRef] [PubMed]
6. Weinhold, B. Conservation Medicine: Combining the Best of All Worlds. *Environ. Health Perspect.* **2003**, *111*, A524–A529. [CrossRef]
7. Stoskopf, M.K.; Paul-Murphy, J.; Kennedy-Stoskopf, S.; Kaufman, G. American College of Zoological Medicine recommendations on veterinary curricula. *J. Am. Vet. Med. Assoc.* **2001**, *219*, 1532–1535. [CrossRef]
8. Delarada, R.S. Challenges in wildlife conservation and management. The contribution of veterinary doctors. *Cienc. Vet.* **2020**, *22*, 181–188. [CrossRef]
9. Schwabe, C.W. *Veterinary Medicine and Human Health*, 1st ed.; Williams & Wilkins: Baltimore, MD, USA, 1964.
10. Kock, M.D. Wildlife, people and development: Veterinary contributions to wildlife health and resource management in Africa. *Trop. Anim. Health Prod.* **1996**, *28*, 68–80. [CrossRef]
11. One Health. Available online: https://www.avma.org/resources-tools/one-health (accessed on 28 December 2022).
12. Palacios-Díaz, M.D.P.; Mendoza-Grimón, V. Environment in Veterinary Education. *Vet. Sci.* **2023**, *10*, 146. [CrossRef]
13. Morgado García, A.J. Conocer a Los Animales: Historia Natural, Coleccionismo y Mascotas en la Edad Moderna Española. Silex. 2017. Available online: http://dialnet.unirioja.es/servlet/articulo?codigo=6974591 (accessed on 28 December 2022).

14. The Editors of Encyclopaedia Britannica. Pet. Available online: https://www.britannica.com/animal/pet (accessed on 15 December 2022).
15. FEDIAF. European Pet Food Annual Report 2022. 2022. Available online: https://europeanpetfood.org/about/annual-report/ (accessed on 20 October 2022).
16. U.S Pet Market Focus. Available online: https://www.freedoniagroup.com/packaged-facts/fish-small-mammal-herptile-bird-products-pet-trends-opportunities (accessed on 28 December 2022).
17. Goins, M.; Hanlon, A.J. Exotic pets in Ireland: 2. Provision of veterinary services and perspectives of veterinary professionals' on responsible ownership. *Ir. Vet. J.* **2021**, *74*, 13. [CrossRef]
18. Toland, E.; Bando, M.; Hamers, V.; Cadenas, V.; Laidlaw, R.; Martínez-Silvestre, A.; Van Der Wielen, P. Turning negatives into positives for pet trading and keeping: A review of positive lists. *Animals* **2020**, *10*, 2371. [CrossRef]
19. Parker, M. The genealogy of the zoo: Collection, park and carnival. *Organization* **2020**, *28*, 604–620. [CrossRef]
20. Fernandes, D.R.N.; Pinto, M.L.R. Veterinarian's Role in Conservation Medicine and Animal Welfare. In *Veterinary Anatomy and Physiology*; IntechOpen: London, UK, 2000. Available online: www.intechopen.com (accessed on 12 May 2023).
21. Slatch, A.K. *Landscape Immersion-Understanding Zoo Designs*; ResearchGate: Berlin, Germany, 2015. [CrossRef]
22. Njeru, G. Hope of saving rhino from extinction remains alive. *New Sci.* **2021**, *249*, 16. [CrossRef]
23. Vaughan, A. Back from the brink. *New Sci.* **2021**, *249*, 42–45. [CrossRef]
24. Pérez Garrido, A.J. Medio Ambiente, Fauna Silvestre y Ciencias Veterinarias. 2017. Available online: https://www.researchgate.net/publication/350637173 (accessed on 12 May 2023).
25. Daszak, P.; Cunningham, A.A.; Hyatt, A.D. Emerging Infectious Diseases of Wildlife—Threats to Biodiversity and Human Health. *Science* **2000**, *287*, 443–449. [CrossRef] [PubMed]
26. Smith, D.A. Zoological medicine education in Canada: Options and opportunities. *J. Vet. Med. Educ.* **2006**, *33*, 394–400. [CrossRef]
27. Chomel, B.; Marano, N. Essential veterinary education in emerging infections, modes of introduction of exotic animals, zoonotic diseases, bioterrorism, implications for human and animal health and disease manifestation. *OIE Rev. Sci. Tech.* **2009**, *28*, 559–565. [CrossRef] [PubMed]
28. Bocanegra, G.I.; Casas, A.A.; Rodríguez, C.B.; Martínez, A.C.; Terriza, D.C.; Ruiz, S.J.; García, I.A.; Rodríguez, F.M.; Plaza, A.D.; Lloret, J.M.N.; et al. Desarrollo de ompetencias y contenidos sobre fauna silvestre en el Grado de Veterinaria y Máster en Medicina, Sanidad y Mejora Animal. *Rev. Innovación Buenas Prácticas Docentes* **2018**, *5*, 11–17. Available online: https://journals.uco.es/ripadoc/article/view/10964/10106 (accessed on 12 May 2023). [CrossRef]
29. Norris, S. A New Voice in Conservation. *Bioscience* **2009**, *51*, 7–12. [CrossRef]
30. Mazet, J.A.; Hamilton, G.E.; Dierauf, L.A. Educating veterinarians for careers in free-ranging wildlife medicine and ecosystem health. *J. Vet. Med. Educ.* **2006**, *33*, 352–360. [CrossRef]
31. Frölich, K.; Grabitzky, S.E.; Walzer, C.; Delahay, R.J.; Dorrestein, G.M.; Hatt, J.-M. Zoo and wildlife medical education: A European perspective. *J. Vet. Med. Educ.* **2006**, *33*, 401–407. [CrossRef] [PubMed]
32. Ritzman, T.K. New Veterinary Graduates: Spreading their wings and exploring career paths in avian and EXOTIC animal medicine. *J. Avian Med. Surg.* **2014**, *28*, 168–172. [CrossRef] [PubMed]
33. Goins, M.; Hanlon, A.J. Exotic pets in Ireland: 1. Prevalence of ownership and access to veterinary services. *Ir. Vet. J.* **2021**, *74*, 14. [CrossRef]
34. Ostović, M.; Sabolek, I.; Piplica, A.; Žaja, I.Ž.; Menčik, S.; Nejedli, S.; Mesić, Ž. A survey study of veterinary student opinions and knowledge about pet reptiles and their welfare. *Animals* **2021**, *11*, 3185. [CrossRef] [PubMed]
35. Roopnarine, R.; Regan, J.-A. Faculty Perceptions: A Qualitative Study of the Perceived Need, Opportunities, and Challenges of Developing "One Health-One Medicine" in the Medical, Veterinary, and Public Health Curricula. *J. Contin. Educ. Health Prof.* **2021**, *41*, 16–23. [CrossRef]
36. Lepe-Lopez, M.; Guerra-Centeno, D. Wild pets in the veterinary practice of Guatemala. *Rev. Investig. Vet. Perú (RIVEP)* **2018**, *29*, 840–847. [CrossRef]
37. Sigirci, B.D.; Ikiz, S.; Celik, B.; Ak, S. A survey study on self-evaluations of small pet practitioners about exotic pets in Istanbul in 2016. *Acta Vet. Eurasia* **2019**, *45*, 9–15. [CrossRef]
38. Aguirre, A. Essential veterinary education in zoological and wildlife medicine: A global perspective. *OIE Rev. Sci. Tech.* **2009**, *28*, 605–610. [CrossRef] [PubMed]

Disclaimer/Publisher's Note: The statements, opinions and data contained in all publications are solely those of the individual author(s) and contributor(s) and not of MDPI and/or the editor(s). MDPI and/or the editor(s) disclaim responsibility for any injury to people or property resulting from any ideas, methods, instructions or products referred to in the content.

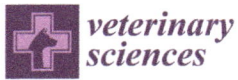

Article

Using Machine Learning in Veterinary Medical Education: An Introduction for Veterinary Medicine Educators

Sarah E. Hooper [1,*], Kent G. Hecker [2,3] and Elpida Artemiou [4]

1. Department of Biomedical Sciences, Ross University School of Veterinary Medicine, P.O. Box 334, Basseterre KN0101, Saint Kitts and Nevis
2. Faculty of Veterinary Medicine, University of Calgary, Calgary, AB T2N 4Z6, Canada; kghecker@ucalgary.ca
3. International Council for Veterinary Assessment, Crystal Lake, IL 60014, USA
4. School of Veterinary Medicine, Texas Tech University, 7671 Evans Drive, Amarillo, TX 79106, USA; elpida.artemiou@ttu.edu
* Correspondence: shooper@rossvet.edu.kn or sarahdvm.ugamizzou@gmail.com

Simple Summary: Machine learning (ML) is subfield of artificial intelligence that enables computers to learn from data and improve their performance without being explicitly programmed by a human. ML has the potential to enhance veterinary medical education by improving learning, teaching, and assessments. This primer introduces ML concepts to veterinary educators and administrators, highlighting their similarities and differences with classical statistics. It then provides a step-by-step example using simulated veterinary student data to address a specific question: which records in the simulated veterinary student data will predict a student passing or failing a specific course. The example demonstrates the use of the Python programming language to create a random forest ML prediction model, a type of ML algorithm which is composed of many decision trees and each of these trees is composed of nodes and leaves. During the creation of the random forest model, we emphasize specific considerations such as managing student records which may have missing information. The results show how decisions made by veterinary educators during ML model creation may impact which type of records are shown to be most important. While this form of ML may prove to be beneficial, transparency in creating ML models is crucial, and further research is needed to establish best practices and guidelines for veterinary medical education ML projects.

Abstract: Machine learning (ML) offers potential opportunities to enhance the learning, teaching, and assessments within veterinary medical education including but not limited to assisting with admissions processes as well as student progress evaluations. The purpose of this primer is to assist veterinary educators in appraising and potentially adopting these rapid upcoming advances in data science and technology. In the first section, we introduce ML concepts and highlight similarities/differences between ML and classical statistics. In the second section, we provide a step-by-step worked example using simulated veterinary student data to answer a hypothesis-driven question. Python syntax with explanations is provided within the text to create a random forest ML prediction model, a model composed of decision trees with each decision tree being composed of nodes and leaves. Within each step of the model creation, specific considerations such as how to manage incomplete student records are highlighted when applying ML algorithms within the veterinary education field. The results from the simulated data demonstrate how decisions by the veterinary educator during ML model creation may impact the most important features contributing to the model. These results highlight the need for the veterinary educator to be fully transparent during the creation of ML models and future research is needed to establish guidelines for handling data not missing at random in medical education, and preferred methods for model evaluation.

Keywords: machine learning; veterinary medical education; random forest; medical education; artificial intelligence; Python; R; veterinary educators; educational data mining; learning analytics

Citation: Hooper, S.E.; Hecker, K.G.; Artemiou, E. Using Machine Learning in Veterinary Medical Education: An Introduction for Veterinary Medicine Educators. *Vet. Sci.* **2023**, *10*, 537. https://doi.org/10.3390/vetsci10090537

Academic Editors: Simona Sacchini and Ayoze Castro-Alonso

Received: 20 July 2023
Revised: 15 August 2023
Accepted: 19 August 2023
Published: 23 August 2023

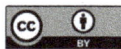

Copyright: © 2023 by the authors. Licensee MDPI, Basel, Switzerland. This article is an open access article distributed under the terms and conditions of the Creative Commons Attribution (CC BY) license (https://creativecommons.org/licenses/by/4.0/).

1. Introduction

In recent years, the field of health professions education has witnessed significant advances with the integration of machine learning (ML). ML, a subfield of artificial intelligence (AI), involves the development of algorithms and models that enable computers to learn from data and make predictions or decisions without being explicitly programmed. ML holds tremendous potential in creating adaptive learning platforms and intelligent tutoring systems, and has shown promise in the assessment and analysis of large-scale datasets including clinical records [1], diagnostic images [2], etc.

ML also offers the potential to enhance the learning, teaching, and assessments within veterinary medical education and may be incorporated across all aspects of veterinary medical education including admissions processes as well as student progress evaluations. Accordingly, veterinary educators must adapt to these rapid upcoming advances in technology and data science. As the field of veterinary medical education increasingly embraces data-driven approaches and evidence-based practices, understanding the fundamental differences and similarities between ML and classical statistics is paramount. Equally important is the recognition of the benefits, risks, and ethical dilemmas that may arise when utilizing machine learning within the veterinary education field. While a full discussion of machine learning ethics is outside the scope of this manuscript, veterinary educators should be aware of ongoing recommendations in the medical field to provide "machine learning literacy" to medical students and medical school faculty [3].

The purpose of this primer is to (i) introduce veterinary educators and veterinary college administrators to ML concepts, (ii) highlight similarities/differences between ML and classical statistics, and (iii) describe important considerations when using ML prediction models to answer hypothesis driven veterinary education questions.

This manuscript is divided into two sections. The first section defines educational data mining (EDM) and provides an overview of classical statistics commonly used in the veterinary medical education field. Information is presented alongside basic ML concepts and workflow to help illustrate the similarities and differences between these two main methodology categories. The second section provides a step-by-step worked example using simulated veterinary student data to answer a hypothesis driven question. Python syntax with explanations is provided within the text to create a random forest ML prediction model and within each step, specific considerations are highlighted when applying ML algorithms within the veterinary education field. A brief discussion follows highlighting additional considerations during the decision-making processes and interpretation of the random forest models after the initial models are constructed.

1.1. Introduction to Educational Data Mining and Machine Learning

Educational data mining (EDM) uses educational and student data and can potentially inform educational issues and learning environments [4,5]. Specifically, one of the key applications of ML within EDM is to better understand student progression in a degree program or course [5] and to develop prediction models to identify students at risk of not completing their degree program or a specific course [5,6]. EDM methodologies can be classified into three general methods, (1) classical statistical analysis (e.g., regression analysis), (2) artificial intelligence (e.g., neural computing), and (3) machine learning (e.g., random forests) [6]. This paper focuses on ML models and highlights uses of this methodology, although it is important to note that methodologies should be selected based upon the educational question that needs to be addressed.

The premise behind the use of ML is that it (1) enables computers to "learn" without requiring an individual to directly program it to do so [7,8] and (2) most often to build predictive models using big data or large, high-dimensional datasets [8]. A predictive model is a model which predicts future events or outcomes based upon the patterns found in the input data. The concept of big data can be viewed as large sized datasets (also known as large volume); datasets which contain diverse data such as numeric, text, graphics, etc. (also called wide variety); and allow quick generation of the data (also known as high velocity) [9]. For example, in a study assessing a medical school's curricula, clustering ML techniques were employed to visualize the relationship between the learning objectives of courses and required competencies of medical students [10]. This type of question cannot be answered using classical statistical analysis. Statistical analysis may refer to the descriptive use, "to present and summarize data" [11] or the inferential use, "the process of drawing conclusions which have a wider applicability than solely to the sample of observations or measurements obtained", and described in terms of probability or the likelihood of the occurrence of an event [11].

1.2. Comparison of Classical Statistical Analysis and Machine Learning Models

To help understand the difference between ML models and classical statistical analysis, assumptions, and the approach used to build such models or analyses, we discuss a recently published example of logistic regression that was used to evaluate if veterinary school admissions variable(s) would serve as predictors for students at risk of academic difficulty in the professional program. The statistical model building was structured following three main steps, (1) model specification, (2) parameter estimation, and (3) parameter probability distribution derivation [12].

During model specification, the authors calculated zero-order correlations [13], which means that the authors pre-determined potential correlations between two independent variables and only selected variables with zero-order correlations to include when building a single logistic regression model. The data included in the model adhered to specific assumptions including (1) the relationship between the logit (also known as log-odds) of the outcome and each of the included continuous independent variables were all linear, (2) there were no highly influential outlier data points, (3) there were no highly correlated independent variables (i.e., absence of multicollinearity), (4) the observations were independent of each other, and (5) the sample size was sufficient which is typically considered at least 10 observations of the least frequent outcome for each independent variable [14]. The parameter estimation was completed using a method such as maximum likelihood estimation (MLE), and subsequently tested the significance of each regression parameter based on the parameter distribution calculated previously [12].

While there are many different ML algorithms, the steps for constructing a model are quite similar and involve (1) model specification and (2) parameter estimation steps (i.e., training of the model). The approach to model specification and parameter estimation is different for ML algorithms as the model specification typically is data-driven rather than theory-driven [15]. This means that often, the parameter probability distribution derivation is not specified before training the ML model which results in ML models having better prediction power [12]. Furthermore, during the training of the ML model, many different empirical models need to be built using the ML algorithm. These initial models are built by the ML algorithm based on the relationships between the input and output variables using training sets of data. While the algorithm completes this step, the veterinary educator will need to make educated decisions when specifying the parameters for the final, best performing ML model. For example, the educator will need to specify certain parameters such as how many iterations should be performed for optimal performance of the trained model, and in response, the outputs of the ML models created from the training dataset will provide these answers. Furthermore, when constructing a ML model, it is important to note that each ML algorithm will have different assumptions or have no assumptions about the data. For example, with logistic regression models, five assumptions were listed above whereas many commonly used ML models do not make any assumptions about the data. Due to few to no assumptions about the data and because the training of the model typically consists of multiple datasets or resampling of the same dataset to form multiple datasets during parameter estimation within the ML model, highly correlated variables and outliers may be able to be included in the ML model. The same cannot be included in a logistic regression model [12,16,17] which could be disadvantageous for addressing some veterinary education and curricula questions.

In part 2 of this primer, we describe step by step, (i) how a training model is built, (ii) the different parameters of these models can be specified based upon the training of the model, and (iii) the specific assumptions for the algorithm selected in support of the working example.

1.3. Overview of the Main Types of Machine Learning Algorithms and Random Forest Machine Learning Models

Within ML, the algorithms employed are commonly categorized into four main categories, (1) supervised learning, (2) unsupervised learning, (3) semi-supervised learning, and (4) reinforcement learning [18]. In supervised ML, the veterinary educator serves as the "teacher" and the training data contain a range of predictors while the outcome is known. Following the veterinary school admissions example presented earlier, if each student was assigned a set of admissions variables and if it was known whether the student had academic difficulties (defined as dismissed from the DVM program or put on academic probation) or no academic difficulties, this could be used in the supervised model. In unsupervised ML, the outcome is unknown and instead the algorithm focuses on identifying relationships and groupings within the data [8]. In semi-supervised ML, the outcome is known for some of the dataset [18]. As such, utilizing the same veterinary school admissions example, the model would be trained only using student data with the known outcomes of academic difficulties or no academic difficulties. Immediately following, we would then iteratively apply the model to data with many unknown student academic difficulty outcomes. Reinforcement learning refers to the process when the machine/computer learns about its environment and chooses the optimal behavior to gain the greatest reward. The ML algorithm learns the behavior through trial and error, with some behaviors receiving rewards while other behaviors not deserving to receive rewards [18].

Selection of the ML algorithm is typically based upon the data structure type and the question being asked. In veterinary education, most data could be considered structured or unstructured. Briefly defined, structured data are typically stored in tabular format and follow a standard order such as student names, addresses, grades, etc. Unstructured data have no pre-defined format or organization, such as videos, audio files, presentations, and e-mails.

The example in this primer focuses on using structured data, which are simulated student records. We opted to use random forest as the example ML algorithm to help illustrate the steps for creating and evaluating a ML model. This model is one of the most utilized supervised learning algorithms and offers numerous benefits such as handling non-parametric data and being robust to outliers [6,19–23], both of which are commonly observed in veterinary educational data.

A random forest model is composed of decision trees as shown in Figure 1. Each decision tree is composed of nodes and leaves. The root node sits at the top of the decision tree and is the first division where the dataset is divided based upon whether the data are true or false. For example, if we asked whether a student practiced suture tying more than 15 h, if true, the data on the student move to the true decision node and if false, then they are assigned to the false decision node. At each subsequent node, the same division occurs with the student's data being classified as "true" or "false" based upon that specific node's statement (e.g., the student has more than 250 h of working as a surgical technician). The leaf node is the final output of the decision tree. Furthermore, Figure 1 shows how decision trees are a type of bagging (also known as bootstrap aggregating) ML algorithm. Bagging or bootstrapping is a method used to create smaller, random datasets out of the full dataset with replacement to estimate a population parameter [24].

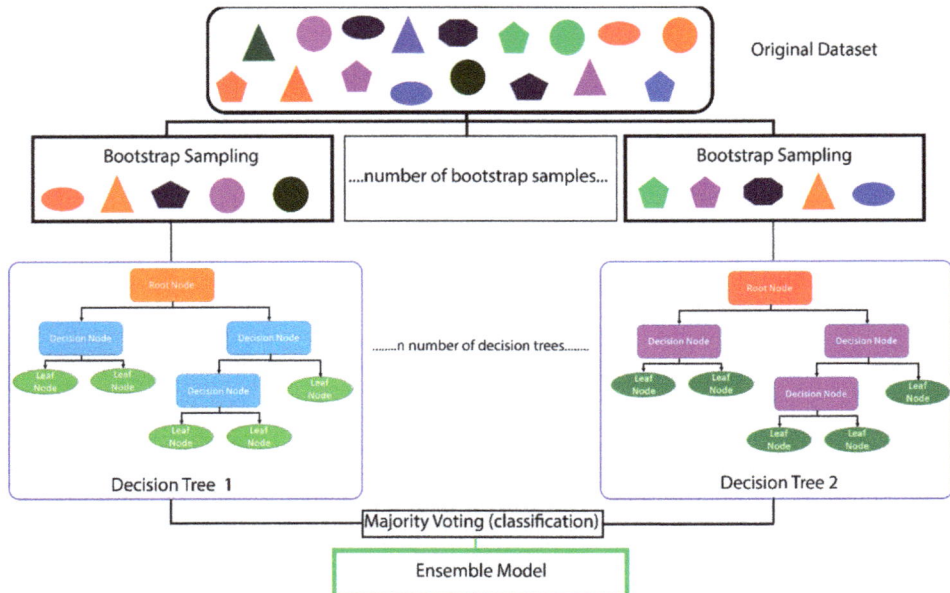

Figure 1. The original dataset is subset into many smaller, random datasets by the process known as bootstrap sampling. The number of bootstrap samples is equal to the number of decision trees that are created. Each decisions tree consists of a root node. If the data are true to the statement within the root node (e.g., a student's Graduate Record Exam (GRE) > 300), all true data will go to the decision node on the left whereas all false data will go to the decision node on the right. The terminal nodes are known as leaf nodes. After the creation of each decision tree, the results of each decision tree are averaged (bagging) and the final prediction is the ensemble model as it is based upon the results of all the generated decision trees.

Random forest models are a type of ensemble learning algorithm because the model contains many different decision trees which are then combined to produce the most effective optimal prediction model (Figure 1). In other words, rather than using a single hypothesis, an ensemble learning method will construct a set of hypotheses [25]—in our case, multiple decision trees. These hypotheses are assigned weights and voted upon by the ML algorithm which ultimately will result in providing the most important features contributing to the random forest models [20,22,25]. By creating many trees with a subset of the data, then combining the output of all trees, it helps to reduce over-fitting (i.e., the algorithm model trains the data too well and fails to be predictive for the testing data), reduces variance, and ultimately improves the model's performance [20,22,25].

1.4. Programming Languages and Tools

When constructing ML models, there are several different programming languages, tools, and software that can be used, each with different strengths. Here, we recommend veterinary educators use Anaconda Distribution, an open-source repository and toolkit. Anaconda is a platform that provides Python and R programming languages as well as a range of packages including a package management system [26]. An R or Python package is a collection of functions, compiled codes, sample data, and documentation in a well-defined format and is used to complete specific tasks or analysis. Within Anaconda, a designated environment is created specifically for a research study to avoid executing an installation or update that would disrupt packages or other frameworks such as integrated development environments (IDEs) (Figure 2). IDEs such as Spyder combine common developer tools with a single graphical user interface (GUI) and as such, not every action requires a line of code. Another way to think about Anaconda is to equate it to a mansion and a toolbox. Anaconda provides rooms where you can dedicate that room to a specific type of work or theme. Many times, the packages (i.e., the tools) will interact with each other or cause problems, which is why it is important to dedicate a specific "room" in the mansion for each project you are working on, as then, once your model is complete, it will always run within that room without issues. If you update or install a new package for a different project, it will not affect the other projects. This highlights that it is essential to report the version of the IDE, the programming language and the package version, used in creation of the ML models as not all versions may be compatible [27].

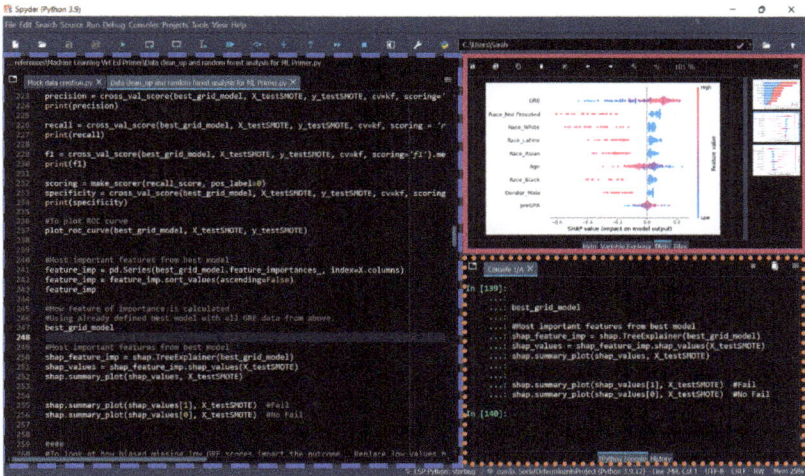

Figure 2. A screenshot showing the IDE Spyder with a few of the available panes or windows available. The Editor panel is outlined in a blue dashed line wherein the educator can create, open, and modify files with features such as autocompletion and syntax highlighting. The IPython console is outlined in an orange dashed line wherein the code is executed (Python code is run). The Plots window is outlined in a solid pink line and displays a beeswarm plot. Spyder is the IDE preferably utilized by the authors for Python projects and the IDE RStudio for R projects.

2. Simulation of Dataset and Creation of a Random Forest Machine Learning Model

In this second part of the primer, we provide a working example of creating a ML model using simulated data and Python programming language to answer a hypothesis driven research question. Figure 3 shows a visual workflow of the working example. Within each step of the process, important considerations for the veterinary educator community will be discussed and it will be illustrated how data quality and decisions by the educator may impact the ML model.

2.1. Defining the Project Goals

The first step requires defining the problem or hypothesis and determining the data needed to answer the question. Here, we explore two project goals. The first project goal is to demonstrate a ML Python pipeline for creating a random forest classification model from simulated data. The purpose of this ML model is to identify the most important predictors utilizing a simulated dataset that contributes to students failing a course during the pre-clinical years of veterinary school training. Our hypothesis suggests that students' GRE scores are the most important predictor for determining if a student will pass or fail a course in the Doctor of Veterinary Medicine (DVM) program. Our second project goal delineates specific considerations for building ML models which incorporate veterinary student data.

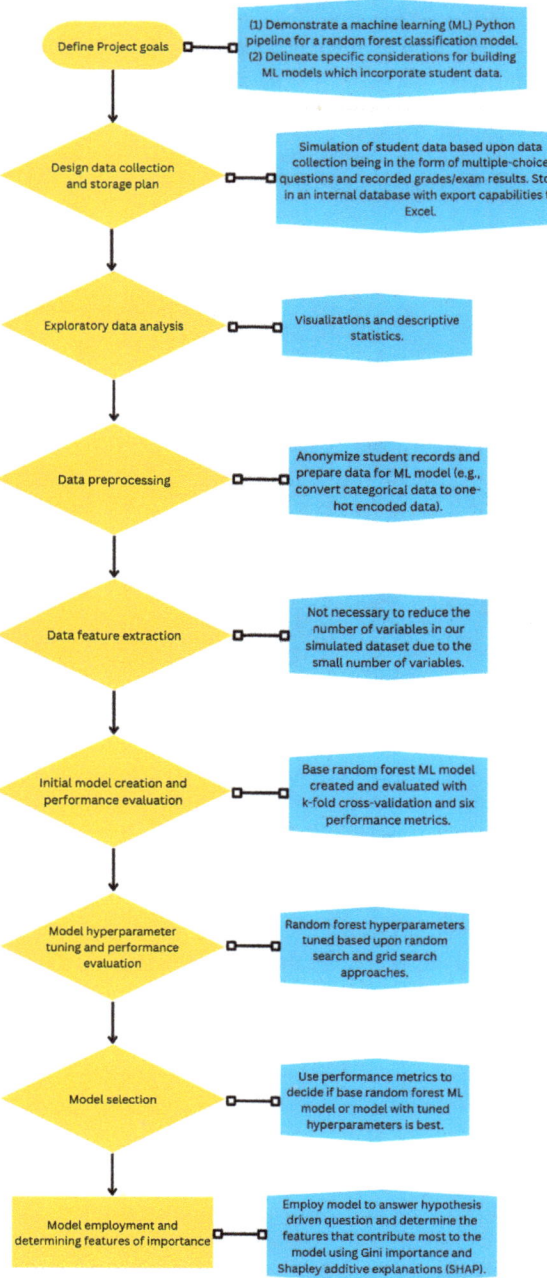

Figure 3. A flowchart highlighting the key steps for a machine learning project which are detailed in this primer is shown in orange. In blue describes the specific outcomes or processes that we will describe in our working example.

2.2. Data Collection and Storage Plan

After defining the project goals, it is critical to design a data collection and storage plan. The quality and performance of the ML models depends on the quality of data that are collected [28]. A good data collection strategy and well-designed storage medium for the dataset is essential for appropriate analyses and interpretation (i.e., database or Excel spreadsheets). For this to occur, the veterinary educator should have a basic understanding about the model being used. This requires educators to determine if the raw data can be used in the model or if different transformation processes will need to be used first. For example, a random forest model cannot handle non-numeric data; therefore, if a student's demographic data are collected, they will need to be transformed (transformations are discussed in Section 2.4). When collecting the demographic data, it is important to decide if it should be collected by multiple choice options or free-text entry. Multiple choice may limit responses if a student does not identify with the options, but if free-text entry is used, then the veterinary educator will need to ensure that all answers entered are identical in format and spelling (i.e., the programming languages will view "black" and "Black" as two different ethnicities) and have pre-defined groups (e.g., Will Hispanic and Latinx be grouped together or separately?). Additionally, some random forest models cannot handle missing data, and so the veterinary educator should establish a plan for how to deal with an incomplete student record. By addressing these considerations, we can prevent a variety of problems that arise from poorly defined or poorly collected datasets such as ensuring the data collected are adequate to answer the hypothesis or question [12,29].

2.2.1. Simulated Data Collection and Storage

The dataset format is based upon OutReach IQ [30], an internal database of students enrolled at Ross University School of Veterinary Medicine (RUSVM) where all data can only be viewed by faculty with approved Institutional Review Board (IRB) protocols or IRB exemptions to maintain student confidentiality. For this example, three simulated datasets were created, and each contains 400 simulated student records. To keep the analysis simple, the number of variables in the simulated datasets are limited to: Full name, gender, ethnicity/race, age, pre-admission GPA, and GRE (Table 1). All three datasets are imbalanced, meaning those passing and failing a course are not equal. All three datasets have 10% of the students failing a course and 90% not failing a course. All three datasets have identical values except for the GRE value as this will represent commonly missing GRE values, a result of not being an admission requirement for many veterinary schools. In the dataset named "BiasedGRE1", we removed the lowest GRE from 14 of the students who experienced failure and from 71 of the students who did not experience failure. In the dataset named "BiasedGRE2", we randomly removed GRE scores from 200 student records. The simulated datasets and all code for the models created in this manuscript are available at https://github.com/RUSVMCenter4/Veterinary_Education_ML_Tutorial (accessed on 14 May 2023) [31].

2.2.2. Importing the Dataset

The first step to creating a ML model is to load the required Python packages and the dataset(s). We used Python version 3.11.1 within Spyder version 5.1.5 for all coding. To load our datasets, we used a package called pandas [32], version 1.4.3. Any characters or text after a pound sign (#) are not read by Python and this provides a way to insert notes into the Python code.

```
#Import required packages:
Import pandas as pd
#Import the dataset using the function pd.read_excel().
Dataset = pd.read_excel(r'C:\location_of_data\name_of_excell_datafile.xlsx', sheet_name = 'name')
#To view the first 10 rows of the dataset with the column names:
Dataset.head(10)
```

Table 1. All simulated variables for the student records are shown with the range of values or potential options. As an introductory primer for educators, some variables displayed in the table were limited to reduce the complexity of the analysis. The fail variable is the target variable with 0 describing a student who did not fail the veterinary school course (0 = no) and 1 describing a student who did fail the veterinary school course (1 = yes).

Variable Name	Range of Values	Type of Data
Full Name	400 randomly generated female and male names	Categorical
Gender	Male or Female	Categorical
Race/Ethnicity	Asian, Black, Latinx, Not Provided, White	Categorical
Age	20–40 years	Numeric
Pre-Vet School GPA	3.00–4.00	Numeric
GRE	260–330	Numeric
Fail	0–1	Numeric

2.3. Exploratory Data Analysis

Once the dataset is loaded, we recommend that data visualization and descriptive statistics are completed prior to moving to the next step. This helps the veterinary educator to understand if the data contain outliers, missing data, the distribution of variables, and much more. We are limited in further expanding upon this critical step considering that we randomly generated our small dataset and selected the distribution of the values.

2.4. Data Preprocessing

Data preprocessing describes the process of when the raw data are prepared for training and testing the ML model. As a first step in protecting student confidentiality, we recommend that student records be assigned a randomized ID, and the list of names along with the assigned random IDs be stored safely per IRB standards at your institution. This can be easily done in Python using a for loop with a random number generator function from the random module which is built-in to Python. A for loop in Python is a line of code which repeatedly uses, or iterates, a function, and in this case, we repeat the function 400 times. This is equal to the number of student records in our dataset. All python code for this step is available at https://github.com/RUSVMCenter4/Veterinary_Education_ML_Tutorial (accessed on 14 May 2023) and shows how to generate random student IDs and then add the IDs as a column to the dataset [31]. This step is not included here because we simulated the entire datasets. Additionally, in this manuscript, we do not address all steps and considerations when making a dataset completely anonymous, and therefore we recommend an expert be consulted if outcomes of the ML project are made public.

We use the random forest algorithm provided in the Python package scikit-learn [33]. To begin to prepare the datasets for this ML algorithm, categorical data such as gender and ethnicity/race must be converted to numerical values. This is accomplished through one-hot encoding or dummy encoding. One-hot encoding ensures a rank is not assigned to categorical variables while the variable is converted into numerical data. One-hot encoding adds a new binary variable for each unique categorical value and the original encoded variable is removed (Figure 4). Dummy encoding uses binary variables and creates the number of columns equal to the number of categories minus 1 (Figure 4).

	One-hot Encoding					Dummy Encoding			
Raw Data Race/Ethnicity	Asian	Black	Latinx	Not Provided	White	Black	Latinx	Not Provided	White
Asian	1	0	0	0	0				
Black	0	1	0	0	0	1	0	0	0
Latinx	0	0	1	0	0	0	1	0	0
Not Provided	0	0	0	1	0	0	0	1	0
White	0	0	0	0	1	0	0	0	1

Figure 4. The race/ethnicity raw data is composed of categorical variables which are converted to numerical values using one-hot encoding. There are now five columns for race with one-hot encoding as one-hot encoding adds a new binary column for each category. Students who identify as Asian will have a 1 in the Asian column and a 0 in all other columns.

#To one-hot encode for race column, use the get_dummies() from the pandas package
#We assign this transformed data to a new variable called dataset_OneHot
#We also need the argument drop_first to not be true in order to perform one-hot
#encoding.
Dataset_OneHot = pd.get_dummies(dataset, columns = ["Race"], drop_first = False)
dataset_OneHot.head() #To view the first several rows and column names

It is important to note that Python functions have different arguments or parameters, and when these arguments have an assigned value, they are used when the function is performed. To perform dummy encoding (Figure 4, we will need to set the argument drop_first to true.

#To dummy encode the gender column
dataset_OneHot = pd.get_dummies(dataset_OneHot, columns = ["Gender"], drop_first = True)
print(dataset_OneHot.head()) #To view the first several rows and column names

For continuous variables such as age, pre-admission GPA, and GRE, scaling the variables, commonly known as feature scaling, or standardizing the variables may need to occur. When employing feature scaling techniques, our goal is to make sure that all the variables are on the same scale or nearly the same scale. This will not change the distribution of the data. This means this step will not transform non-parametric data into normally distributed data. For example, within our dataset, age ranges from 20 to 40 whereas GPA ranges from 3.00 to 4.00 and GRE ranges from 260 to 330. If we were using a ML model that was unsupervised and cluster based upon relationships and groupings [8], leaving these values unscaled could impact the results due to many models being based upon Euclidean Distance, or the distance between two data points.

We kept age as a continuous variable as random forests are not a distance-based classifier, robust to outliers, and do not need parametric data [23]. We also kept pre-admission GPA and GRE scores continuous because random forests handle high non-linearity between independent variables [34]. Non-linear parameters typically do not affect the performance of the decision tree models because the splitting of the decision nodes is based upon absolute values, "yes" or "no" (Figure 4), and the branches are not based upon a numerical value of the feature [20,21,23,34,35].

GRE is a continuous variable, with two of the simulated datasets containing missing GRE scores. It is important to determine if the data are missing not at random (MNAR) due to a specific reason (i.e., a student does poorly on the GRE and so does not report the result), or if the missing data are missing at random (MAR) or missing completely at random (MCAR). MAR data are missing and while randomly missing, can be explained by another observed variable (i.e., a dataset contains information on medical absences and course exam grades, a student with a missing course exam grade could be explained if they had a medical absence). MCAR data refer to missing data that are randomly distributed across the variable and is not related to the other variables (i.e., if the dataset contained a few student records without GPA scores due to human error inputting the scores into the student record database). GRE was chosen as an example variable for missing data because the GRE is recommended or no longer required for many veterinary professional programs as there are concerns the GRE may hinder diversity and inclusion efforts and may be a burden for low-income students [36,37]. How the veterinary educator decides to handle these data will impact the results of the ML model. This will be shown when reviewing the results of the ML models created using the three datasets.

Unfortunately, currently there are no established methods for handling MNAR data in medical education, and therefore there are no guidelines on imputation methods, or the action of replacing missing values in the dataset with an alternative or predicted value. Our code below demonstrates loading 1 of the 2 biased GRE datasets and use listwise deletion (deletion of the student recording containing NAs) and substitution (the mean or median value for the column) [38,39], which are two common methods reported in education and often are the default methods in R and Python packages.

#Import the first dataset with missing GRE values using the function pd.read_excel().
Biased_dataset = pd.read_excel(r'C:\location_of_data/name_of_excell_datafile.xlsx', sheet_name = 'name')
#Code to drop delete each student record that does not have a GRE score reported
#The "empty" GRE value will be noted as an "na" in Python, therefore we use the
#dropna()
#The argument axis = 0 means the row with the "na" will be dropped.
#The argument how = 'any' means that any "na" will result in the row being deleted
#The argument inplace = True means that a new dataframe will not be created
biased_dataset_OneHot.dropna(axis = 0, how = 'any', inplace = True)
#Code to replace each missing GRE score with the mean of the GRE value
biased_dataset_OneHot.fillna((biased_dataset_OneHot['GRE'].mean()), inplace = True)

The full code to create the base random forest models using the two missing GRE datasets is available on Github [31]. These datasets with missing GRE were created to illustrate NMAR and MCAR data and how commonly accepted methods for handling these data types in the literature have the potential to affect the model; therefore, only base random forest models were created and no hyperparameter search was conducted.

2.5. Data Feature Extraction

Feature extraction, also commonly referred to as feature selection or dimension reduction, refers to when different techniques are used such as principal component analysis (PCA) or stepwise regression to reduce the number of variables into the model [40]. Our original datasets contained 5 variables after removing the student names. After one-hot encoding, our datasets expanded to 9 variables. These datasets are quite small and do not need to undergo dimension reduction or reducing the number of variables (i.e., feature selection). However, veterinary educators need to be aware that having datasets with high dimensionality will require higher computational power to run the ML algorithm [41]. More importantly, some ML algorithms may have lower predictive performance and have the potential to fail to provide meaningful results when there are a large number of variables [41,42].

2.6. Model Creation and Performance Evaluation

ML algorithms learn from the input dataset which is typically divided into training and testing datasets. The training dataset is used to train the ML model followed by evaluating the model with the testing dataset. Splitting the dataset is commonly done to help reduce the risk of over-fitting. If over-fitting occurs, this means the model only performs well on the data used to train it, and the model's performance is reduced when it is applied on new data [43]. We recommend that multiple models be trained with different parameters and compared to find the best candidate model for the identified educational research question. This is commonly done by what is termed as a ML pipeline. The parameters within the pipeline can be adjusted in any of the steps, (1) data pre-processing, (2) feature extraction, (3) model training, and (4) model evaluation. Model evaluation is completed by comparing a variety of different metrics which may include accuracy, F-scores, receiver operating characteristic (ROC) curves, and others which we will expand upon more in the experimental section.

2.6.1. Generation of Base Random Forest Model

The first step of creating a ML model, including random forests, is to take the dataset and separate the variables into one dataframe (a table with rows and columns) and the target column in a second dataframe. The target column is the outcome we wish to predict. Within our example, we are creating a classification model, so the outcome is a binary outcome, either a "Pass" or a "Fail. In the "Fail" target column, a 0 indicates a student did not fail a course and 1 indicates a student failed a course.

#X is our variable dataframe and y is our target dataframe
#create dataframe without target, [rows, columns], the : indicates to select all rows
X = dataset_OneHot.loc[: , dataset_OneHot.columns != 'Fail']
y = dataset_OneHot['Fail'] #target variable for prediction

We are most interested in determining what variables lead to the outcome or target column. Considering that the simulated dataset is composed of a majority and minority class (target variable does not have an equal number of 0 s and 1 s), the dataset has an imbalance bias, one of the three main types of recognized biases in ML [44]. The two main approaches to deal with imbalanced target variables is to use an oversampling technique which creates additional minority classes (student records with a course failure) or undersampling techniques to randomly delete majority classes (student records without a course failure). We selected to turn our dataset into a balanced dataset by using an oversampling method called synthetic minority oversampling technique (SMOTE) which is a common method for dealing with models predicting student success in higher education [45–47]. After performing SMOTE, our dataset will result in students who failed a course being equal to the number of students who did not fail a course.

#Import required python function of SMOTE from Python package imbalanced-learn
#version 0.10.1from imblearn.over_sampling import SMOTE,
#Oversampling to allow 0 and 1 target to be equal
#Assigning a value to the random state argument ensures that anyone can generate
#the same set of random numbers again
X_resampled, y_resampled = SMOTE(random_state = 23).fit_resample(X, y)

With a balanced target variable, we are now ready to split our dataset into training data and testing data. Splitting the dataset is commonly done to help reduce the risk of over-fitting. As our code shows below, we used train_test_split() from scikit learn Python package (version 1.1.1) to split our dataset. We also provide code showing the data structure as the length dataframes containing the variables must be the same length as its counterpart containing the target, otherwise the random forest model will not be constructed.

#Import required functions:
from sklearn.model_selection import train_test_split
#Use the balanced data to create testing and training datasets with 70% of the data
#being training and 30% of the data being testing.
X_trainSMOTE, X_testSMOTE, y_trainSMOTE, y_testSMOTE = train_test_split(X_resampled, y_resampled, stratify = y_resampled, test_size = 0.3, random_state = 50)
#Check sizes of arrays to make sure it they match each other
print('Training Variables Shape:', X_trainSMOTE.shape)
print('Training Target Shape:', y_trainSMOTE.shape)
print('Testing Variables Shape:', X_testSMOTE.shape)
print('Testing Target Shape:', y_testSMOTE.shape)

Once we have our training and testing dataset, we are ready to construct the base random forest model with the arguments, or parameters, being left at their default values. The model must first be built and then trained using the training data.

#Import required functions:
from sklearn.ensemble import RandomForestClassifier
#Build base model without any changes to default settings
forest_base = RandomForestClassifier(random_state = 23)
#Train the model via fit()
forest_base.fit(X_trainSMOTE, y_trainSMOTE) #using training data

2.6.2. Evaluation of the Base Random Forest Model

Once the base ML model is created, then we evaluate how well the model performs when it is shown new data, the test data. ML model performance can be assessed using different techniques which are discussed individually below. Each of the model performance methods uses a range from zero to one, with one indicating perfect performance and zero indicating all predictions were wrong. We recommend that cross-validation (CV) be included in each of the performance metric calculations.

CV is used to help detect overfitting while evaluating the performance of the ML model on new data. We used k-fold cross validation, which is one of the most common cross validation techniques [48]. In k-fold cross validation, the dataset is divided into folds (consider these as subset datasets) based upon the assigned k-value. One fold is saved as a validation dataset and the other folds are used to train the model. As Figure 5 shows, this process is repeated multiple times with each repeat holding out a different fold for validation of the model. The results from each validation set are averaged to produce the final performance value. Typical k-values are 3, 5, and 10, but there are no established rules guiding the selection of these values.

Example of k-fold cross-validation, k = 5

	Fold 1	Fold 2	Fold 3	Fold 4	Fold 5
Iteration 1 of 5	Test	Train	Train	Train	Train
Iteration 2 of 5	Train	Test	Train	Train	Train
Iteration 3 of 5	Train	Train	Test	Train	Train
Iteration 4 of 5	Train	Train	Train	Test	Train
Iteration 5 of 5	Train	Train	Train	Train	Test

Figure 5. An example of a k-fold cross validation with k = 5. Five iterations of the training dataset are evenly divided into five folds, four of which are used for training and the last one for testing the model. This is repeated five times. The final validation would take place using the testing dataset (not shown).

To prepare our model for the performance metrics, we must define the k-value for the CV and input our testing dataset into the trained random forest model. The trained random forest ML model will predict the target category or outcome of whether a student failed a course or not based upon what it learned from the training dataset.

#Make predictions using testing data set
y_predictions = forest_base.predict(X_testSMOTE)
y_trueSMOTE = y_testSMOTE #Rename the test target dataframe
#Import required function
from sklearn.model_selection import KFold

#Defining the cross-validation to be able to compute the performance metrics using
#the k-fold CV
kf = KFold(shuffle = True, n_splits = 5)

Overall accuracy, recall (i.e., sensitivity or true positive rate), specificity (i.e., true negative rate), precision, F-score (i.e., F1-score), and receiver operating characteristic (ROC) curves are performance metrics which are computed using the true negative (TN), false negative (FN), false positive (FP), and true positive (TP) values. A confusion matrix summarizes the results of the random forest classification algorithm and defines these values as shown in Table 2.

Table 2. A confusion matrix defines the true negative (TN), false negative (FN), false positive (FP), and true positive (TP) values used in the calculation of the performance metrics. As shown in the chart, a TN outcome is when the model correctly predicts the student did not fail the course; a TP outcome is when the model correctly predicts the student failed a course; a FN outcome is when the model incorrectly predicts the student did not fail, but in reality the student did fail the course; and a FP outcome is when the model incorrectly predicts a student failed a course, but in reality the student did not fail the course.

	Actual Negative Class: 0, Student Who Did Not Fail	Actual Positive Class: 1, Student Who Did Fail
Predicted negative Class: 0, student who did not fail	True negative (TN)	False negative (FN)
Predicted positive Class: 1, student who did fail	False positive (FP)	True positive (TP)

The *overall accuracy* is determined by the proportion of the total number of student predictions that were correct over all type of predictions made, and can be calculated using Equation (1):

$$Overall\ accuracy = \frac{(TN + TP)}{(TP + TN + FP + FN)} \quad (1)$$

#Import required function
from sklearn.model_selection import cross_val_score
#To calculate the accuracy of the model using k-fold cross validation
score_accuracy_mean = cross_val_score(forest_base, X_testSMOTE, y_trueSMOTE, cv = kf, scoring = 'accuracy').mean()
print(score_accuracy_mean) #View the mean of the CV validation results for
#accuracy of the model.

The true positive rate (*TPR*), also known as sensitivity or recall, is defined as the proportion of students who failed a course which were correctly classified as having failed a course and was calculated using Equation (2):

$$recall\ or\ sensitivity\ or\ TPR = \frac{TP}{(TP + FN)} \quad (2)$$

#To calculate the recall of the model using k-fold cross validation
recall = cross_val_score(best_grid_model, X_testSMOTE, y_testSMOTE, cv = kf, scoring = 'recall').mean()
print(recall) #View the mean of the CV validation results for recall of the model

The true negative rate (*TNR*), also known as specificity, is defined as the proportion of students who did not fail a course which were classified correctly as not failing and was calculated using Equation (3):

$$specificity \text{ or } TNR = \frac{TN}{(TN + FP)} \quad (3)$$

There is no *specificity or TNR* option in the cross_val_score() and so we must define specificity using the make_scorer() function.
#Import required function
from sklearn.metrics import make_scorer
#Define specificity
scoring = make_scorer(recall_score, pos_label = 0)
#Use our defined specificity as the type of score that is calculated
score_specificity_mean = cross_val_score(forest_base, X_testSMOTE, y_trueSMOTE, cv = kf, scoring = scoring).mean()
cross_val_score(forest_base, X_testSMOTE, y_trueSMOTE, cv = kf, scoring = scoring)
print(score_specificity_mean) #View the mean of the CV validation results for
#specificity of the model

Precision is the number of correct predictions a student failure out of all students that were classified as experiencing a failure and was calculated using Equation (4):

$$Precision = \frac{TP}{(TP + FP)} \quad (4)$$

# To calculate the precision of the model using k-fold cross validation
score_precision_mean = cross_val_score(forest_base, X_testSMOTE, y_trueSMOTE, cv = kf, scoring = 'precision').mean()
print(score_precision_mean) #View the mean of the CV validation results for
#precision of the model

The *F-score* (*F1*) is a weighted harmonic average of precision and recall and is calculated using Equation (5):

$$F\text{-}score \text{ or } F1 = 2 \times \frac{(precision \times recall)}{(precision + recall)} \quad (5)$$

#To calculate the *F-score* of the model using k-fold cross validation
score_f1_mean = cross_val_score(forest_base, X_testSMOTE, y_trueSMOTE, cv = kf, scoring = 'f1').mean()
print(score_f1_mean) #View the mean of the CV validation results for precision of
#the model

Receiver operating characteristic (ROC) curves are created by plotting the sensitivity versus the specificity at different cut points for binary classification models [49]. The area under the ROC curve (AUC) is calculated from the ROC curves and is the last validation method we will use to assess each model. This single numerical score is considered a superior method compared to accuracy when evaluating the performance of prediction models [50].
#To calculate the ROC curve AUC of the model using k-fold cross validation
#score_auc_mean = cross_val_score(forest_base, X_testSMOTE, y_trueSMOTE, cv = kf, scoring = 'roc_auc').mean()
print(score_auc_mean)) #View the mean of the CV validation results for ROC curve
#AUC of the model

2.6.3. Tuning of the Random Forest Model

Now that we know our model results, we can try to use data-driven approaches to improve the performance of our model. This means we will try to tune our model's hyperparameters to improve the performance of the model. First, we will define a list of hyperparameters, or the parameters that are specific before training the model. This will help determine the best parameters that are learned during the training process of the model. We will demonstrate two common data-driven hyperparameter approaches, (1) Random search [51] and (2) Grid Search [52]. We first use random search as it requires lower computational power and will test a user-specified random number of combinations in the hyperparameter grid. Once we have the best estimates using random search, we will define a new hyperparameter grid with values closer to the selected output values from the random search. We will then use grid search, which will look at every possible combination in the hyperparameter grid.

##Assess hyperparameters to try to improve upon base model:
#Import required functions:
from sklearn.model_selection import RandomizedSearchCV
from sklearn.model_selection import GridSearchCV
# Create the hyperparameter grid for first the random search function
hyper_grid = {# Number of trees to be included in random forest
    'n_estimators': [150, 200, 250, 300, 350, 400],
Number of features to consider at every split
    'max_features': ['sqrt'],
#Maximum number of levels in a tree
    'max_depth': [10, 20, 40, 60, 80, 100, 120, 140, 160, 180, 200],
Minimum number of samples required to split a node
    'min_samples_split': [2, 4, 6, 8, 10],
Minimum number of samples required at each leaf node
    'min_samples_leaf': [1, 2, 4, 6, 8, 10],
Method of selecting samples for training each tree
    'bootstrap': [True, False]}
#Initiate random forest base model to tune
best_params = RandomForestClassifier(random_state = (23))
#Use random grid search to find best hyperparameters, uses k-fold validation as cross
#validation method
#Search 200 different combinations
best_params_results = RandomizedSearchCV(estimator = best_params,
 param_distributions = hyper_grid, n_iter = 200, cv = kf, verbose = 5, random_state = (23))
#Fit the random search model
best_params_results.fit(X_trainSMOTE, y_trainSMOTE)
#Find the best parameters from the grid search results
Print(best_params_results.best_params_)
#Build another hyperparameter grid using narrowed down parameter guidelines
#from above
#Then use GridSearchCV method to search every combination of grid
new_grid = {'n_estimators': [250, 275, 300, 325, 332, 350, 375],
    'max_features': ['sqrt'],
    'max_depth': [160, 165, 170, 175, 180, 185, 190, 195],
    'min_samples_split': [1, 2, 3, 4, 5, 6],
    'min_samples_leaf': [1, 2, 3],
    'bootstrap': [True]}
#Initiate random forest base model to tune
best_params = RandomForestClassifier(random_state = (23))
#Use GridSearchCV method to search every combination of grid
best_params_grid_search = GridSearchCV(estimator = best_params, param_grid = new_grid, cv = kf, n_jobs = −1, verbose = 10)
#Fit the gridsearch model
best_params_grid_search.fit(X_trainSMOTE, y_trainSMOTE)
#Get the results of the search grid form the random forest model

best_params_grid_search.best_params_
#Using the results of the best parameters, we will create a new model and show the
#specific arguments.
best_grid_model = RandomForestClassifier(n_estimators = 375, max_features = 'sqrt',
max_depth = (160), min_samples_split = 2, min_samples_leaf = 2, bootstrap = True)
#Best model based upon grid
best_grid_model.fit(X_trainSMOTE, y_trainSMOTE)

After creation of the model, the performance metrics can be calculated, and the veterinary educator will need to decide which model is best, the base model or the model using the new parameters.

2.6.4. Determining the Most Important Features of the Random Forest Model

After selecting the best model based upon the performance metrics, we need to determine which features contribute most to the model being able to predict the outcome of a student. Each feature has a score. A higher score means it contributes more to the model's prediction whereas a lower score indicates the feature has a lower contribution to the model's prediction. There are a variety of approaches to calculating the feature importance values, and some approaches depend on the ML algorithm selected whereas others can be used for a variety of ML algorithms [12].

We will use two methods to assess the features of importance, the Gini importance (or mean decrease Gini) and the visual Shapley additive explanations (SHAP) (Shap python package version 0.40.0). Gini importance is the most common method used to determine the relative depth or rank of a feature used as a decision node within the random forest model [20,53]. The most important features have a larger value and will be located most often at decision nodes near the top of the individual trees (Figure 1). By being near the top of the tree, a larger percentage of the input samples are utilized by that specific decision node. This means that the feature contributes more to the final prediction decision compared to decision nodes lower on the tree [33,53]. Features of importance determined by SHAP are based upon classic game-theoretic Shapley values. SHAP measures local feature interaction effects and helps provide a better understanding of the overall model [54] based on combining the explanations for each student outcome that is predicted.

#Most important features from best performing random forest model, Gini im
#portance
feature_imp = pd.Series(best_grid_model.feature_importances_, index = X.columns)
feature_imp = feature_imp.sort_values(ascending = False)
print(feature_imp)
#Import required package
import shap
#Most important features from best performing random forest model, SHAP values
shap_feature_imp = shap.TreeExplainer(best_grid_model)
shap_values = shap_feature_imp.shap_values(X_testSMOTE)
shap.summary_plot(shap_values, X_testSMOTE) #Shows results in a plot

Model employment:
The best performing model is selected and used to address the educational research question or problem.

3. Results

In the methods, we describe how a total of five random forest models were created. The full code provided resulted in the production of two random forest models, a model using the default parameters and a model with parameters selected after hyperparameter tuning. Table 3 shows the performance metrics for both models which were built from the complete dataset without any missing values.

Table 3. The performance metrics calculated when the random forest base model and the tuned random forest model was given the testing dataset.

Performance Metric	Random Forest Base Model	Radom Forest Tuned Model
Accuracy	87.07%	86.61%
Recall/Sensitivity/TPR	89.61%	89.77%
Specificity/TNR	87.15%	88.11%
Precision	86.46%	86.21%
F1-Score	86.24%	88.40%
ROC curve AUC	87.15%	88.11%

The most important features, as ranked by the Gini criterion, varied depending on which dataset was used to train and test the model as well as the imputation or replacement method selected to address the missing values. The full list of most important features from each model are in Table 4.

Table 4. The Gini criterion ranking of all features from each of the five random forest models created using the datasets. All GRE records dataset contained no missing values, whereas the missing low GRE values removed dataset removed any incomplete student records or were replaced by the mean values (missing low GRE values replaced with mean). The most important features for the randomly removed GRE scores with all student records eliminated that were incomplete is shown in the random missing GRE values removed columns and when those missing scores were replaced with the mean, the most important features are shown in the respective column.

All GRE Records	Feature Importance Score	Missing Low GRE Values Removed	Feature Importance Score	Missing Low GRE Values Replaced with Mean	Feature Importance Score	Random Missing GRE Values Removed	Feature Importance Score	Random Missing GRE Values Replaced with Mean	Feature Importance Score
GRE	0.241850	GRE	0.370290	GRE	0.357720	GRE	0.291419	preGPA	0.218575
Age	0.150457	Race_Not Provided	0.131981	preGPA	0.152793	preGPA	0.199777	GRE	0.181400
Race_Not Provided	0.146913	preGPA	0.106498	Age	0.146683	Age	0.163021	Age	0.180350
preGPA	0.130455	Age	0.100696	Race_Not Provided	0.096973	Race_Not Provided	0.071514	Race_Not Provided	0.117902
Race_White	0.078924	Race_White	0.093832	Race_Latinx	0.062529	Race_Asian	0.062693	Race_White	0.073569
Race_Latinx	0.067359	Gender_Male	0.082514	Race_White	0.057276	Race_White	0.059140	Race_Black	0.071190
Gender_Male	0.063287	Race_Latinx	0.047706	Race_Asian	0.044694	Race_Black	0.051953	Race_Asian	0.062513
Race_Black	0.063043	Race_Black	0.041844	Gender_Male	0.042020	Gender_Male	0.050608	Race_Latinx	0.060454
Race_Asian	0.057713	Race_Asian	0.024639	Race_Black	0.039311	Race_Latinx	0.049876	Gender_male	0.034048

GRE and three of the one-hot encoded categorical variable levels from the race/ethnicity column were identified by SHAP values as the most important features of the best-performing random forest model without any missing values. The results are plotted as summary beeswarm plots in Figure 6. Figure 7 shows the SHAP-determined most important features of the four random forest models with missing GRE values and are visually displayed as summary bar plots ranking the most important features at the top of the y-axis.

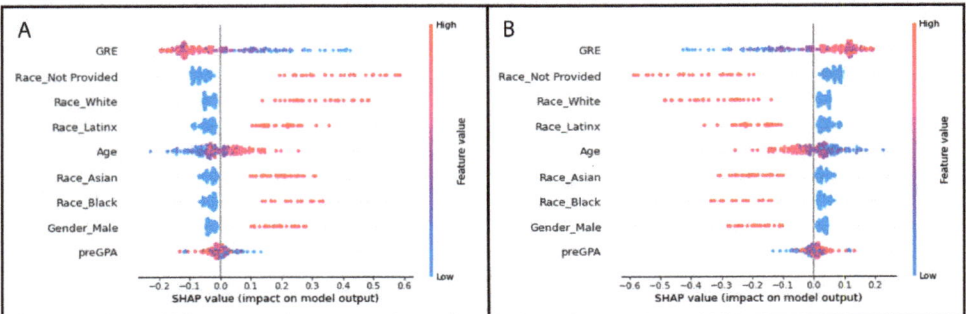

Figure 6. Beeswarm plots of the simulated dataset containing no missing GRE values. Each dot represents a student record with the feature value represented by a color. As the feature value color bar shows, a higher value is pink and a lower value is blue. The *x*-axis shows the SHAP values for the most important features listed along the *y*-axis. The *y*-axis values represent the features of importance with the top variable being the most important and the subsequent ones organized in descending rank of importance. (**A**) shows the SHAP values for students who did not fail any course, (**B**) shows the SHAP values for students who failed a course.

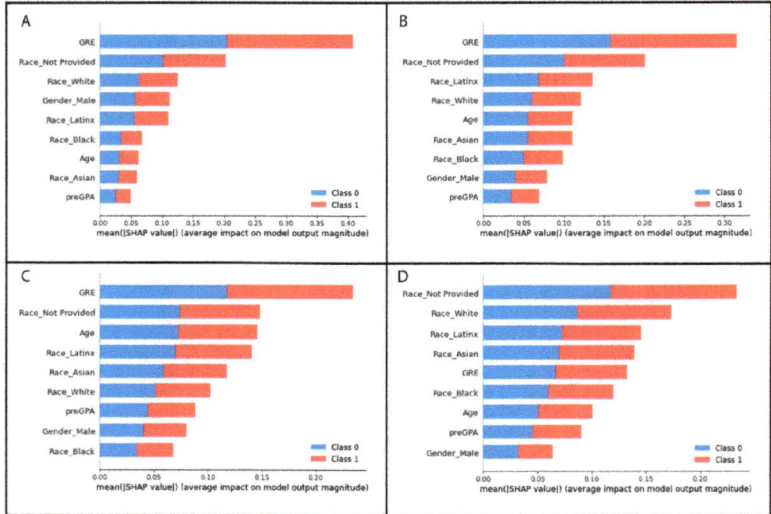

Figure 7. Global feature importance plots based on SHAP values for the datasets with missing GRE values. The *y*-axis values represent the features of importance with the top variable being the most important and the subsequent ones organized in descending rank of importance. The mean absolute value for each feature for all student records in the dataset is displayed on the *x*-axis. (**A**) Shows the features of importance for the simulated data where student records were eliminated with missing low GRE values. (**B**) Shows the features of importance for the simulated data where student records with missing low GRE scores were replaced with the mean GRE score of all applicants. (**C**) Shows the features of importance for the simulated data where student records were eliminated with random missing GRE values. (**D**) Shows the features of importance for the simulated data where student records with randomly missing GRE scores were replaced with the mean GRE score of all applicants.

4. Discussion

ML has the potential to become a powerful tool in veterinary education; however, ML algorithms have yet to be tapped by veterinary educators. This manuscript focuses on making ML more accessible by providing a practical overview of ML and the creation of a supervised ML algorithm, a random forest ML model. As an emerging tool, there are some important considerations that veterinary educators must be aware of when employing ML models. We further highlight some of these considerations below which we initially present in the working example section when creating the models by discussing the results of the different models created by the different datasets.

Two of the most important considerations are the quality of a dataset and when it contains incomplete records. As previously discussed, missing data can be categorized into three main types. In education studies, often, the missing data will be MAR (e.g., a student who is sick misses an exam and can be explained by a leave of absence) or NMAR (e.g., a student chooses to not participate in an active learning exercise or chooses to not complete a teaching evaluation). NMAR data are non-ignorable data, meaning simply eliminating these students from the analysis will result in bias. In the literature, there are well accepted methods for handling MCAR or MAR data in education [6,38,39,55,56], but there are not commonly accepted methods for NMAR data in medical or veterinary education fields.

We utilized two pre-replacing methods that have been reported to be two of the most frequently encountered techniques in the higher education literature [6,57], listwise deletion and imputation (i.e., replacement). While there are many different imputation methods, we selected a single imputation method over multiple imputation (the creation of many datasets with the model results averaged). Our decision in part was to help maintain the simplicity of our model for this introductory manuscript and to emphasize to the reader the importance of recognizing and handling NMAR and MAR data. In Table 4, our random forest model without missing data revealed that GRE, age, and race/ethnicity not reported were the top three features that contributed most to our prediction model when Gini criteria were used. When approximately 20% of the lower GRE values were eliminated, listwise deletion resulted in GRE contributing more to the model with race/ethnicity not provided and pre-vet school GPA being the second and third most important feature. When we used single imputation with the mean, our top three most important features were GRE, pre-vet school GPA, and age. Keeping in mind that our dataset has very few variables, and on a dataset with more features, it is possible to see even more of a dramatic effect. The two random forest models created with the MAR or MCAR GRE dataset shows listwise deletion and single imputation were more similar than the NMAR GRE dataset. However, our simulation shows that both listwise deletion and replacement with the mean still impacted the random forest model with only the top two of the three top contributing variables being the same. This supports that in the education field, there is a large gap of knowledge in how to deal with missing data within student records and should be an area of future research. Until this can be addressed, we recommend that any veterinary education studies choosing to use ML clearly state why they selected the reported method for handling missing data, and to consider using multiple replacement methods to compare the results between models and provide a better understanding of the impacts of each replacement method.

Another important consideration that must be made when constructing ML models is to decide how the decision trees are constructed and how the features of importance will be determined. We opted to use the Gini index as the impurity function within our code. This is the default option in the random forest function within the scikit learn package [33]; however, in random forest models, permutation importance is also commonly used [20]. While a full discussion between these methods is beyond the scope of this manuscript, we selected the most commonly reported method in the EDM literature and, if we accept a greatly oversimplified explanation, the Gini index (or Gini impurity criterion) can be considered a robust and reliable impurity function and in part, it has been attributed to helping to reduce the errors in prediction when combining the individual decision trees into the random forest [16,20]. It is important to recognize that the Gini impurity criterion is not perfect, and in our veterinary education datasets where there is a mix of continuous variables, binary variables, and categorial variables, the Gini impurity criterion tends to overestimate the importance of continuous variables [20].

We can see how the continuous variables of GRE, age, and pre-vet GPA are in the top four most important features based upon the Gini criterion (Table 4), but this changes when we evaluate our model using the SHAP method to determine the features of most importance. The SHAP method for estimating the features of importance in decision trees, which uses the game-theoretic Shapley values as a basis, was proposed in 2020 [54], and is beginning to gain popularity due to the SHAP method results relying heavily on a very visual based report. The visual aspects of the SHAP method help to communicate the models to non-technical stakeholders and provide a way for us to view the contribution of each variable in the model for each row of student data (Figure 6).

The bar plots (Figure 7) show the mean absolute SHAP value with the most important feature having the largest value and being at the top of the plot. As the SHAP value, or feature importance, decreases, it descends along the y-axis. The beeswarm plots are similar with the y-values representing the features of importance with the top variable being the most important and the subsequent ones organized in descending rank of importance. Beeswarm plots must be plotted for a single target variable, in our case a student with a failure or a student without a failed course. In Figure 7, each dot represents a student record with the feature value represented by a color. As the feature value color bar shows, a higher value is pink and a lower value is blue. This helps us understand how the points are distributed and how the value of the variable may impact our model's prediction. In the case of Figure 7, the most important feature on average is a student's GRE scores, with students who passed all their courses tending to have lower GRE scores compared to students who failed a course (Figure 7B) tending to have higher GRE scores based upon the simulated data.

As we can see, the features of importance are different when using the SHAP approach. SHAP values did not rank age or pre-vet GPA as contributing to the model as greatly as the Gini criterion method did (Figures 6 and 7 and Table 4). This may be explained by SHAP values not being as biased towards overestimating the importance of continuous variables, although it has been reported that in some datasets under certain conditions, SHAP has the potential to still be biased towards certain feature types such as numerical features with many unique values and categorical features with high cardinality [58]. Additionally, there is some discussion in the data science community about adding up the SHAP values for categorial variables that have been transformed with one-hot encoding to truly understand the categorical variable's contribution to the model (e.g., https://towardsdatascience.com/shap-for-categorical-features-7c63e6a554ea (accessed on 1 May 2023)).

While our categorical data contained only five levels, one-hot encoding and dummy encoding may not be appropriate for handling categorical data with many different categorical levels (aka high-cardinality categorical variables). High cardinality categorical variables can lead to statistical problems [59], "dilute" the features of importance, and reduce the predictive performance of ML algorithms [59,60]. This means that other encoding methods such as hashing may need to be explored, or reducing or limiting the number of unique categories that are one-hot encoded.

Our mock dataset contained a low number of variables; however, often, academic datasets will contain a large number of variables. Feature selection, a way to reduce high dimensionality datasets, is routinely completed during the data preparation phase in order to reduce computation power, improve the performance of the ML algorithm, and to help with model interpretation [40]. It is important to consider the overall project goal as in veterinary education, it may be just as important to understand which variables are contributing only at a low level. Therefore, it may be best to consider developing models that undergo a feature selection step as well as a model which does not undergo feature selection.

It is important to recognize that this practical introduction to ML provides veterinary educators a basic knowledge of ML and to recognize how certain decisions, such as how to handle missing data, can impact ML models such as our example random forest model. While we cannot cover every aspect of building a ML model, there is one final consideration which is often overlooked, but has begun to be recognized in clinical datasets, and that is inclusion of under-represented populations. When demographic variables have categories that are highly underrepresented, this can result in bias [61,62] and provide potentially misleading conclusions. Consider our veterinary student population. Most colleges of veterinary medicine have a primarily white, female student population [63]; therefore, when incorporating demographic data, it is important to realize that low numbers of students from underrepresented minority groups, students who are or identify as male, and/or students who identify as LGTBQIA+ are some potential variables to consider may result in a biased model. Certain research questions, such as seeking to identify at-risk students, may need to be answered by incorporating a double prioritized bias correction technique which was recently published to correct bias in prognostic ML models where the dataset contained underrepresented racial and age groups [62]. In this approach to eliminating bias, custom ML models were built for each underrepresented group in addition to an all-encompassing ML model. This may be suitable for helping eliminate the under-representation bias that is present in the veterinary student population. Furthermore, this highlights one of many research priorities as ML begins to be incorporated into veterinary education.

Prediction models, such as the model described in this manuscript, are one of the primary uses of ML in higher education as the goal of predictive analytics is to identify students at-risk in mastering knowledge and successful course completion—enabling timely interventions [21,64]. Other potential uses of ML surrounding personalizing learning experiences for veterinary students include adaptive learning platforms. These platforms have been employed in medical education programs and use ML to analyze students' performance and tailor the content based upon the identified strengths and weaknesses of the learner [65]. Furthermore, much interest exists in assessing veterinary skills and being able to provide objective, consistent, and immediate feedback to students. There is ongoing work to train AI on visual and physiologic data such as surface electromyographical (sEMG) data to use ML to help assess surgical skills of veterinary students [66].

5. Conclusions

Without established guidelines for handling data (i.e., MNAR) within the medical education field nor preferred methods for model evaluation, our results using simulated veterinary student data highlight the need for the veterinary educator to be fully transparent during the creation of ML models. We suggest future research efforts be directed toward establishing best practices within the education field for handling MNAR data and the other critical considerations.

Author Contributions: Conceptualization, S.E.H., E.A. and K.G.H.; methodology, S.E.H.; software, S.E.H.; validation, S.E.H., E.A. and K.G.H.; formal analysis, S.E.H.; investigation, S.E.H.; resources, S.E.H.; data curation, S.E.H.; writing—original draft preparation, S.E.H.; writing—review and editing, S.E.H., E.A. and K.G.H.; visualization, S.E.H.; supervision, S.E.H.; project administration, S.E.H.; funding acquisition, S.E.H. and E.A. All authors have read and agreed to the published version of the manuscript.

Funding: This research was funded by Ross University School of Veterinary Medicine Center for Research and Innovation in Veterinary and Medical Education, intramural grant numbers 44019-2023 and 44026-2024.

Institutional Review Board Statement: Not applicable as all student data were simulated.

Informed Consent Statement: Not applicable as all student data were simulated.

Data Availability Statement: All simulated datasets and Python code is at https://github.com/RUSVMCenter4/Veterinary_Education_ML_Tutorial (accessed on 14 May 2023).

Conflicts of Interest: Kent Hecker (K.G.H.) is Chief Assessment Officer of the International Council for Veterinary Assessment. S.E.H. and E.A. declare no conflicts of interest. The funders had no role in the design of the study; in the collection, analyses, or interpretation of data; in the writing of the manuscript; or in the decision to publish the results.

References

1. Basran, P.S.; Appleby, R.B. The unmet potential of artificial intelligence in veterinary medicine. *Am. J. Vet. Res.* **2022**, *83*, 385–392. [CrossRef] [PubMed]
2. Hennessey, E.; DiFazio, M.; Hennessey, R.; Cassel, N. Artificial intelligence in veterinary diagnostic imaging: A literature review. *Vet. Radiol. Ultrasound* **2022**, *63*, 851–870. [CrossRef] [PubMed]
3. Katznelson, G.; Gerke, S. The need for health AI ethics in medical school education. *Adv. Health Sci. Educ.* **2021**, *26*, 1447. [CrossRef]
4. Calvet Liñán, L.; Juan Pérez, Á.A. Educational Data Mining and Learning Analytics: Differences, similarities, and time evolution. *Int. J. Educ. Technol. High. Educ.* **2015**, *12*, 98–112. [CrossRef]
5. Algarni, A. Data mining in education. *Int. J. Adv. Comput. Sci. Appl.* **2016**, *7*, 456–461. [CrossRef]
6. Alyahyan, E.; Düştegör, D. Predicting academic success in higher education: Literature review and best practices. *Int. J. Educ. Technol. High. Educ.* **2020**, *17*, 1–21. [CrossRef]
7. Samuel, A.L. Some studies in machine learning using the game of checkers. *IBM J. Res. Dev.* **1959**, *3*, 210–229. [CrossRef]
8. Bi, Q.; Goodman, K.E.; Kaminsky, J.; Lessler, J. What is Machine Learning? A Primer for the Epidemiologist. *Am. J. Epidemiol.* **2019**, *188*, 2222–2239. [CrossRef]
9. Von Davier, A.A.; Mislevy, R.J.; Hao, J. Introduction to Computational Psychometrics: Towards a Principled Integration of Data Science and Machine Learning Techniques into Psychometrics. In *Computational Psychometrics: New Methodologies for a New Generation of Digital Learning and Assessment: With Examples in R and Python*; von Davier, A.A., Mislevy, R.J., Hao, J., Eds.; Springer International Publishing: Cham, Switzerland, 2021; pp. 1–6.
10. Khamisy-Farah, R.; Gilbey, P.; Furstenau, L.B.; Sott, M.K.; Farah, R.; Viviani, M.; Bisogni, M.; Kong, J.D.; Ciliberti, R.; Bragazzi, N.L. Big Data for Biomedical Education with a Focus on the COVID-19 Era: An Integrative Review of the Literature. *Int J Env. Res Public Health* **2021**, *18*, 8989. [CrossRef]
11. Peers, I. *Statistical Analysis for Education and Psychology Researchers: Tools for Researchers in Education and Psychology*; Routledge: London, UK, 2006.
12. Nie, R.; Guo, Q.; Morin, M. Machine Learning Literacy for Measurement Professionals: A Practical Tutorial. *Educ. Meas. Issues Pract.* **2023**, *42*, 9–23. [CrossRef]
13. Van Vertloo, L.R.; Burzette, R.G.; Danielson, J.A. Predicting Academic Difficulty in Veterinary Medicine: A Case-Control Study. *J. Vet. Med. Educ.* **2022**, *49*, 524–530. [CrossRef] [PubMed]
14. Stoltzfus, J.C. Logistic Regression: A Brief Primer. *Acad. Emerg. Med.* **2011**, *18*, 1099–1104. [CrossRef] [PubMed]
15. Wang, S.; Mo, B.; Zhao, J. Theory-based residual neural networks: A synergy of discrete choice models and deep neural networks. *Transp. Res. Part B Methodol.* **2021**, *146*, 333–358. [CrossRef]
16. Dass, S.; Gary, K.; Cunningham, J. Predicting Student Dropout in Self-Paced MOOC Course Using Random Forest Model. *Information* **2021**, *12*, 476. [CrossRef]
17. He, L.; Levine, R.A.; Fan, J.; Beemer, J.; Stronach, J. Random forest as a predictive analytics alternative to regression in institutional research. *Pract. Assess. Res. Eval.* **2018**, *23*, 1.
18. Sarker, I.H. Machine Learning: Algorithms, Real-World Applications and Research Directions. *SN Comput. Sci.* **2021**, *2*, 160. [CrossRef]
19. Romero, C.; Ventura, S. Educational Data Mining: A Review of the State of the Art. *IEEE Trans. Syst. Man Cybern. Part C (Appl. Rev.)* **2010**, *40*, 601–618. [CrossRef]
20. Louppe, G. Understanding random forests: From theory to practice. *arXiv* **2014**, arXiv:1407.7502.
21. Spoon, K.; Beemer, J.; Whitmer, J.C.; Fan, J.; Frazee, J.P.; Stronach, J.; Bohonak, A.J.; Levine, R.A. Random Forests for Evaluating Pedagogy and Informing Personalized Learning. *J. Educ. Data Min.* **2016**, *8*, 20–50. [CrossRef]
22. Choudhary, R.; Gianey, H.K. Comprehensive Review On Supervised Machine Learning Algorithms. In Proceedings of the 2017 International Conference on Machine Learning and Data Science (MLDS), Noida, India, 14–15 December 2017; pp. 37–43.
23. Kumar, N. Advantages and Disadvantages of Random Forest Algorithm in Machine Learning. Available online: http://theprofessionalspoint.blogspot.com/2019/02/advantages-and-disadvantages-of-random.html (accessed on 11 February 2022).
24. Altman, N.; Krzywinski, M. Ensemble methods: Bagging and random forests. *Nat. Methods* **2017**, *14*, 933–935. [CrossRef]
25. Dietterich, T.G. Ensemble Learning. In *The Handbook of Brain Theory and Neural Networks*, 2nd ed.; Arbib, M.A., Ed.; MIT Press: Cambridge, MA, USA, 2002.
26. Anaconda Software Distribution. v22.9.0. October 2022. Available online: https://www.anaconda.com/download (accessed on 13 November 2022).
27. Wang, Y.; Wen, M.; Liu, Y.; Wang, Y.; Li, Z.; Wang, C.; Yu, H.; Cheung, S.-C.; Xu, C.; Zhu, Z. Watchman: Monitoring dependency conflicts for python library ecosystem. In Proceedings of the ACM/IEEE 42nd International Conference on Software Engineering, Seoul, Republic of Korea, 27 June–19 July 2020; pp. 125–135.
28. Gudivada, V.; Apon, A.; Ding, J. Data quality considerations for big data and machine learning: Going beyond data cleaning and transformations. *Int. J. Adv. Softw.* **2017**, *10*, 1–20.
29. Hao, J.; Mislevy, R.J. A Data Science Perspective on Computational Psychometrics. In *Computational Psychometrics: New Methodologies for a New Generation of Digital Learning and Assessment: With Examples in R and Python*; von Davier, A.A., Mislevy, R.J., Hao, J., Eds.; Springer International Publishing: Cham, Switzerland, 2021; pp. 133–158.

30. Adtalem Global Education. *OutReach IQ*; Adtalem Global Education: Chicago, IL ,USA, 2022.
31. MicroBatVet. Rusvmcenter4/veterinary_education_ml_tutorial: Vet Ed ML Primer V1.1. *Zenodo* **2023**. [CrossRef]
32. McKinney, W. Data structures for statistical computing in python. In Proceedings of the 9th Python in Science Conference, Austin, TX, USA, 28 June 28–3 July 2010; pp. 51–56.
33. Pedregosa, F.; Varoquaux, G.; Gramfort, A.; Michel, V.; Thirion, B.; Grisel, O.; Blondel, M.; Prettenhofer, P.; Weiss, R.; Dubourg, V. Scikit-learn: Machine learning in Python. *J. Mach. Learn. Res.* **2011**, *12*, 2825–2830.
34. Cutler, A.; Cutler, D.R.; Stevens, J.R. Random Forests. In *Ensemble Machine Learning: Methods and Applications*; Zhang, C., Ma, Y., Eds.; Springer: Boston, MA, USA, 2012; pp. 157–175.
35. Horning, N. Random Forests: An algorithm for image classification and generation of continuous fields data sets. In Proceedings of the International Conference on Geoinformatics for Spatial Infrastructure Development in Earth and Allied Sciences, Osaka, Japan, 9–11 December 2010; pp. 1–6.
36. Sullivan, L.M.; Velez, A.A.; Longe, N.; Larese, A.M.; Galea, S. Removing the Graduate Record Examination as an Admissions Requirement Does Not Impact Student Success. *Public Health Rev.* **2022**, *43*, 1605023. [CrossRef] [PubMed]
37. Langin, K. A Wave of Graduate Programs Drops the GRE Application Requirement. Available online: https://www.science.org/content/article/wave-graduate-programs-drops-gre-application-requirement (accessed on 28 May 2023).
38. Peng, J.; Harwell, M.; Liou, S.M.; Ehman, L.H. Advances in missing data methods and implications for educational research. *Real Data Anal.* **2006**, *3178*, 102.
39. Pigott, T.D. A Review of Methods for Missing Data. *Educ. Res. Eval.* **2001**, *7*, 353–383. [CrossRef]
40. Khalid, S.; Khalil, T.; Nasreen, S. A survey of feature selection and feature extraction techniques in machine learning. In Proceedings of the 2014 Science and Information Conference, London, UK, 27–29 August 2014; pp. 372–378.
41. Chizi, B.; Maimon, O. Dimension Reduction and Feature Selection. In *Data Mining and Knowledge Discovery Handbook*; Maimon, O., Rokach, L., Eds.; Springer: Boston, MA, USA, 2010; pp. 83–100.
42. Brownlee, J. *Data Preparation for Machine Learning: Data Cleaning, Feature Selection, and Data Transforms in Python*; Machine Learning Mastery: Vermont, Australia, 2020.
43. Jabbar, H.; Khan, R.Z. Methods to avoid over-fitting and under-fitting in supervised machine learning (comparative study). *Comput. Sci. Commun. Instrum. Devices* **2015**, *70*, 163–172.
44. Gu, J.; Oelke, D. Understanding bias in machine learning. *arXiv* **2019**, arXiv:1909.01866.
45. Ashfaq, U.; Poolan Marikannan, B.; Raheem, M. Managing Student Performance: A Predictive Analytics using Imbalanced Data. *Int. J. Recent Technol. Eng.* **2020**, *8*, 2277–2283. [CrossRef]
46. Flores, V.; Heras, S.; Julian, V. Comparison of Predictive Models with Balanced Classes Using the SMOTE Method for the Forecast of Student Dropout in Higher Education. *Electronics* **2022**, *11*, 457. [CrossRef]
47. Revathy, M.; Kamalakkannan, S.; Kavitha, P. Machine Learning based Prediction of Dropout Students from the Education University using SMOTE. In Proceedings of the 2022 4th International Conference on Smart Systems and Inventive Technology (ICSSIT), Tirunelveli, India, 20–22 January 2022; pp. 1750–1758.
48. Berrar, D. Cross-Validation. In *Encyclopedia of Bioinformatics and Computational Biology*, Ranganathan, S., Gribskov, M., Nakai, K., Schönbach, C., Eds.; Academic Press: Oxford, 2019; pp. 542–545. [CrossRef]
49. Hanley, J.A.; McNeil, B.J. The meaning and use of the area under a receiver operating characteristic (ROC) curve. *Radiology* **1982**, *143*, 29–36. [CrossRef] [PubMed]
50. Jin, H.; Ling, C.X. Using AUC and accuracy in evaluating learning algorithms. *IEEE Trans. Knowl. Data Eng.* **2005**, *17*, 299–310. [CrossRef]
51. Bergstra, J.; Bengio, Y. Random search for hyper-parameter optimization. *J. Mach. Learn. Res.* **2012**, *13*, 281–305.
52. Belete, D.M.; Huchaiah, M.D. Grid search in hyperparameter optimization of machine learning models for prediction of HIV/AIDS test results. *Int. J. Comput. Appl.* **2022**, *44*, 875–886. [CrossRef]
53. Feature Importance Evaluation. Available online: https://scikit-learn.org/stable/modules/ensemble.html (accessed on 1 August 2022).
54. Lundberg, S.M.; Erion, G.; Chen, H.; DeGrave, A.; Prutkin, J.M.; Nair, B.; Katz, R.; Himmelfarb, J.; Bansal, N.; Lee, S.-I. From local explanations to global understanding with explainable AI for trees. *Nat. Mach. Intell.* **2020**, *2*, 56–67. [CrossRef] [PubMed]
55. Aljuaid, T.; Sasi, S. Proper imputation techniques for missing values in data sets. In Proceedings of the 2016 International Conference on Data Science and Engineering (ICDSE), Cochin, India, 23–25 August 2016; pp. 1–5.
56. Newgard, C.D.; Lewis, R.J. Missing Data: How to Best Account for What Is Not Known. *JAMA* **2015**, *314*, 940–941. [CrossRef]
57. Sawilowsky, S.S. *Real Data Analysis*; Information Age Pub.: Charlotte, NC, USA, 2007.
58. Baudeu, R.; Wright, M.N.; Loecher, M. *Are SHAP Values Biased Towards High-Entropy Features?* Springer Nature: Cham, Switzerland, 2023; pp. 418–433.
59. Seger, C. An Investigation of Categorical Variable Encoding Techniques in Machine Learning: Binary Versus One-Hot and Feature Hashing. Master's Thesis, KTH Royal Institute of Technology School of Electrical Engineering and Computer Science, Stockholm, Sweden, 25 September 2018.
60. Cerda, P.; Varoquaux, G.; Kégl, B. Similarity encoding for learning with dirty categorical variables. *Mach. Learn.* **2018**, *107*, 1477–1494. [CrossRef]
61. Huang, J.; Galal, G.; Etemadi, M.; Vaidyanathan, M. Evaluation and Mitigation of Racial Bias in Clinical Machine Learning Models: Scoping Review. *JMIR Med. Inf.* **2022**, *10*, e36388. [CrossRef]

62. Afrose, S.; Song, W.; Nemeroff, C.B.; Lu, C.; Yao, D. Subpopulation-specific machine learning prognosis for underrepresented patients with double prioritized bias correction. *Commun. Med.* **2022**, *2*, 111. [CrossRef]
63. American Assocation of Veterinary Medical Colleges. *Annual Data Report 2022–2023*; American Assocation of Veterinary Medical Colleges: Washington, DC, USA, 2023; pp. 1–67.
64. Boyajian, M.Y. Student Intervention System Using Machine Learning. Ph.D. Thesis, American University of Beirut, Beirut, Lebanon, 2019.
65. Yakin, M.; Linden, K. Adaptive e-learning platforms can improve student performance and engagement in dental education. *J. Dent. Educ.* **2021**, *85*, 1309–1315. [CrossRef]
66. Kuzminsky, J.; Phillips, H.; Sharif, H.; Moran, C.; Gleason, H.E.; Topulos, S.P.; Pitt, K.; McNeil, L.K.; McCoy, A.M.; Kesavadas, T. Reliability in performance assessment creates a potential application of artificial intelligence in veterinary education: Evaluation of suturing skills at a single institution. *Am. J. Vet. Res.* **2023**, *84*, 1–11. [CrossRef] [PubMed]

Disclaimer/Publisher's Note: The statements, opinions and data contained in all publications are solely those of the individual author(s) and contributor(s) and not of MDPI and/or the editor(s). MDPI and/or the editor(s) disclaim responsibility for any injury to people or property resulting from any ideas, methods, instructions or products referred to in the content.

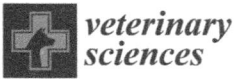

Article

The Use of Simulation Models and Student-Owned Animals for Teaching Clinical Examination Procedures in Veterinary Medicine

Ricardo Marcos [1,*], Sónia Macedo [2,3], Macamen de Vega [3] and Pablo Payo-Puente [3,4]

[1] Cytology and Hematology Diagnostic Services, Laboratory of Histology and Embryology, Department of Microscopy, ICBAS—School of Medicine and Biomedical Sciences, University of Porto (U.Porto), Rua de Jorge Viterbo Ferreira, 228, 4050-313 Porto, Portugal
[2] Centro de Investigação Vasco da Gama (CIVG), Escola Universitária Vasco da Gama (EUVG), Campus Universitário, Av. José R. Sousa Fernandes, 3020-210 Coimbra, Portugal
[3] GIIPEV-Grupo Investigação em Ensino de Medicina Veterinária, Rua de Jorge Viterbo Ferreira 228, 4050-313 Porto, Portugal
[4] Department of Veterinary Clinics, School of Medicine and Biomedical Sciences ICBAS-UP, Rua de Jorge Viterbo Ferreira 228, 4050-313 Porto, Portugal
* Correspondence: rmarcos@icbas.up.pt

Simple Summary: Clinical examination procedures (CEPs) are cornerstone skills for veterinarians that are taught in all veterinary faculties. CEPs include procedures that are well tolerated by animals and others that are not. In a classical teaching approach, institutional animals which are kept in kennels at the university are used to teach and practice CEPs. Undergraduate students (n = 231) from four consecutive years were assigned to two groups that used institutional animals only (AO) or a combination of students' owned animals and simulation models (model–animal, MA) to teach and practice CEPs. The latter comprised stuffed dogs and handmade molding silicone models. The learning outcome of each system was compared through questionnaires, grades, and pass rates in objectively structured clinical examinations. Most veterinary students had their own animals, and it was easy to have a dog per group of two students in class. All the students' owned animals adapted well to this environment. The interest in the practical activities with the simulation models was comparable to that exhibited in the AO system, and students reported to learn more with the MA method. No differences existed in the final grades and pass rates. The MA system was effective for learning CEPs. Beyond animal welfare advantages, the MA system increased out-of-school training and had financial saving benefits.

Abstract: Clinical examination procedures (CEPs) are cornerstone clinical skills for veterinary practitioners, being taught in all veterinary faculties. CEPs include innocuous procedures that are well tolerated by animals as well as more distressful and less tolerated ones. In a classical approach, institutional animals are used to teach and practice CEPs. Two hundred and thirty-one undergraduate students from four consecutive years were assigned to two groups that used institutional animals only (AO) or a combination of students' owned animals and simulation models (model–animal, MA) to teach and practice CEPs. This latter comprised stuffed teddy dogs, eye and ear models made of molding silicone, as well as skin models. The learning outcome of each system was compared through questionnaires (throughout classes and at the end of course), grades, and pass rates in objectively structured clinical examinations. Most veterinary students had their own animals, being easy to have a dog per group of two students in class. All the students' owned animals adapted well to this environment. The interest in the practical activities with the simulation models was comparable to that exhibited in the classical AO system. Students reported to learn more with the MA system than with the AO, while the interest on the subjects and the relevance were appraised similarly in both systems. No differences existed in the final grades and pass rates. The MA system was effective for learning CEPs. Beyond animal welfare advantages, this system increased the out-of-school training and had financial saving benefits, being a valuable option for the teaching and training of CEPs.

Citation: Marcos, R.; Macedo, S.; de Vega, M.; Payo-Puente, P. The Use of Simulation Models and Student-Owned Animals for Teaching Clinical Examination Procedures in Veterinary Medicine. *Vet. Sci.* 2023, 10, 193. https://doi.org/10.3390/vetsci10030193

Academic Editor: Simona Sacchini

Received: 24 January 2023
Revised: 23 February 2023
Accepted: 2 March 2023
Published: 4 March 2023

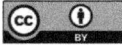

Copyright: © 2023 by the authors. Licensee MDPI, Basel, Switzerland. This article is an open access article distributed under the terms and conditions of the Creative Commons Attribution (CC BY) license (https://creativecommons.org/licenses/by/4.0/).

Keywords: educational methodology; simulator; clinical examination

1. Introduction

Clinical examination procedures (CEPs) are cornerstone clinical skills for veterinary practitioners and serve as a baseline for all internal medicine and clinical activities. These procedures are taught in all veterinary faculties, being mandatory practical competences for all veterinary students [1]. Depending on the veterinary curricula, CEPs may be taught either in the second or third year of the veterinary degree. CEPs are needed to recognize signs of illness in animals. CEPs include innocuous procedures that are fairly well tolerated by animals, such as auscultation or lymph node palpation, as well as distressful and less tolerated procedures, such as otoscopy, fine needle aspiration (FNA), or many ophthalmology tests.

It is well recognized that a major investment in learning basic skills, such as CEPs, will save many hours of auxiliary teaching in future practical contexts and offers major benefits by developing the practical confidence of students [2]. In fact, the lack of self-confidence by students has been described as the most common source of negative emotions when a practical skill must be performed [3]. Learning CEP (e.g., exploring the clinical signs of an animal within a reasonable time) is similar to any other practical knowledge such as music, sculpture, or even surgery. Besides knowing how things are performed in an abstract way (knowledge), students need to spend their time "learning how to do" (skills learning) and repeatedly practice the procedures, so that the CEP can be performed systematically and quickly (intrinsic skills). To analyze the learning effectiveness of CEP, the Kirkpatrick's training evaluation framework can be used [4]. This model comprises distinct levels of evaluation, from assessing the students' reactions and learning in the first and second levels, to addressing changes in the behavior and output results at the third and fourth levels, respectively. The first and second levels are also called internal criteria, being the focus of most studies on training programs, in opposition to the third and fourth levels, the so-called external criteria, that typically occur after the program [5].

For teaching CEPs, two main sets of items are usually needed: exploration tools (e.g., thermometers, otoscopes, ophthalmoscopes, reflex hammers, containment systems, stethoscopes) and animals, which serve as "models" for the skill learning. Currently, there is a trend towards reducing the use of animals in teaching procedures in many veterinary faculties [6–8]. It is estimated that up to 10% of the animals listed for experimental purposes are used for education and training [9]. Traditionally, live animals used for education purposes have been derived from three sources: animals seen at the university clinics, shelter animals, and purpose-bred animals [10,11]. Universities frequently buy dogs of specific breeds (e.g., Beagles) [10] from authorized breeders that are used for both animal research and learning activities. This has important ethical connotations because animals will be forced to live all, or almost all, of their existence in a university kennel, which often has limited space.

In recent years, there has been intense research on the use of non-animal models for learning various subjects [6]. Some universities around the globe, from the Ankara University to the University of Hannover or the University of California Davis, for example, already have a long history of the so-called "Clinical Skill Labs", where plastic models and full-body manikins are used to learn and practice various procedures [8]. Even if it has been shown that the learning outcomes with non-harmful teaching methods can be similar to the use of harmful animal models [12], it is still advocated among veterinary educators that practicing on living animals is needed for proper learning [7]. For learning purposes, model-based and animal-based approaches are often grounded on polarized opinions, according to their advantages and drawbacks [7]. To the best of our knowledge, there are no studies focusing on the use of a mixed model–animal (MA) system, which, at least in theory, could incorporate the best factors of each polarized opinion.

The aim of this study was to evaluate the use of an innovative solution for teaching CEPs to veterinary students and compare it with a traditional "animals only" (AO) solution. The mixed MA system was comprised of simulation models used for harmful and distressful procedures and student-owned animals used for non-stressful activities.

2. Materials and Methods

2.1. Experimental Design

To evaluate the performance of the MA system, a case-control monocentric study was performed. Two hundred and thirty-one undergraduate third-year students in a Doctorate in Veterinary Medicine (DVM) program were assigned to two groups in four consecutive years (N1 to N4). In the control group, [N1(2018/19) 57 students and N2(2019/20) 53 students] only institutional animals (Beagles) were used in practical "learning-by-doing" classes. In this AO group, all in-class CEPs were practiced only with institutional animals. The case group [N3(2020/21) 61 students and N4 (2021/22) 60 students] adhered to the MA approach, using low-cost models for distressful procedures (Figure 1), whilst conducting non-stressful procedures using student-owned dogs (Figure 2). These four consecutive years were comparable in terms of gender distribution [17% and 15% males in N1(2018/19) and N2(2019/20), respectively, and 21% and 23% males in N3(2020/21) and N4 (2021/22), respectively] and age of students [21 years old in both groups, range 20 to 34 years old].

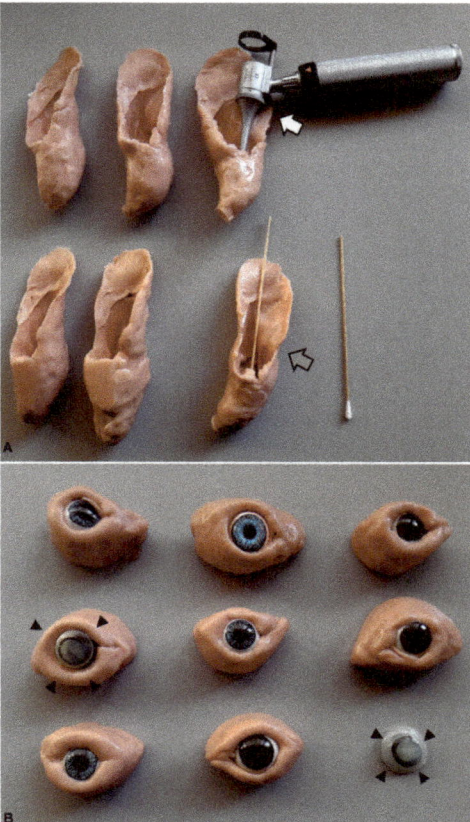

Figure 1. Ear (**A**) and eye (**B**) models made with moldable silicone. The ear models are at scale (medium sized dog) and allowed otoscopy (white arrow) and ear cytology (grey arrow) procedures. The eye models included the eye and eyelids; the corneas could be changed to represent various clinical conditions, such as corneal edema (arrowheads).

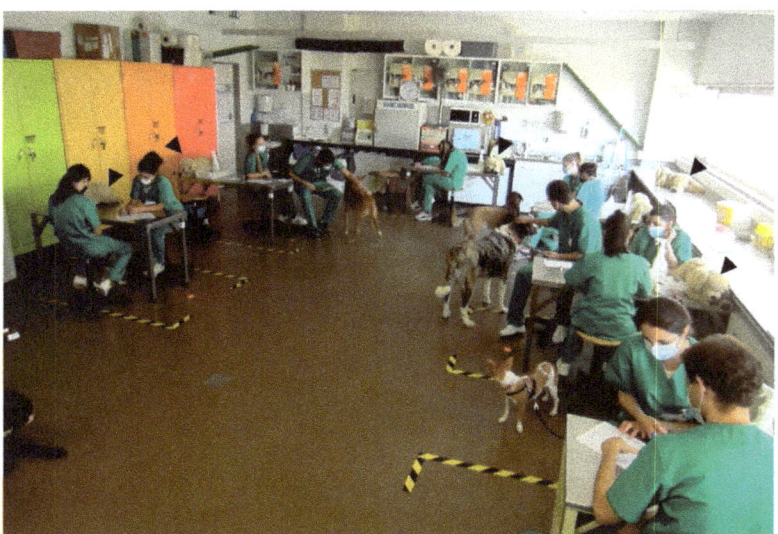

Figure 2. Students in class with their own animals of different sizes and breeds. Each group of two or three students first practiced the procedures with a stuffed teddy dog (arrowheads) and then with their own dog.

To assess the students' perception of the learning methodology, anonymous questionnaires were obtained. Two types were used: brief questionnaires with a single question, which were distributed after each class, and long questionnaires that were filled after the final examination. Both questionnaires included questions with Likert scales (1 to 5 scale, 3 being the average) which appraised the amount of learning, the interest and relevance of classes, as well as issues regarding the final examination (difficulty, stringency, and fairness). Answers to the questionnaires were always voluntary and anonymous, and personal data were never collected.

In both the case (MA) and control (AO) groups, an objectively structured clinical examination (OSCE) was performed at the end of the semester using the same evaluator (PP), who has more than 20 years of experience with OSCE evaluations. The same type of OSCE evaluations were performed for the two groups (case and controls). The use of institutional animals in classes was always preceded by the authorization of the Institutional Animal Welfare Committee (P328/2019/ORBEA and P347/2020/ORBEA). The collection of data from students was authorized by competent local authorities [Comissão de Ética 2022/CE(413/2023/CETI)].

2.2. Simulation Models

The simulation models comprised stuffed teddy dogs (Gosig Golden, IKEA, Almhult, Sweden), which were used in basic procedures (restraints and positioning for different types of exams) and in some painful procedures and tests (e.g., cystocentesis, deep sensitivity tests). For ophthalmology and otoscopy procedures, eye and ear models were built in-house, made of molding silicone (Herbitas Blanda Blanda, Nakamor Gel Corporation, Valencia, Spain) (Figure 1). The ear model allowed the practice of sampling for cytology purposes, as well as for otoscopy, with different scenarios, such as inflammation and ruptured tympanum and the presence of foreign bodies. Regarding the eye models, these included the eyelids and eye, with interchangeable corneas that simulated various clinical conditions, such as corneal edema (Figure 1), cornea stromal hemorrhage with neovascularization, and anterior chamber hemorrhage (hyphema). For dermatology, skin models were used to teach skin biopsies and skin scrapings, as well as models for FNA [13]. The latter comprised two types of models, namely, boxes covered with artificial fur, with paintball munitions of different size, so that students could practice the sample collection using FNA [13], and small, soft plastic containers with pork-fat and bovine thymus, in which students could not only practice the FNA procedure, but also stain the retrieved cells and observe them using a microscope.

2.3. Student-Owned Animals

Students could bring their own companion animals to practical classes, voluntarily, without any age, sex, or breed requirements, if they were vaccinated and dewormed. Animals had to bear a leash to avoid eventual conflicts and muzzles were provided if needed. For ethical reasons, no painful or stressful manipulations were performed on students' animals during classes. These practical classes are not considered as animal experimentation by current European and National Legislations (Law 113/2013). For the initial CEP (e.g., holding and restraining the animal), students first practiced with stuffed teddy dogs (Gosig Golden) and only utilized their own companion animals afterwards, assisted by the teacher. As previously mentioned, all possibly painful procedures were practiced only in simulation models.

2.4. Comparison between Model–Animal and Animal-Only Systems

Answers to the questionnaires and the exam pass rates in the final practical examination were compared. Regarding the latter, it was performed using Beagle dogs (AO) or with simulation models and their own animals (MA). An OSCE scoresheet was filled during the practical evaluation, and the comparison between groups focused on pass rates and final grades. Once students took their practical exam and received their grades, they answered a final questionnaire anonymously. This assessed the students' own perception regarding the learning process, the importance of the knowledge acquired, and the degree of difficulty of the practical test.

Upon request, students were allowed to use the classroom facilities during out-of-school time. The number of requests per semester was compared in both systems.

2.5. Statistical Analysis

SPSS26 statistics software, version 26.0.0.0 (IBM, Armonk, NY, USA) was used for analysis. Normally distributed continuous data (final grades and number of requests to use the classroom out of school time) were analyzed using Student's *t*-test, whereas other data were analyzed using the Mann–Whitney U test (questionnaire answers). A value of $p < 0.05$ was considered statistically significant.

3. Results

Most veterinary students had their own animals (62%) or had dogs from friends or family that could be taken to classes; therefore, it was easy to obtain one dog per group of two students during class. By adjusting the students' class schedules, the animals came happily with their owners and stayed during classes without signs of stress. There were no conflicts between students' animals in the MA system. Animals adapted fairly well to the class environment with other dogs and became more sociable over time. Furthermore, some students reported that these periods of socialization were beneficial for the animal's behavior at home.

For most students, this was their first contextualized practical experience with different animals (young/old, thin/obese, calm/nervous) from various breeds. This contrasted to the practical classes of previous years (AO groups), which included only institutional Beagles, which were very similar to each other.

The evaluation by students during the semester with the mixed system (MA) was positive, and their general impression improved over time, as assessed by using the brief questionnaires (Figure 3).

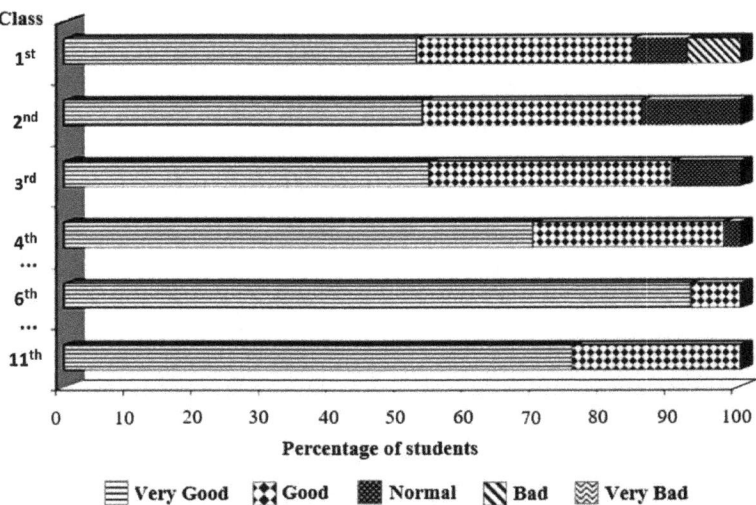

Figure 3. Students' general evaluation of the classes using the mixed model system, as assessed using brief questionnaires in N3 (2020/21) and N4 (2021/22). In the first class, 8% of students rated the class as "Bad", and another 8% rated it as "Normal". By the fourth class, this percentage was reduced to 2%, and, thereafter, students appraised the classes as "Good" or "Very Good".

In the final questionnaire, when students appraised the amount of learning (1 to 5 Likert scale, 3 being the average), it was rated 4.71 ± 0.40 in the MA, which was superior ($p < 0.001$) to the AO classical system (4.31 ± 0.59) (Table 1). The interest was similar, being rated as 4.52 ± 0.49 in the MA and 4.47 ± 0.54 in the AO groups. Regarding the relevance of classes for their clinical activity as DVMs, as perceived by students, it was rated as 4.88 ± 0.21 in the MA group, similar to that of the AO system (4.79 ± 0.45). Regarding the final examination (difficulty, stringency, and fairness), no differences existed between the systems. The perception of students regarding the level of demand and difficulty of the exam were comparable for both groups of students. The pass rates obtained on the exam were similar: 81% to 88% in the AO system and 87% to 92% in the MA (Table 1). In this vein, the blended learning system was robust and maintained high standards of student learning, even under atypical conditions imposed by the recent COVID-19 pandemic.

Table 1. Comparison between students enrolled in the animal only system (AO), corresponding to 110 students from N1(2018/19) and N2(2019/20), and the students using the model–animal (MA) approach, comprising 121 students from N3(2020/21) and N4 (2021/22).

	Animal-Only (AO)	Model–Animal (MA)
Final questionnaire (Likert scale)		
Amount of learning	4.31 ± 0.59	4.71 ± 0.40 *
Interest	4.47 ± 0.54	4.52 ± 0.49
Relevance of classes	4.79 ± 0.45	4.88 ± 0.21
Pass rates at final exam	81–88%	87–92%

* $p < 0.001$.

Regarding the simulation models, it was possible to create low-cost and accessible models with very high performances (Figure 4). All models could and were used by students in and out of school hours. The models (stuffed animals, soft silicone devices) were robust and suffered no apparent deterioration from repeated use by students during these two curricular years. The interest in the practical activities with the simulation models was comparable to that exhibited in the classical AO system. In some activities, such as the otoscopy and ophthalmology procedures, it was even greater, since students had higher chances of repeating more difficult procedures out of school hours, which was not possible with institutional animals in the AO system. During the two years, we had over 250 requests from students during the semester to use the classroom facilities out of school time in the MA system (compared with 80 requests in the previous years). In this facility, they could use the stuffed teddy dogs and silicone models and could bring their own animals, working in small groups (Figure 5). After the fourth week, students already recognized that they were using the models and animals regularly out of school time. More than half of the students had used more than one animal of different breeds to learn CEP (40% used two animals, 12% used three, and 2% had used more than three different animals). Despite having their own live animals available, a third of students used the models to practice out of school time. During the vacation periods, students also requested the models so that they could be used for learning at home. The number of requests was significantly higher in the MA system compared to AO.

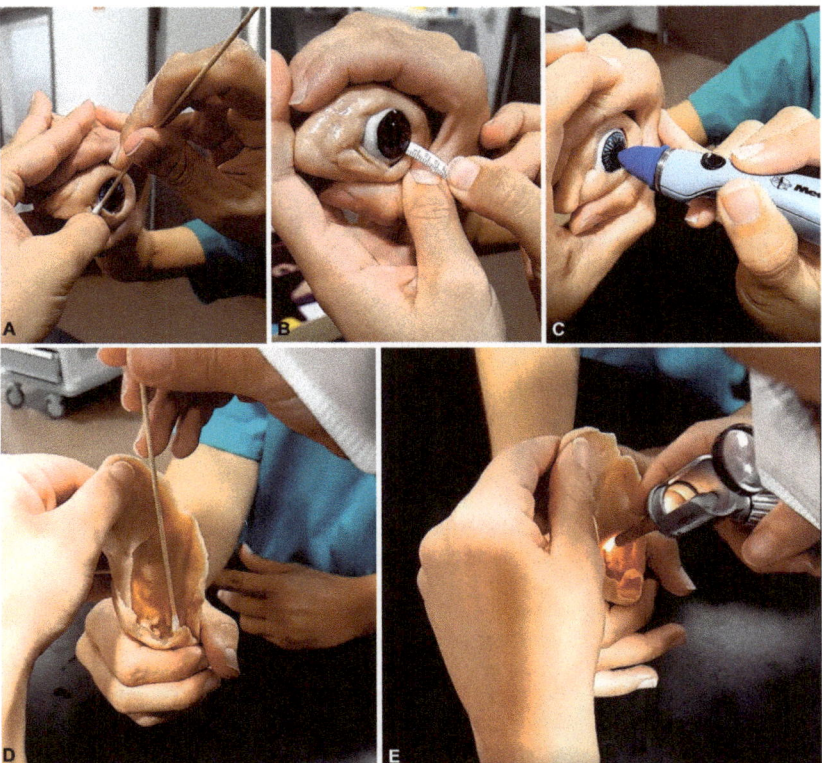

Figure 4. Students using the models to practice ophthalmology (**A–C**) and otoscopy procedures (**D**,**E**). By working in pairs, students obtained conjunctival swabs (**A**), performed the Shirmer's test (**B**), and used the tonometer to assess the intraocular pressure (**C**). They also obtained ear canal swabs (**D**) and used the otoscope (**E**). In the ear canal, the tympanic membrane could be changed to represent simulated clinical conditions (inflammation and ruptured tympanum).

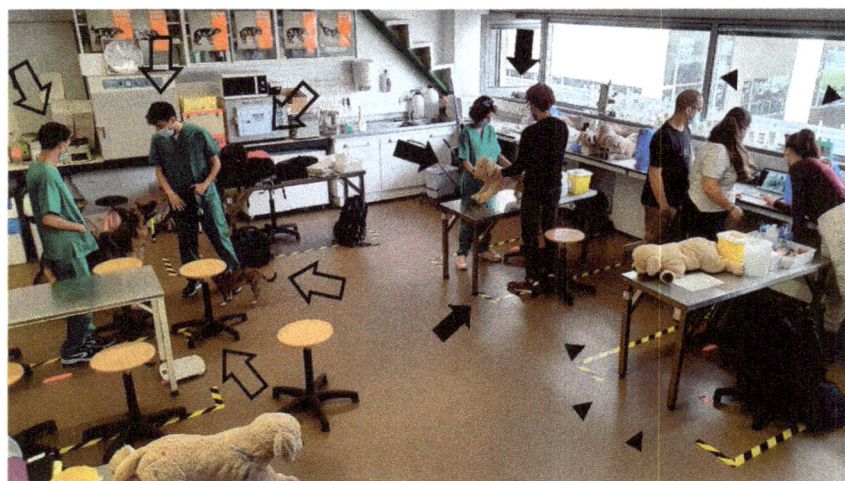

Figure 5. Students practicing out of school time, either using their own animals (block arrows) or stuffed teddy dogs (arrows and arrowheads). The group of students on the right (arrowheads) is also using video resources (supporting class material).

4. Discussion

Currently, veterinary teaching stands in a crossroad between the classical perspective of using live animals and the more modern approach of using simulators and "Clinical Skills Labs" [6,8,14–17]. The use of live animals as "learning instruments" evokes ethical and financial dilemmas. Veterinary training itself seems to reverse the natural empathic and compassionate character of students and, probably, of later veterinarians. It has been described that veterinary students at the end of their 5 years of training tend to be less compassionate towards fear, boredom, hunger, and pain in animals [18], being less likely to treat animal pain than junior students [19]. Moreover, it has been shown that moral reasoning declines during the 5 years of veterinary education [20]. In the MA system, veterinary students tended to view the animals used in classes as their companion animals and not just as learning instruments imposed by teachers and administrators [20]. This reasoning probably accounts for the smooth transition from institutional animals to their own companion animals.

Using the students' animals also has financial and animal welfare advantages. In our faculty, Beagles were used only for ≈26 weeks per year, meaning that the animals spend more time housed in kennels than in pedagogical activities. Regardless of the ethical issue that this entails, the pedagogical profitability of these animals is low, and the cost of food/personnel is very high. The cost of kenneling a dog varies substantially between countries, and marked differences may even exist within a country; still, it may cost between 4000 EUR (as in our institution, data not shown) to 6000 EUR per year [21]. Beyond the financial advantages of the MA system, there are animal welfare issues that must be considered. Spatial restriction is one of the factors that generates more stress [22–24], contributing to a decrease in animal welfare in kennels [24]. Numerous studies have already highlighted that dogs housed in kennel facilities for long periods of time experience suboptimal living conditions [22,25–28]. For instance, a higher incidence of chronic stress-related behavior problems has been described in dogs 4 to 8 weeks after admission to a kennel facility [22,28]. In this context, issues regarding the animal welfare of institutional animals can legitimately be raised, and there is a current "public opinion" advocating for a decrease in the use of animals among higher education institutions [7,11].

Shelter animals would be another alternative source, which has been assessed previously for teaching clinical-based subjects [10]. However, this would still require an established protocol with nearby shelters and would demand further logistics, such as the transport of students and a classroom facility at the shelter. Moreover, using shelter animals would still raise concerns regarding the repetition of painful or stressful procedures for learning purposes.

Many veterinary faculties in the world are reducing the number of animals used for teaching purposes, moving towards using simulation strategies and developing simulation devices [6,8,14]. Recently, the use of simulation-based methods in veterinary education has been reviewed, and many studies have shown that simulation prototypes reduce students' stress when faced with real situations involving animals [29–33]. Repetitive practice is a major advantage of using simulators, and it has been shown that a repetitive practice in a model, prior to reproducing the task in a live animal, increases the self-confidence of students, develops their dexterity and motor skills, and reduces their levels of anxiety [33]. The use of complex simulators is not necessarily a prerequisite, since it has been shown in the surgical field that simple suture models can be as effective as more expensive devices [34–37]. Some high-tech simulation devices can be highly expensive, and some studies have been devoted to evaluating simpler and more economic solutions [16,17]. To the best of our knowledge, there are few experiences with low-cost and custom-based models in the context of veterinary semiology. Our simulation models cost from 7 EUR (Gosig Golden) to 90 EUR (more sophisticated eye and ear models) (Figure 1) and were endurable enough for students' manipulation under intensive use (during classes and out of school time). The use of models beyond classes was also beneficial, since it has been shown that the learning of practical skills is enhanced if the tasks can be repeated in the following days [38]. This may account for the increased amount of learning reported by the students in the final questionnaire. Still, we are currently unable to disclose if such an effect was due to the use of models, their own companion animals, or both. If, on one hand, they practiced more on the models, then this probably helped to strengthen their self-confidence on the learned skills; on the other hand, the students became actively involved in the learning process by using their own companion animals, and this may have helped establishing a nurturing environment, in which students felt satisfied and may have learned more effectively. Furthermore, we may not exclude that the novelty effect may have led to an overvaluation of the students towards the practical skills they were learning. We cannot rule out the consequences of the Hawthorne effect, i.e., students behaving differently because they are being included in a study. The consequences of research participation for behaviors being investigated do exist, although little can be known for sure about the conditions under which they operate, their mechanisms, and their magnitudes [39]. Therefore, we will extend the present study to include more curricular years and will test this MA system in other institutions to have a wider global scope.

Our study has some limitations related to its single-center nature and learning outputs. Regarding the former, students were evaluated by a single instructor, not blinded to treatment/control status during the OSCEs, and this may be considered as a potential source of bias. Even if the eventual contribution towards the MA system cannot be excluded, this bias should be minimal considering that: (1) the instructor had a long experience in OSCE assessments, performing these evaluations for more than 20 years; (2) the students' feedback assessed by questionnaires was comparable in both systems; (3) out-of-class deliberate practice by students increased significantly using the MA system. Deliberate practice sets the path to mastering clinical skills and probably increased students' self-confidence in their practical skills, which will be needed later on in their fourth and fifth years of the DVM degree. It should be stressed that this study focused mostly on the first and second levels of the Kirkpatrick's learning model, since we mostly analyzed the reaction and learning, dismissing the third and fourth levels, behavior and results, which are influenced by many external factors, such as economic and organizational contexts [5]. Even if it may be assumed that the MA system may have changed the students' behavior, with students more compassionate towards fear, boredom, and pain in animals, we failed to assess this level. As for the fourth level, this could be addressed by evaluating the skills' maintenance [40], which could have been achieved by repeating some of the OSCE evaluations in the following years or by evaluating their performance as veterinary practitioners later on [5].

5. Conclusion

In conclusion, we have shown that the MA system is as effective for learning and practicing CEPs in dogs as the classical AO model. Further studies are needed to elucidate the specific effects of the models included herein; however, the finding that the MA system is effective should be highlighted, as it may set the path towards a more "animal welfare"-driven veterinary education, which could improve the training and humane condition of veterinary students and, consequently, of future veterinary practitioners.

Author Contributions: Conceptualization, R.M. and P.P.-P.; methodology, S.M., M.d.V. and P.P.-P.; software, R.M. and P.P.-P.; validation, R.M. and P.P.-P.; formal analysis, R.M. and P.P.-P.; investigation, S.M. and P.P.-P.; resources, S.M., M.d.V. and P.P.-P.; data curation, R.M. and P.P.-P.; writing—original draft preparation, R.M. and P.P.-P.; writing—review and editing, R.M. and P.P.-P.; visualization, P.P.-P.; supervision, P.P.-P.; project administration, P.P.-P.; funding acquisition, R.M. All authors have read and agreed to the published version of the manuscript.

Funding: This research received no external funding.

Institutional Review Board Statement: The study was conducted in accordance with the Declaration of Helsinki, and approved by the Institutional Review Board (or Ethics Committee) of CHUP/ICBAS—Centro Hospitalar da Universidade do Porto and School of Medicine and Biomedical Sciences (2022/CE/P17(P395/CETI/ICBAS) and (413/2023/CETI), approved on 12 October) for studies involving humans, and Institutional Animal Welfare Committee [(P328/2019/ORBEA) and (P347/2020/ORBEA)—Órgão Responsável pelo Bem-Estar dos Animais, ICBAS, approved on 5 March 2020) for the studies involving animals.

Informed Consent Statement: Informed consent was obtained from all subjects involved in the study. Written informed consent has been obtained from the patients to publish this paper.

Data Availability Statement: All data generated or analyzed during this study are included in this published article.

Conflicts of Interest: The authors declare no conflict of interest.

References

1. European Association of Establishments for Veterinary Education (EAEVE). European Coordination Committee for Veterinary Training (ECCVT) Day One Competences—Adopted 26 March 2015. EAEVE: Vienna, Austria. Available online: https://www.eaeve.org/fileadmin/downloads/eccvt/2015_2_D1C_Adopted_Annex_5.4.1.pdf (accessed on 3 March 2021).
2. Brown, S.; Glasner, A. *Evaluar en la Universidad. Problemas y Nuevos Enfoques*; Narcea Ed: Madrid, Spain, 2003.
3. Langebæk, R.; Eika, B.; Tanggaard, L.; Jensen, A.L.; Berendt, M. Emotions in Veterinary Surgical Students: A Qualitative Study. *J. Vet. Med. Educ.* **2012**, *39*, 312–321. [CrossRef]
4. Kirkpatrick, D.L.; Kirkpatrick, J.D. *Evalutating Training Programs*, 3rd ed.; Berrett-Koehler Publishers, Inc.: San Francisco, CA, USA, 2006; ISBN 9781576753484.
5. Alsalamah, A.; Callinan, C. Adaptation of Kirkpatrick's four-level model of training criteria to evaluate training programmes for Head Teachers. *Educ. Sci.* **2021**, *11*, 116. [CrossRef]
6. May, S. Developing Veterinary Clinical Skills: The Pedagogy. In *Veterinary Clinical Skills Manual*; Coombes, N., Silva-Fletcher, A., Eds.; CAB International: Wallingford, UK, 2018; pp. 3–6.
7. Zemanova, M.; Knight, A.; Lybaek, S. Educational use of animals in Europe indicates reluctance to implement alternatives. *ALTEX* **2021**, *38*, 490–506. [CrossRef]
8. Zambelli, D.; Canova, M.; Ballotta, G.; Ferrari, A.; Cunto, M. Innovative models for teaching reproduction in small animals: The experience at DIMEVET of Bologna University. *Theriogenology* **2023**, *196*, 244–253. [CrossRef] [PubMed]
9. Akbarsha, M.A.; Zeeshan, M.; Meenakumari, K.J. Alternatives to animals in education, research, and risk assessment: An overview with special reference to Indian context. *ALTEX Proc.* **2013**, *2*, 5–19.

10. Smeak, D.D. Teaching veterinary students using shelter animals. *J. Vet. Med. Educ.* **2008**, *35*, 26–30. [CrossRef]
11. Ward, S.L.; Osenkowski, P. Dog as the experimental model: Laboratory use of dogs in the United States. *ALTEX* **2022**, *39*, 605–620. [CrossRef] [PubMed]
12. Knight, A. The effectiveness of humane teaching methods in veterinary education. *ALTEX* **2007**, *24*, 91–109. [CrossRef]
13. Pires, J.L.; Payo, P.; Marcos, R. The Use of Simulators for Teaching Fine Needle Aspiration Cytology in Veterinary Medicine. *J. Vet. Med. Educ.* **2022**, *49*, 39–44. [CrossRef]
14. Hart, L.A.; Wood, M.W. Uses of animals and alternatives in college and veterinary education at the University of California, Davis: Institutional commitment for mainstreaming alternatives. *Altern. Lab. Anim.* **2004**, *32*, 617–620. [CrossRef]
15. Patronek, G.J.; Rauch, A. Systematic review of comparative studies examining alternatives to the harmful use of animals in biomedical education. *J. Am. Vet. Med. Assoc.* **2007**, *230*, 37–43. [CrossRef] [PubMed]
16. Langebaek, R.; Toft, N.; Eriksen, T. The SimSpay—Student perceptions of a low-cost build-it-yourself model for novice training of surgical skills in canine OVH. *J. Vet. Med. Educ.* **2015**, *42*, 166–171. [CrossRef]
17. Motta, T.; Carter, B.; Silveira, C.; Hill, L.; McLoughlin, M. Development and validation of a low-cost surgical simulator to teach canine ovariohysterectomy. In Proceedings of the InVeST 2015: International Veterinary Simulation in Teaching Conference, Hannover, Germany, 14–16 September 2015; German Medical Science GMS Publishing House: Düsseldorf, Germany, 2015.
18. Paul, E.S.; Podberscek, A.L. Veterinary Education and Students' Attitudes towards Animal Welfare. *Vet Rec.* **2000**, *146*, 269–272. [CrossRef] [PubMed]
19. Hellyer, P.W.; Frederick, C.; Lacy, M.; Salman, M.D.; Wagner, A.E. Attitudes of veterinary medical students, house officers, clinical faculty, and staff toward pain management in animals. *J. Am. Vet. Med. Assoc.* **1999**, *214*, 238–244.
20. Arluke, A. The use of dogs in medical and veterinary training: Understanding and approaching student uneasiness. *J. Appl. Anim. Welf. Sci.* **2004**, *7*, 197–204. [CrossRef] [PubMed]
21. "How Much Does It Cost to Board a Dog?" HomeGuide. Available online: https://homeguide.com/costs/dog-boarding-cost (accessed on 1 June 2022).
22. Beerda, B.; Schilder, M.B.; Bernadina, W.; Van Hooff, J.A.; De Vries, H.W.; Mol, J.A. Chronic stress in dogs subjected to social and spatial restriction. II. Hormonal and Immunological Responses. *Physiol. Behav.* **1999**, *66*, 243–254. [CrossRef]
23. Markowitz, H.; Woodworth, G. Experimental analysis and control of group behavior. In *Behavior of Captive Wild Animals*; Markowitz, H., Stevens, V.J., Eds.; Nelson-Hall: Chicago, IL, USA, 1978; pp. 107–131.
24. Morris, C.L.; Grandin, T.; Irlbeck, N.A. Companion animals symposium: Environmental enrichment for companion, exotic, and laboratory animals. *J. Anim. Sci.* **2011**, *89*, 4227–4238. [CrossRef]
25. Protopopova, A. Effects of sheltering on physiology, immune function, behavior, and the welfare of dogs. *Physiol. Behav.* **2016**, *159*, 95–103. [CrossRef]
26. Hubrecht, R.C.; Serpell, J.A.; Poole, T.B. Correlates of pen size and housing conditions on the behaviour of kennelled dogs. *Appl. Anim. Behav. Sci.* **1992**, *34*, 365–383. [CrossRef]
27. Beerda, B.; Schilder, M.B.H.; Van Hooff, J.A.; De Vries, H.W.; Mol, J.A. Behavioural and hormonal indicators of enduring environmental stress in dogs. *Anim. Welf.* **2000**, *9*, 49–62. [CrossRef]
28. Stephen, J.M.; Ledger, R.A. An audit of behavioral indicators of poor welfare in kenneled dogs in the United Kingdom. *J. Appl. Anim. Welf. Sci.* **2005**, *8*, 79–95. [CrossRef] [PubMed]
29. Badman, M.; Tullberg, M.; Hoglund, O.V.; Hagman, R. Veterinary student confidence after practicing with a new surgical training model for feline OVH. *J. Vet. Med. Educ.* **2016**, *43*, 427–433. [CrossRef]
30. Fahie, M.; Cloke, A.; Lagman, M.; Levi, O.; Schmidt, P. Training veterinary students to perform ovariectomy using theMOOSE spay model with traditional method versus the dowling spay retractor. *J. Vet. Med. Educ.* **2016**, *43*, 176–183. [CrossRef] [PubMed]
31. Read, E.K.; Vallevand, A.; Farrell, R.M. Evaluation of veterinary student surgical skills preparation for ovariohysterectomy using simulators: A pilot study. *J. Vet. Med. Educ.* **2016**, *43*, 190–213. [CrossRef]
32. Bradley, C.; Edwards, G.; Carlson, A. A synthetic abdominal model for teaching basic veterinary surgical techniques. In Proceedings of the InVeST 2015: International Veterinary Simulation in Teaching Conference, Hannover, Germany, 14–16 September 2015; German Medical Science GMS Publishing House: Düsseldorf, Germany, 2015.
33. Wetzel, C.M.; Kneebone, R.L.; Woloshynowych, M.; Moorthy, K. The effects of stress on surgical performance. *Am. J. Surg.* **2006**, *191*, 5–10. [CrossRef]
34. Gopinath, D.; McGreevy, P.D.; Zuber, R.M.; Klupiec, C.; Baguley, J.; Barrs, V.R. Developments in undergraduate teaching of small-animal soft-tissue surgical skills at the University of Sydney. *J. Vet. Med. Educ.* **2012**, *39*, 21–29. [CrossRef] [PubMed]
35. Chen, T.M.; Mellette, J.R. Surgical pearl: Tomato-an alternative model for shave biopsy training. *J. Am. Acad. Dermatol.* **2006**, *54*, 517–518. [CrossRef]
36. Kneebone, R.; Kidd, J.; Nestel, D.; Asvall, S.; Paraskeva, P.; Darzi, A. An innovative model for teaching and learning clinical procedures. *Med. Educ.* **2002**, *36*, 628–634. [CrossRef]
37. Yag-Howard, C. Making and Using a Mouse Pad Model of Skin to Practice Suturing Techniques. *Dermatol. Surg.* **2013**, *39*, 1947–1949. [CrossRef]
38. Malone, E. Evidence-Based clinical skills teaching and learning: What do we really know? *J. Vet. Med. Educ.* **2019**, *46*, 379–398. [CrossRef]

39. McCambridge, J.; Witton, J.; Elbourne, D. Systematic review of the Hawthorne effect: New concepts are needed to study research participation effects. *J. Clin. Epidemiol.* **2014**, *67*, 267–277. [CrossRef] [PubMed]
40. McGaghie, M.C.; Issenberg, S.B.; Petrusa, E.R.; Scalese, R.J. A critical review of simulation-based medical education research: 2003-2009. *Med. Educ.* **2010**, *44*, 50–63. [CrossRef] [PubMed]

Disclaimer/Publisher's Note: The statements, opinions and data contained in all publications are solely those of the individual author(s) and contributor(s) and not of MDPI and/or the editor(s). MDPI and/or the editor(s) disclaim responsibility for any injury to people or property resulting from any ideas, methods, instructions or products referred to in the content.

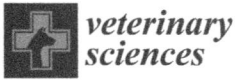

Article

Environment in Veterinary Education

María del Pino Palacios-Díaz and Vanessa Mendoza-Grimón *

Instituto de Estudios Ambientales y Recursos Naturales, Universidad de Las Palmas de Gran Canaria, 35017 Las Palmas, Spain
* Correspondence: v.mendozagrimon@ulpgc.es

Simple Summary: Environmental education is an important pillar for responding and adapting to climate change. The EU's common agricultural policy (CAP) has evolved from rules which supported the farming sector after years of famine and has become oriented towards looking at environmental aspects. The CAP policies oriented towards optimizing natural resource use, residue management, antimicrobial use reduction, the decrease in greenhouse gas (GHG) emissions, and animal welfare, need educational programs linked to the environmental problems. In this context, veterinarians are experts in animal production, welfare, food safety, and its technology and in public health under the One Health concept. Unfortunately, they are barely trained in environmental aspects, which would help them to understand and face the consequences of climate change in the rural world. Veterinarians must be able to quantify the effects of animal production in the environment by using different analysis tools, which need to be included in their learning programs. In addition, they must be able to optimize the use of natural resources, minimize GHG emissions, and manage the risks associated with climate change.

Abstract: Environmental concerns have become priority issues over the last third of the 20th century. The EU's common agricultural policy (CAP) has gone from rules which supported the farming sector after years of famine to being oriented towards looking at environmental aspects. Therefore, it has evolved not only to react to a changing market and consumer demands but also to respond to climate change and the need for sustainable development. Environmental education is an important pillar for responding and adapting to climate change. The CAP policies oriented towards optimizing the use of natural resources, residue management, antimicrobial use reduction, the decrease of greenhouse gas emissions (GHG), and animal welfare need linked educational programs. In this context, veterinarians, being experts in animal production, welfare, and food safety and its technology and public health under the One Health concept, are scarcely informed in environmental aspects, which would help them to understand and face the consequences of climate change in the rural world. Future veterinarians must be able to quantify the effects of animal production on the environment, optimizing the use of natural resources, minimizing GHG emissions, and managing the risks associated with climate change by using different analysis tools that need to be included in their learning programs.

Keywords: environment; climate change; veterinarian education; one health; soil food web; GHG emissions; climate change

Citation: Palacios-Díaz, M.d.P.; Mendoza-Grimón, V. Environment in Veterinary Education. *Vet. Sci.* **2023**, *10*, 146. https://doi.org/10.3390/vetsci10020146

Academic Editor: Annamaria Passantino

Received: 26 December 2022
Revised: 3 February 2023
Accepted: 9 February 2023
Published: 10 February 2023

Copyright: © 2023 by the authors. Licensee MDPI, Basel, Switzerland. This article is an open access article distributed under the terms and conditions of the Creative Commons Attribution (CC BY) license (https://creativecommons.org/licenses/by/4.0/).

1. Introduction

Environmental concern has become a priority issue over the last third of the 20th century. The policy's original goals are included in the Treaty of Rome. Launched in 1962, the EU's common agricultural policy (CAP) supports farmers and ensures Europe's food security [1]. While the CAP originally introduced rules for member states which would support the farming sector after years of devastating war and famine [2], it has progressively been re-oriented to look at environmental aspects. Therefore, it has evolved not only to react to a changing market and consumer demands but also to respond to climate change, biodiversity loss, and the need for sustainable development. Animals will feel the impact of climate change through multiple, often interacting, means, including changing patterns of infectious diseases, increased exposure to heat, contaminants, and extreme weather, changes in access to the natural resources they need for daily living, and shifts in animal ecology, sociobiology, and population dynamics [3].

The new concept of animal production has created environmental problems in certain geographical locations, which has led many countries to review their regulations with regard to intensive livestock farming and its inclusion in such regulations. This review aims to limit the direct effect of the livestock facilities themselves on the environment; it also considers the regulation of waste removal from livestock farms, with adequate management technologies to dispose of all the generated waste in an environmentally friendly manner. In Europe there is a payment for practices beneficial to the climate and the environment; this is also known as the "green payment". This allows an annual payment to be granted for each admissible hectare linked to a basic payment right, if certain environmental practices are respected, and depending on the structure of the farm. Therefore, veterinarians need to know how to advise the farmers on how to proceed in exercising this right.

In this context, veterinarians who conduct their activities in rural zones must deeply understand these environment-related concepts. However, it is not clear whether veterinarian teaching programs are touching on these subjects, nor is it clear whether the veterinarians' investigation aims are related to the discussed environmental issues. Hence, the purpose of this study was to determine: (i) what the main environmental issues are that veterinarians must know, particularly those working in the European context; (ii) whether there is enough content regarding the mentioned issues on the veterinary students' syllabus, which is crucial to achieving sustainable rural development; and (iii) whether there are veterinarian publications related to environmental aspects; these are needed when proper education is encouraged.

2. Materials and Methods

To develop and justify the issues that veterinarians must know, we made a scientific (taking into account articles and projects) and normative review, including some tools useful to managing some of the concepts related to climate change. In addition, a study of the skills described by the Spanish Government to develop a veterinarian degree related to environmental issues was incorporated.

To demonstrate whether the above-mentioned issues were taught in veterinary schools, we presented (i) a scientific review; (ii) the results of an anonymous survey made of veterinarians from the USA and Canada to identify any educational gaps regarding veterinary medicine and climate change; (iii) the ideas exposed on some websites regarding veterinary education and veterinarian practices and climate change; and (iv) the results from a study of subjects related to the environmental issues of nine veterinary faculties in Europe: Alfort (France), Bologna (Italy), Budapest (Hungary), Hannover (Germany), Liège (Belgium), Liverpool (England, UK), Nantes (France), Uppsala (Sweden), and Utrecht (Netherlands). The original study included all the subjects taught in the selected veterinarian schools. As a criterion, at least one representative faculty per country was included; the faculty of Budapest was included as being representative of a European country not yet belonging to the EU, although of imminent entry; in the case of France, two centers (Alfort and Nantes) with recent changes in the structure of their degrees and different levels of application were included. Finally (v), a survey was carried out by the authors among the teachers from the Veterinary Medicine Faculty of the University of Las Palmas de Gran Canaria (ULPGC), asking whether environmental issues, climate change and the One Health (OH) concept were explicitly included in their teaching program and about the time spent during classes on these topics.

Finally, to describe the veterinary scientific publications related to environmental issues: (i) the scientific communications from the last (7th) OH congress related to these topics were analyzed (this congress was selected because OH is the environmental concept most related to veterinarian practices), and (ii) a mini-review was performed to describe the publications related to environmental issues and veterinarians. For this review, we initially evaluated the search strategy by considering the public databases of the peer-reviewed literature included in Academic Search Complete and PubMed from 2000 to the present, using keyword algorithms. Additionally, the same was performed from 2012 to the present, calculating the contribution from the last ten years and expressing it as a percentage of the published total. The following combinations of words were used: veterinary medicine + microbial + reduction or decrease; environment + veterinary; veterinary medicine + residue + environment; veterinary medicine + residue + water; antibiotics/antibacterial/antimicrobials + residue + environment; veterinary medicine + one health + environment; animal production + one health + environment; animal production + GHG (greenhouse gas); veterinary medicine + GHG; animal production + animal welfare + climate change; and veterinary medicine + animal welfare + climate change.

3. Results and Discussion

3.1. Environmental Issues That Veterinarians Must Know

One of the veterinarian practices is to advise the farmers on how to manage their livestock and residues and in the twenty-first century; sustainability and technology are critical factors in relation to these activities; so, they are going to be analyzed in this section. In the European context, the CAP indicates the activities which can be subsidized, and European farmers can rely on a more stable income through the CAP direct payments, weathering the impact of fluctuating prices and demand. Therefore, all the concepts included in the CAP must be known by European veterinarians. In this sense, special attention must be paid to GHG emissions and the use of technological tools. Since the early 2000s, farmers have received payments according to the area that they farm and not its output. Moreover, to protect the environment and safeguard Earth's resources, direct payments remunerate environmentally friendly farming and public services which are not normally paid for by the markets, such as taking care of the countryside, preserving landscapes, protecting biodiversity, and helping to mitigate the impacts of climate change [2]. Thanks to the CAP, the European agricultural sector maintains some of the world's highest safety and environmental standards. EU farmers are forced to practice environmentally sustainable farming. Therefore, they have to produce food whilst simultaneously protecting nature and safeguarding biodiversity. In this context, optimizing the use of natural resources to adaptively allocate them is essential for food production, guaranteeing the quality of life for current and future generations.

Once the new CAP comes into effect, we should see an increased contribution of EU agriculture to the environment and climate with the establishing of new schemes (so-called 'eco-schemes'). The Green Deal objectives are extremely ambitious for EU farms and food systems, setting quantitative reduction targets by 2030 for pesticides, fertilizers, and antibiotics and aiming at a quantitative increase in organic farming, agricultural areas with high-diversity landscape features, and protected areas, focusing on the three related issues of climate, environment (notably biodiversity), and health [4]. The new CAP seeks to enhance the contribution of agriculture to the EU environmental and climate goals, to provide more targeted support to smaller farms, and to allow greater flexibility for member states in adapting measures to local conditions [5]. Fahad et al. [6] concluded that heat and drought are the two most important abiotic stresses that are exacerbated by climate change, with enormous impact on the growth and productivity of the crops. Consequently, animal productions are also affected by climate change; so, veterinarians need to properly understand and manage these changes. Conversely, climate change in temperate zones increases the vegetation period. Therefore, changes in agricultural systems and practices are needed to take advantage of the production growth during the more prolonged vegetative periods in temperate climates [7]. Rather than focus on risk management only, the programs will need to include capacity building for healthy, resilient animal populations and animal health systems [3]. In addition, the budget for the modernization of farming, which has grown consistently over the years in developed countries, is also used to help connect farmers with researchers and universities to fully unlock knowledge sharing. This partnership between agriculture and society has its complement in EU research priorities. Inter-professional education is needed to dissolve the siloes that have historically discouraged collaboration among professionals with different degrees and to increase the ability to solve the problems that frequently arise in rural zones.

The green practices which farmers can adopt include crop rotation or diversification and the maintenance of ecologically rich landscapes with a minimum amount of permanent grassland, as well as organic farming and carbon farming. The European Union countries are key producers and exporters of various agricultural products, such as pork, poultry, honey, milk, and eggs. Several of these agricultural products are covered by the Single Common Market Organisation, which provides one market [5]. The CAP policies oriented towards (i) antimicrobial use reduction, (ii) GHG emissions decrease (one of the main climate change goals), and (iii) animal welfare need educational programs. In addition, the role of ruminant livestock, the main extensive livestock system, and food security, with a particular emphasis on animal source foods and environmental sanitation, need to be taught in veterinarian programs.

Livestock models, which are mainly developed in Western Europe, lack the specific sustainability themes, which hinders the further rural development [8]. The authors highlight that model development would benefit from networks and multidisciplinary collaboration. In this sense, new tools based on the integration of geographical information systems (GIS) and multi-criteria are proposed to assess the risk of livestock farms, considering sectorial, social, and environmental criteria [9]. As an example, this overview is necessary to improve the surveillance systems, which are now based on compulsory notification to health authorities and are rather fragmented and limited with regard to the most severe diseases and only marginally consider the non-scientific community, while the initiatives characterized by trans-disciplinary collaboration may be more effective for the surveillance and prevention of transmitted diseases [10].

Specifically related to climate change and GHG emissions, the EX-Ante Carbon-balance Tool (EX-ACT) [11] has been developed by the FAO based on the Intergovernmental Panel on Climate Change (IPCC) methodology for GHG emission inventories by rural activities. This web tool (currently available in its v. 9.3.4) provides its users with a consistent way to estimate and track the outcomes of the agricultural interventions regarding GHG emissions. EX-ACT is the only GHG accounting tool to cover the entire agricultural sector, including agriculture, forestry, and other land use (AFOLU,) inland and coastal wetlands, fisheries and aquaculture, agricultural inputs, and infrastructure. Recently, an extension tool has been developed to account for the value chains (EX-ACT VC) [12]. At the EU level, there are also web tools related to environmental aspects and farming, such as the AGRIADAPT tool [13]. The objective of the AGRIADAPT project, developed under the LIFE program of the European Commission, was twofold: to assess the vulnerability of the main European agricultural products to climate change and to propose sustainable adaptation plans allowing these systems to become more resilient. The tool was based on the monitoring results of more than 120 pilot farms located in France, Spain, Germany, and Estonia, aiming to strengthen the agroclimatic knowledge of the users and to support them in moving towards a more adapted agriculture. Additionally, and as an example, the Spanish Government has recently established an ECOGAN web tool, as farm owners are responsible for estimating their emissions and applying the best available techniques (BATs), to avoid or, when this is not possible, reduce emissions and the impact on the whole environment. These tools will improve future veterinarians' skills.

To address the effect of climate change on health in a broader context, some authors have described the link between humans, animals, and their environmental and social contexts [14,15]. The conceptual framework of One Health (OH) provides a strategy for the promotion of collaboration across the nexus of animal, human, and environmental health, which is essential for tackling emerging disease threats [16]. Rweyemamu et al. [17] concluded that the lessons learnt from recent zoonotic epidemics clearly indicate the need for coordinated research, interdisciplinary centers, response systems and infrastructures, integrated surveillance systems, and workforce development strategies. The authors pointed out the importance of initiatives such as "The SACIDS", a One Health African initiative linking southern African academic and research institutions with international research institutions; it strives to strengthen Africa's capacity to better manage the risks posed by infectious diseases and to improve the research capacity in investigating the biologic, socio-economic, ecologic, and anthropogenic factors responsible for the emergence and re-emergence of infectious diseases. A successful "One Health" strategy was implemented in Mongolia under the concept of "Healthy Animal-Healthy Food-Healthy People" [18], integrating not only the veterinary and public health sectors but also incorporating more work on food safety, emergency management, and the effects of climate change on zoonotic diseases. As concluded by Zinsstag et al. [19], "A One Health approach to climate change adaptation may significantly contribute to food security with emphasis on animal source foods, extensive livestock systems, particularly ruminant livestock, environmental sanitation, and steps towards regional and global integrated syndromic surveillance and response systems".

The soil food web (SFW) is an essential component of a healthy ecosystem, as it naturally supports plant health by providing protection against pests and diseases and provides fundamental ecosystem goods and services. The spread of antibiotic resistance genes (ARGs) represents a major threat to public health in which the SFW can play an important role by providing an additional treatment against this contamination. For instance, Han et al. (2022) [20] studied the field application of organic fertilizers (the long-term fertilization of swine manure or sewage sludge), which may promote the spread of ARGs in farmland ecosystems. The plant phyllosphere is a tough habitat for microbes with limited nutrients, high radiation, and frequent alteration of relative humidity, temperature, and wind speed. Their results demonstrated that the long-term application of swine manure and sewage sludge differently impacts the ARGs in soil and the phyllosphere, which has implications for sustainable agricultural management.

The American Veterinary Medical Association (AVMA) asserts that veterinary expertise in toxicology, epidemiology, and ecology are vital to understanding, controlling, preventing, diagnosing, and treating the environment-associated diseases that affect both people and animals. Although these concepts, as well as animal production, are included in all of the veterinarian students' programs, there is a lack of global vision and a more holistic approach should be included to properly include environmental issues. The most actualized document defined by the Spanish Government, called "*Libro Blanco de Veterinaria*" [21], which is to evaluate Spanish veterinarian studies and in which the main disciplinary competences to be known by the students are established, describes the following skills regarding environmental issues (Table 1).

Therefore, veterinarians must be able to quantify the effects of animal production in the environment using different tools, which must be included in their learning programs. Furthermore, they must be able to optimize the use of natural resources, in order to minimize GHG emissions and to manage the risks related to climate change through different strategies, including the ones derived by One Health knowledge.

3.2. Is Enough Knowledge Taught in Veterinary Schools to Familiarize Their Students with Environmental Issues?

Once we determine the main environmental issues that veterinarians must know, a question arises with regard to their coverage in existing teaching programs. Roopnarine et al. [16] pointed out that there is no accreditation requirement for One Health to prepare students across the professions for collaborative practice. Environmental studies seem to be barely developed in veterinarian programs, although veterinarians usually collaborate with other professionals related to environmental studies. Although the soil food web is an essential component of a healthy ecosystem, soil is scarcely included in the veterinarian view of One Health. An anonymous survey was made of veterinarians from the USA and Canada to identify any educational gaps regarding veterinary medicine and climate change. Although the veterinarians agreed that the profession needs to be involved with climate change advocacy, most reported having had no educational opportunities within their veterinary medicine curriculum or access to continuing education on climate change. The study concluded that there is a need to develop educational programs on the topic of climate change such that veterinarians are equipped to address their concerns about current and future animal health threats [22]. In this sense, some websites, such as that of the Michigan State University College of Veterinary Medicine, raise awareness about climate change by explaining the role of veterinary medicine and encouraging their students to sign up for the Environmental Wellness Committee. In addition, the Global Consortium on Climate and Health Education [23] was created by Columbia Public Health. Moreover, the American Veterinary Medical Association (AVMA) [24] encourages research and education to improve the understanding of the impacts of climate change on animal, human, and ecosystem health on its website, under the "Global Climate Change and One Health" tab.

Table 1. Skills described by Spanish Government to develop veterinarian degree and its relation to environmental issues.

	Skills	Mentioned	Related
Discipline	6. Know the basics of the different biological agents of veterinary interest (veterinary medicine/animal production and health)		X
	8. Knowledge and diagnosis of the different animal diseases, individual and collective, and their prevention measures, with special emphasis on zoonoses and notifiable diseases (all)		X
	10. Knowledge of the bases of the operation and optimization of animal production systems and their repercussions on the environment (animal production and health)	X	
Professional	5. Identify, control, and eradicate animal diseases, with special attention to notifiable diseases and zoonoses (animal production and health/veterinary medicine)		X
	9. Advise and carry out epidemiological studies and therapeutic and preventive programs in accordance with the standards of animal welfare, animal health and public health (animal production and health)		X
	11. Manage specific protocols and technologies aimed at modifying and optimizing the different animal production systems (animal production and health)		X
	14. Carry out risk analysis, including environmental and biosafety risks, as well as their assessment and management (hygiene, safety and food technology/animal production and health/others)	X	
	16. Advice and management, technical and economic, of companies in the veterinary field in a context of sustainability (all)		X

The Association for Prevention Teaching and Research (APTR) [25] invited the American Association of Veterinary Medical Colleges (AAVMC) [26] to develop a One Health educational framework as a part of the Healthy People Curriculum Task Force (HPCTF). A working group comprising representatives from the AAVMC, the APTR, the American Association of Colleges of Nursing, the Association of American Medical Colleges, and other groups has established a program to develop case studies in inter-professional education and to nominate One Health scholars. In addition, Rabinowitz et al. [27] concluded that, while many medical educators may not yet be familiar with the concept, the One Health approach has been endorsed by several major medical and public health organizations and that it is beginning to be implemented in several medical schools. As an example, a massive open access online course: "One Health: Connecting Humans, Animals and the Environment" [28] has 10,523 enrolled students. In addition, many open access documents of OH resources for public health educators are available in the One Health Commission web page [29]. Finally, there are some articles requesting the expansion of education for veterinary professionals and students in policy and advocacy; calls to action are established to address climate change and planetary health issues [30].

In the last study carried out for the Government of Spain on the curricula of veterinary schools in Europe [21], a total of nine centers were analyzed, including the basic structure of the subjects developed by their programs. There was no subject which mentioned climate change or One Health in either of the faculties, while the subjects related to environmental issues are described in Table 2.

Table 2. Subjects related to environmental issues of nine Veterinary Faculties in Europe.

University	Subject	Mandatory	Optional	Clinical Studies
Alfort	Environmental Toxicology			X
Bolonia	-	-	-	-
Liverpool	Animals and Environment	X		
Uppsala	-	-	-	-
Lieja	-	-	-	-
Budapest	-	-	-	-
Hannover	-	-	-	-
Nantes	Environment and Toxicological Clinic	X		
	Environmental Toxicology		X	
Utrecht	Environment	X		

The above-mentioned document [21] also includes the labor insertion of university graduates, and only 0.69% of the veterinarians worked in environmental activities, while 2.08% of them did it as a secondary activity. Of the asked graduates, 0.7% had already had their first work related to these activities.

Despite the fact that environmental issues are not structurally included in veterinarian studies, many of the factors are often taught as stand-alone factors. These factors link medical and public health issues to climate change, such as water-related health issues, the high frequency of extreme weather events, the increasing global temperature, changes in vector-borne diseases, and scarce resources related to food safety/security. As an example, in a survey carried out by these authors among the teachers from the Veterinary Medicine Faculty of the University of Las Palmas de Gran Canaria (ULPGC), 50% of them stated that environmental issues were explicitly included in their teaching program, while 75% incorporated environmental aspects during classes, adding up to more than 10% of the total time being taken by the 50% of the teachers (with only one teacher's answer being that environmental notions were never mentioned). A slightly lower percentage (42%) of the teachers refer specifically to climate change in their teaching programs and, although 67% give some ideas related to this concept, with more than 10% of the teaching time being taken by 33% of the teachers, 25% of them never mention climate change during their lectures (Figure 1). Finally, One Health obtained the same answers as the environmental issues; so, it can be argued that OH is the main environment-related concept perceived by the veterinarian teachers. As concluded in a free webinar to prepare health professionals to meet the needs and challenges of the future, educators worldwide are called upon to integrate climate change studies into health curricula [31].

There is less information on the challenges and training needs of veterinarians in sustainable development and animal production in the face of climate change. However, veterinarians must also be supported and formally trained in animal production and public policies in the face of climate change if they want to maintain their commitment to promoting public health and sustainable development. The new European regulatory requirements incorporate territorial livestock planning as a key element to correct the risks for the sector, for the nearby population, and for the environment. Therefore, GIS and the multi-criteria tools described above should be included in veterinarian learning programs, to allow graduated students that have acquired the new skills to be able to work as private advisers or to allow them to better integrate in multidisciplinary working groups.

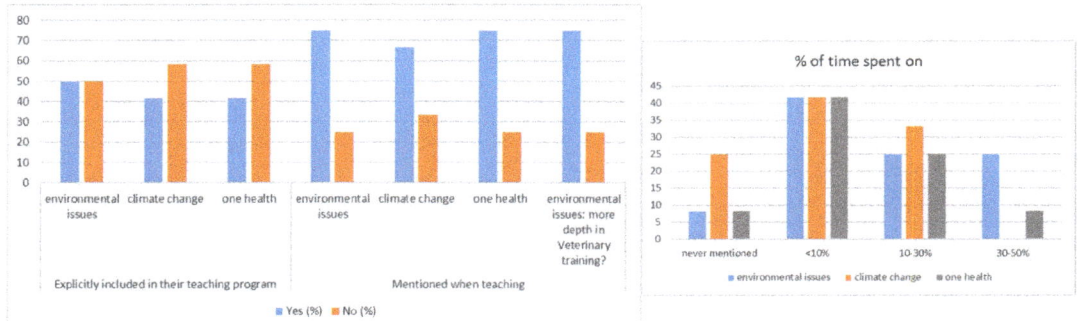

Figure 1. Environmental issues, climate change, and One Health (**left**) and time (%) spent on teaching these issues (**right**), in veterinary studies in Veterinary Medicine Faculty ULPGC.

The veterinarians of the future must have a vision beyond animal health and production and need to understand the links between the different subjects studied. Innovative learning methodologies are very well suited to the introduction of environmental issues in veterinary education. As pointed out by Dooley and Bamford [32], collaborative learning activities in the context of veterinary education can provide an opportunity to scaffold the development of crucial core competencies, including the self-regulated learning skills required to work in collaborative teams and to interpret and act on feedback.

3.3. Veterinarian Scientific Publications Related to Environmental Aspects

Regarding the last aim, veterinarian publications related to the environment, different sources have been consulted: the last (7th) OH congress [33] and two scientific databases: Academic Search Complete and PubMed. In this sense, in the "One Health Science Session of oral presentations and posters" from the 7th One Health congress, more than 70% of communications were strictly linked to environmental aspects. In this congress, analyzing specifically the use of veterinary antimicrobial pharmaceuticals and their residue reduction, 11% of the oral presentations and posters were related to antimicrobial resistance. Finally, 16% of the oral presentations and posters were related to policy, environment and biosecurity. As an example, Magiri et al. [34] describe the fact that there is a considerable overlap in the antibiotic classes sold for use in both human and veterinary medicine, mainly the beta lactam/penicillin, tetracycline, sulfonamide, and macrolide antibiotic classes.

The results of the mini-review, conducted to describe the publications related to environmental issues and veterinarians are presented in Table 3. The combination of words which presents the highest number of publications is: animal production + one health + environment, presenting more than double that of any other combination, showing the deep relation of OH with veterinary practices. The second combination differs between the databases considered: antibiotics/antibacterial/antimicrobials + residue + environment (Academic Search Complete) and environment + veterinary (PubMed). The combination of words which presented the lowest number of publications for both of these databases included GHG plus animal production or veterinary medicine. However, these combinations presented the highest percentage of publications in the last ten years (in a range from 86% to 89% in Academic Search Complete and 95% to 99% in PubMed), showing the increasing importance of this topic nowadays.

Table 3. Results from the mini-review conducted to quantify the number of scientific articles related to environmental issues and veterinarians published in 2000 to 2022 period and them percentage of them published during the last ten years.

	Academic Search Complete		PubMed	
	2000–2022	% (2012–2022)	2000–2022	% (2012–2022)
veterinary medicine + microbial + reduction or decrease	5269	74	3321	84
environment + veterinary	16,465	77	12,380	87
veterinary medicine + residue + environment	4530	70	2176	84
veterinary medicine + residue + water	4800	72	2307	86
antibiotics/antibacterial/antimicrobials + residue + environment	19,570	79	8126	89
veterinary medicine + one health + environment	13,111	74	9003	86
animal production + one health+ environment	56,113	77	35,108	90
animal production + GHG	1081	89	536	99
veterinary medicine + GHG	99	86	59 *	95
animal production + animal welfare + climate change	4674	77	1969	88
veterinary medicine + animal welfare + climate change	1230	75	801	89

* there were no publications before 2010.

4. Conclusions

While veterinary medicine, which plays a critical role in protecting the public from zoonotic infectious diseases, the safety of the food supply, and biomedical research are gaining importance within One Health, the education of veterinarians is currently less linked to the animal production and welfare related to climate change. Expanding their education would help veterinarians understand and face the consequences of climate change in the rural world. Deep changes must come to prepare the students to reduce the effects of animal production on the environment, using different tools which must be included in the learning programs. In addition, they must be able to optimize the usage of natural resources, to minimize GHG emissions, and to manage risks through different strategies. Collaborative learning activities can provide an opportunity to scaffold the development of crucial core competencies, including the self-regulated learning skills required to work in collaborative environmental teams.

Author Contributions: Conceptualization, M.d.P.P.-D. and V.M.-G.; writing—original draft preparation, M.d.P.P.-D. and V.M.-G.; writing—review and editing, M.d.P.P.-D. and V.M.-G. All authors have read and agreed to the published version of the manuscript.

Funding: This research received no external funding.

Institutional Review Board Statement: Not applicable.

Informed Consent Statement: Not applicable.

Data Availability Statement: The data presented in this study are available upon request from the corresponding author.

Acknowledgments: The authors thank Pino Del-Nero for improving the English.

Conflicts of Interest: The authors declare no conflict of interest.

References

1. European Union. 2022. Available online: https://agriculture.ec.europa.eu/common-agricultural-policy/cap-overview/cap-glance_en (accessed on 5 October 2022).
2. European Council. Feeding Europe 60 Years of Common Agricultural Policy. 2022. Available online: https://www.consilium.europa.eu/en/60-years-of-common-agricultural-policy/ (accessed on 11 December 2022).
3. Stephen, C.; Soos, C. The implications of climate change for Veterinary Services. *Rev. Sci. Tech.* **2021**, *40*, 421–430. [CrossRef] [PubMed]

4. Guyomard, H.; Bouamra-Mechemache, Z.; Chatellier, V.; Delaby, L.; Détang-Dessendre, C.; Peyraud, J.L.; Réquillart, V. Review: Why and how to regulate animal production and consumption: The case of the European Union. *Animal* **2021**, *15*, 100283. [CrossRef] [PubMed]
5. European Council. Common Agricultural Policy 2023–2027. 2022. Available online: https://www.consilium.europa.eu/en/policies/cap-introduction/cap-future-2020-common-agricultural-policy-2023-2027/ (accessed on 11 October 2022).
6. Fahad, S.; Bajwa, A.A.; Nazir, U.; Anjum, S.A.; Farooq, A.; Zohaib, A.; Sadia, S.; Nasim, W.; Adkins, S.; Saud, S.; et al. Crop production under drought and heat stress: Plant responses and management options. *Front. Plant Sci.* **2017**, *8*, 1147. [CrossRef] [PubMed]
7. FAO. *Climate Change and Food Security: Risks and Responses*; FAO: Rome, Italy, 2016.
8. van der Linden, A.; de Olde, E.M.; Mostert, P.F.; de Boer, I.J.M. A review of European models to assess the sustainability performance of livestock production systems. *Agric. Syst.* **2020**, *182*, 102842. [CrossRef]
9. Gallego, A.; Calafat, C.; Segura, M.; Quintanilla, I. Land planning and risk assessment for livestock production based on an outranking approach and GIS. *Land Use Policy* **2019**, *83*, 606–621. [CrossRef]
10. Garcia-Vozmediano, A.; De Meneghi, D.; Sprong, H.; Portillo, A.; Oteo, J.A.; Tomassone, L. A One Health Evaluation of the Surveillance Systems on Tick-Borne Diseases in the Netherlands, Spain and Italy. *Vet. Sci.* **2022**, *9*, 504. [CrossRef] [PubMed]
11. EX-ACT. FAO. Available online: https://www.fao.org/in-action/epic/ex-act-tool/suite-of-tools/ex-act/en/ (accessed on 10 December 2022).
12. EX-ACT VC. FAO. Available online: https://www.fao.org/in-action/epic/ex-act-tool/suite-of-tools/ex-act-vc/en/ (accessed on 10 December 2022).
13. AGRIADAPT Web Tool. Available online: https://climate-adapt.eea.europa.eu/en/metadata/tools/agriadapt-webtool-for-adaptation-of-typical-eu-farming-systems-to-climate-change-awa (accessed on 11 December 2022).
14. Charron, D.F. Ecosystem approaches to health for a global sustainability agenda. *Eco Health* **2012**, *9*, 256–266. [CrossRef]
15. Martin-Diaz, J.; Garcia-Aljaro, C.; Pascual-Benito, M.; Galofré, B.; Blanch, A.R.; Lucena, F. Microcosms for evaluating microbial indicator persistence and mobilization in fluvial sediments during rainfall events. *Water Res.* **2017**, *123*, 623–631. [CrossRef]
16. Roopnarine, R.; Regan, J.A. Faculty Perceptions: A Qualitative Study of the Perceived Need, Opportunities, and Challenges of Developing "One Health-One Medicine" in the Medical, Veterinary, and Public Health Curricula. *J. Contin. Educ. Health Prof.* **2021**, *41*, 16–23. [CrossRef] [PubMed]
17. Rweyemamu, M.; Kambarage, D.; Karimuribo, E.; Wambura, P.; Matee, M.; Kayembe, J.M.; Mweene, A.; Neves, L.; Masumu, J.; Kasanga, C.; et al. Development of a One Health National Capacity in Africa: The Southern African Centre for Infectious Disease Surveillance (SACIDS). One Health Virtual Centre Model. *Curr. Top. Microbiol. Immunol.* **2013**, *366*, 73–91. [PubMed]
18. Batsukh, Z.; Tsolmon, B.; Otgonbaatar, D.; Undraa, B.; Dolgorkhand, A.; Ariuntuya, O. One Health in Mongolia. *Curr. Top. Microbiol. Immunol.* **2013**, *366*, 123–137. [CrossRef] [PubMed]
19. Zinsstag, J.; Crump, L.; Schelling, E.; Hattendorf, J.; Maidane, Y.O.; Ali, K.O.; Muhummed, A.; Umer, A.A.; Aliyi, F.; Nooh, F.; et al. Climate change and One Health. *FEMS Microbiol. Lett.* **2018**, *365*, 11. [CrossRef] [PubMed]
20. Han, X.M.; Hu, H.W.; Li, J.Y.; Li, H.L.; He, F.; Sang, W.C.; Liu, Y.H.; Ma, Y.B. Long-term application of swine manure and sewage sludge differently impacts antibiotic resistance genes in soil and phyllosphere. *Geoderma* **2022**, *411*, 115698. [CrossRef]
21. Agencia Nacional de Evaluación y de la Calidad y Acreditación, Libro Blanco. Estudios de Grado en Veterinaria. 2005. Available online: https://www.google.com/url?sa=t&rct=j&q=&esrc=s&source=web&cd=&cad=rja&uact=8&ved=2ahUKEwjoprWntfT8AhWL2aQKHV_RCIcQFnoECAcQAQ&url=https%3A%2F%2Fwww.aneca.es%2Fdocuments%2F20123%2F63950%2Flibroblanco_jun05_veterinaria.pdf%2Feb4a449b-828c-6209-fd3b-5cbc6f53f383%3Ft%3D1654601797301&usg=AOvVaw07NMObAgZhyovpzwtYOOWE (accessed on 1 February 2023).
22. Kramer; Collin, G.; McCaw, K.A.; Zaresky, J.; Duncan, C.G. Veterinarians in a Changing Global Climate: Educational Disconnect and a Path Forward. *Front. Vet. Sci. Sec. Vet. Humanit. Soc. Sci.* **2020**, *7*, 613620. [CrossRef] [PubMed]
23. Global Consortium on Climate and Health Education. Available online: https://www.publichealth.columbia.edu/research/global-consortium-climate-and-health-education (accessed on 11 December 2022).
24. American Veterinary Medical Association (AVMA). Available online: https://www.avma.org/resources-tools/avma-policies/global-climate-change-and-one-health (accessed on 11 December 2022).
25. Association for Prevention Teaching and Research. APTR. Available online: https://www.aptrweb.org/ (accessed on 11 December 2022).
26. American Association of Veterinary Medical Colleges (AAVMC). Available online: https://www.aavmc.org/programs/one-health/ (accessed on 11 October 2022).
27. Rabinowitz, P.M.; Natterson-Horowitz, B.J.; Kahn, L.H.; Kock, R.; Pappaioanou, M. Incorporating One Health into medical education. *BMC Med. Educ.* **2017**, *17*, 45. [CrossRef] [PubMed]
28. One Health: Connecting Humans, Animals and the Environment. Available online: www.futurelearn.com/courses/one-health (accessed on 11 December 2022).
29. One Health Commission. Available online: https://www.onehealthcommission.org/en/resources__services/one_health_education_resources/ (accessed on 11 December 2022).
30. Kiran, D.; Sander, W.E.; Duncan, C. Empow.ering Veterinarians to Be Planetary Health Stewards Through Policy and Practice. *Front. Vet. Sci. Sec. Vet. Humanit. Soc. Sci.* **2022**, *9*, 775411. [CrossRef] [PubMed]

31. IPEC, Inter-Professional Education Collaborative. Strengthening Climate Change Education for the Health Professions. 2022. Available online: https://www.ipecollaborative.org/index.php?option=com_jevents&task=icalevent.detail&evid=44 (accessed on 12 December 2022).
32. Dooley, L.M.; Bamford, N.J. Peer Feedback on Collaborative Learning Activities in Veterinary Education. *Vet. Sci.* **2018**, *5*, 90. [CrossRef] [PubMed]
33. 7th World One Health Congress. Available online: https://worldonehealthcongress2022.miceapps.com/client/sites/view/WOH2022. (accessed on 12 December 2022).
34. Magiri, R.; Dissanayake, C.; Rafai, E.; Gautam, A.; Hayes, K.; Okello, W.; Mutwiri, G.; Iji, P.A. Trends of human and veterinary antimicrobial consumption in fiji from a "one health" perspective. In Proceedings of the 7th World One Health Congress, Singapore, 7–11 November 2022.

Disclaimer/Publisher's Note: The statements, opinions and data contained in all publications are solely those of the individual author(s) and contributor(s) and not of MDPI and/or the editor(s). MDPI and/or the editor(s) disclaim responsibility for any injury to people or property resulting from any ideas, methods, instructions or products referred to in the content.

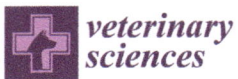

Article

"What If It Was Your Dog?" Resource Shortages and Decision-Making in Veterinary Medicine—A Vignette Study with German Veterinary Students

Kirsten Persson [1,2,*], Wiebke-Rebekka Gerdts [1], Sonja Hartnack [3] and Peter Kunzmann [1]

[1] Applied Ethics in Veterinary Medicine Group, Institute for Animal Hygiene, Animal Welfare and Farm Animal Behaviour, University of Veterinary Medicine Hannover, Foundation, Bischofsholer Damm 15, Geb. 116, 30173 Hannover, Germany

[2] Institute for Biomedical Ethics, University of Basel, Bernoullistrasse 28, 4056 Basel, Switzerland

[3] Section of Epidemiology, Vetsuisse Faculty, University of Zurich, Winterthurerstr. 270, 8057 Zurich, Switzerland

* Correspondence: kirsten.persson@tiho-hannover.de

Simple Summary: The here presented study was part of a survey on ethical decision making among veterinary students at the University of Veterinary Medicine Hannover, Foundation. The students were confronted with challenges in a situation in veterinary practice. Firstly, in the situation, two patients needed a medication but only one dosage was available in the veterinarian's supply. The students based their decision regarding the first challenge, who should (not) get the medication, on the patients' age, general health, life expectancy, the patient owners' wellbeing, and their general knowledge on situations in veterinary practice. Secondly, the students were asked what would change if one of the patients was their own dog. They reacted in four different ways to the question. (1) For a professional, this should not make a difference; (2) they would most likely give the medication to their own dog; (3) they would give the medication to the other dog; and (4) they avoided a decision. Finally, the students judged a list of possible solutions to the dilemma on a scale (from very poor to very good). They preferred those solutions that focused on the animal's wellbeing to those that focused on the owners' wellbeing. Overall, it turned out that in situations of limited medication, students make their decisions for very different reasons, and that a guideline for veterinarians to make decisions in such situations is still missing.

Abstract: The here presented vignette study was part of a survey on ethical judgement skills among advanced veterinary students at the University of Veterinary Medicine Hannover, Foundation. The vignette describes a fictitious dilemma in veterinary practice due to medication supply shortages. First, the students should make an ethically justified decision: who of the two patients in the waiting room gets the last dosage of a medication. Important factors were the animal patients' characteristics (age, state of health, life expectancy), the patient owners' wellbeing, and context-related criteria. Second, the students were asked for decisional changes if one of the patients was their own dog. They reacted in four different ways: (1) for a professional, this should not make a difference; (2) most likely being "egoistic" and preferring their own dog; (3) giving the medication to the other dog; and (4) avoiding a decision. Finally, the students judged a list of possible solutions to the dilemma on a 9-point scale. They preferred patient-related criteria to patient-owner-related criteria in this task. In the overall results, it became obvious that no "gold standard" or guidelines for situations of medication shortages exist, yet, which presents an important subject for future research and veterinary ethics teaching.

Keywords: veterinary ethics; moral reasoning; vignettes; teaching veterinary ethics

Citation: Persson, K.; Gerdts, W.-R.; Hartnack, S.; Kunzmann, P. "What If It Was Your Dog?" Resource Shortages and Decision-Making in Veterinary Medicine—A Vignette Study with German Veterinary Students. *Vet. Sci.* **2023**, *10*, 161. https://doi.org/10.3390/vetsci10020161

Academic Editors: Simona Sacchini and Ayoze Castro-Alonso

Received: 9 January 2023
Revised: 10 February 2023
Accepted: 14 February 2023
Published: 17 February 2023

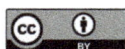

Copyright: © 2023 by the authors. Licensee MDPI, Basel, Switzerland. This article is an open access article distributed under the terms and conditions of the Creative Commons Attribution (CC BY) license (https://creativecommons.org/licenses/by/4.0/).

1. Introduction

It has been observed in recent years that the general public has become increasingly interested in the welfare of animals. This growing awareness not only concerns farm animals, but also companion animals such as dogs, cats, and horses [1]. To the same extent, it can be observed that the moral status of animals is changing and, especially in veterinary medicine, therapies are becoming possible and are also demanded and financed by animal owners, which were previously mostly reserved for human individuals [2]. Animals are no longer seen only as "pets". In large parts of western societies they are often also ascribed the status of a "friend" or "family member" [3]. With new technologies and medications available, further aspects that accompany human medical practice may enter veterinary practice. One of them, the threat of resource shortages, will be dealt with in the here presented study with veterinary students.

Due to the knowledge and skills veterinarians have acquired during their training, they often see themselves as being in a special position of responsibility towards humans and animals. This responsibility is also attributed to veterinarians from external sources [4]. In practice, veterinarians are frequently caught between the individual interests of the owners and the presumed individual interests of the animals. Bernard E. Rollin identified the question of whether a veterinarian's primary obligation is to the animal or to the animal owner as being the "fundamental problem" [5] in veterinary medicine already in 1988 and thus established the basis for the model of the Veterinary Triad [5,6].

Various studies have been conducted on stress levels among veterinarians and these showed that large parts of practicing veterinarians experience their profession as very stressful and morally demanding [7–24]. Primary stress factors mentioned were long working hours and on-call duties, but also fear of treatment errors, customer complaints, and pet owners' claims that veterinarians are the experts in all areas of veterinary medicine. In addition, animal deaths were mentioned, whether from disease or euthanasia, social loneliness, lack of support in decision-making, and ethical challenges in general. A survey of small animal veterinarians in the USA identified ethical dilemmas as a major cause of work-related stress [7].

Accordingly, the conflicts veterinarians are confronted with in their everyday professional life can be of different nature—social or financial, but also moral [7–11,25–29]. Yeates (2009) was the first to analyze ethical conflicts in veterinary practice. He stated that especially with the increasing medical treatment options of veterinarians, the responsibility towards patients, animal owners, colleagues, and society also grows [4]. The fact that veterinarians do not always agree with the procedures of colleagues due to the abundance of treatment methods and that the concept of acting lege artis includes more and more methods, some of which differ greatly from one another, leads to an increasing need for ethical orientation.

All of these study results document the need to prepare veterinary students for ethical challenges in practice. A recent study from North America shows that the cornerstone for stress and depression is already laid during university studies. Among the students surveyed, 49% reported having at least a moderate level of stress, and 66% showed symptoms of mild to moderate depression [17]. For this reason, veterinary medical education institutions were already called to account in 2013. In the context of the Federation of Veterinarians of Europe & European Association of Establishments for Veterinary Education's (FVE & EAEVE) Report on Veterinary Education in Animal Welfare Science, Ethics and Law, the veterinary curriculum should offer a continuous examination of ethical questions that could be relevant to the later professional situations of veterinary students [30].

In response, the German Federal Ministry of Education and Research (BMBF) funded two successive projects on "Teaching veterinary, clinical and ethical skills" (FERTHIK I and II). [31] These projects were carried out consecutively at the University of Veterinary Medicine Hannover, Foundation, Hannover, Germany (TiHo). In particular, teaching in ethics was implemented. As part of this project, Germany's only professorship for applied ethics in veterinary medicine was established in 2015 and corresponding teaching content was integrated into the curriculum [32]. The education in veterinary ethics at the TiHo is not only theory-based, but is also in the form of the concept of "critical guidance" [33]. A special focus is always on the practical applicability of ethical tools and methods. Especially the methodology of applied ethics with a bottom-up and top-down approach, i.e., the development of principles from individual cases and the application of these principles to further individual cases, represents a cornerstone of teaching veterinary ethics [34,35].

Finally, within the framework of the FERTHIK II project, a review of the moral judgement skills of veterinary students should take place. Although veterinary ethics is required in the veterinary curriculum in Germany and part of the First Day Competencies expected of a trained veterinarian according to the FVE and EAEVE, knowledge about tools to assess moral judgement skills is sparse [30]. To put it in Vettical's [36] words: "Further investigation and dissertation on veterinary practice related ethical issues may perk up veterinary instruction and paraphrase of ethics assumption and way of thinking into functional practice." (p. 746). The present article aims to contribute to bridging this gap.

The here presented vignette study was part of a survey on ethical judgements among veterinary students at the TiHo in their fourth year. They had the opportunity to attend all ethics lectures, seminars, and block courses that were established in the new curriculum (for more details on the ethics curriculum see [32]).

The vignette describes a fictitious scenario in veterinary practice and introduces two aspects that call for an ethically justified decision. Two dogs suffering from intestinal cancer and their owners are sitting in the waiting room. The veterinarian has a new medication for intestinal cancer in dogs. However, only one dosage is available due to supply shortages. The first and obvious question is: who should be given the medication? Some additional information on the dogs (age and general health status) and their owners (living circumstances, time available for the dog, further companion animals) is given that might influence the decision. The second question tries to involve the participants personally in the scenario: what if the older dog patient was their own dog? While it is not uncommon that patient owners ask their veterinarian, "What if it was your pet?" this usually comes up in situations of different therapy options for the one animal when the patient owner is looking for help in the decision-making process [37]. In our case, the veterinary students should rather elaborate on the factors that influence their decision, including unexpected personal involvement.

Resource scarcity in the sense of a shortage of medicines and vaccines is not a common phenomenon in Germany. Nevertheless, it regularly happens that vaccines or medicines are not available to the usual extent and are also not available at short notice in other European countries or even worldwide [38–41]. Especially during the corona pandemic and afterwards, pet owners and veterinarians experienced supply problems with medicines and vaccines. A current example is the availability of vaccines against the Equine Herpes Virus (EHV). Due to the herpes outbreak among sport horses in Valencia (Spain) in 2021, vaccination against EHV was introduced as a core vaccination for sport horses in Germany as of 1 January 2023 [39]. In the preliminary discussions, it was argued that the vaccines against EHV were not available at all times in the past and that only strictly limited doses of the vaccine would have been available to veterinarians [40].

Ethics teaching should prepare veterinary students to use and name decision making criteria and, ideally, to develop a professional attitude that leads to consistent ethical judgements. The aim of the vignette study was, firstly, to investigate the participants' skills to identify stakeholders and the ethical conflict, as well as the patterns of their decision-making and justifications. For a more detailed discussion of the classification of different attitudes among our participants, see [32]. Secondly, the focus of this particular vignette was on their reactions to an unconventional problem and to the challenge of personal involvement. Given the recent occurrence of supply shortages in human and veterinary medicine, decision making criteria for such cases should be investigated and sharpened, even though ethics teaching might not have a focus on this specific issue, yet.

2. Materials and Methods

For a detailed description of the complete study, please see [32]. The survey was pilot tested among members of the institute (veterinarians, agricultural scientists, and philosophers) and modified according to their feedback. The animal welfare officer of the TiHo confirmed that the TiHo's ethical requirements for student participation in studies in the form of surveys were met in March 2020.

In summer 2020, the survey was made available online (LimeSurvey GmbH, Hamburg, Germany, www.limesurvey.org (accessed on 2 January 2023)) to a 262-student cohort in their fourth year of veterinary education. The constraints due to the pandemic made it impossible to gather the students for this purpose, as originally planned, in an exam-like situation and hand out a printed version of the survey. Rather, online participation was facultative, advertised via email. After several email reminders and a data collection time of approx. 16 weeks, the return rate was ca. 22% ($n = 87$).

In the survey, four fictional scenarios were presented, one of which is discussed in this article. The first three scenarios dealt with common challenges in veterinary practice (compliance issues in a farm animal case, a conflict due to an expensive treatment in small animal practice, and an animal welfare issue in a jumping horse scenario). The analysis and discussion of the corresponding results are published elsewhere [28]. The here presented fourth scenario asked the students to think about a rather unusual resource allocation problem, combined with a question regarding their general professional attitude.

The scenario reads as follows (translated from German):

"There are delivery shortages for a new medication against intestinal cancer in dogs. The next delivery is not due for several weeks. You only have the amount necessary to treat one dog—but there are two patients in the waiting room that would need the medicine urgently.

Patient 1 is a two-year-old poodle and she was never seriously ill until the diagnosis. She lives in a family with two children and two adults and is alone half the day. Without the administration of the drug, her condition would deteriorate rapidly and she might not survive the wait for the next delivery.

Patient 2 is a nine-year-old terrier who lives with a younger dog with a pensioner. The man is a little frail but devotedly cares for his dogs around the clock. Without the administration of the drug, the dog's condition would rapidly deteriorate and he might not survive the wait for the next delivery".

We asked the participants:

1. What are the ethical conflicts in this case?
2. Who is involved in the conflict (stakeholders)?
3. What information is important? Do you need more information?
4. Which dog would you give the medication to? And why?
5. How would the situation change if patient 2 was your own dog?

After filling in the free-text answers, we presented a list of six statements and asked the participants to indicate their agreement with the statements on a scale from one (very poor) to nine (very good). To avoid any influence of the list of statements on the free-text answers, there was no "back" button in the survey. The statements suggested potential solutions to the case and read as follows:

- You toss a coin and administer the medicine to the dog that "wins".
- You choose the poodle because statistically she will still have a longer lifespan than the older terrier.
- You choose the terrier because he receives better and continuous care and therefore has a better chance of recovery.
- You choose the poodle because an entire family is affected and not just an elderly person who has another dog.
- You openly explain the problem to both owners together and ask them to discuss the decision on their own.

- You have a joint discussion with the owners until a decision is reached that you all agree with.

Answers were exported in Microsoft® Excel (Version 2016). One member of the team (KP) conducted the descriptive statistical analysis. Core quotes, i.e., statements that either represented an opinion that was frequently mentioned or an exceptional, uncommon point of view, were collected, translated verbatim, and are presented in the analysis. The figures were produced with Excel and R.

3. Results

Firstly, we present the results of each free-text answer and secondly, the results of the scale task.

3.1. What Is the Ethical Conflict?

Several participants explicitly reported this to be a challenging decision. First, a weighing process was necessary. Many students identified criteria for each patient: the poodle is younger, the terrier older. The poodle lives with a family who is absent half of the day. The terrier can be taken care of by his owner full-time. The members of the family might be more alert and mobile and better equipped to take care of a sick dog. The elderly patient owner might, however, be willing and be able to sacrifice more time and effort for his dog, as he might not have as much other company and distractions as the family. The difference the loss of each dog makes is equally hard to compare. In the one case, several family members would grieve. In the other case, it is mainly the one owner. However, the loss might be more profound to him as he does not have family members around and his life might be more focused on the dog. One student ascribed more "emotional value" of the dog to the elderly man. Additionally, there is the other dog living with the elderly man, who would suffer from the loss, too, but at the same time comfort his owner in his mourning.

Several students described the problem as having to ascribe more value to one dog's life than to the other dog's, as having to judge which dog "earns" the treatment more, or, more generally, as the burden of having to decide about life and death. Many participants answered with a question to this question, e.g., "Who may live?", "Who should be saved?", "Who is more worthy of a therapy?", "How can I decide here?". At the same time, one student concluded that "it is not my job as a veterinarian to decide on the question which animal has a greater value". A few answers emphasized that this was not only a decision concerning the patient's life, but also that of the patient's owner, which points toward the much-discussed Veterinary Triad ethics between patient, patient owner, and veterinarian [5,6,42–44].

3.2. Who Is Involved in the Conflict (Stakeholders)?

For an overview of the answers to this question, see Figure 1. In line with the above-reported dominant answer that this conflict was mainly an inner decision-making challenge for the veterinarian, our participants identified the latter as the main stakeholder.

The students were familiar with the prominent Veterinary Triad of animal—patient owner—veterinarian [2–4] and mentioned all three stakeholders. However, the patient owner was named as a stakeholder by more than 60% of the students, whereas the animal was only mentioned by a third of all participants. Those who looked beyond the narrow setting in the vignette (7%) also pointed out that the pharmaceutical industry was involved in the conflict.

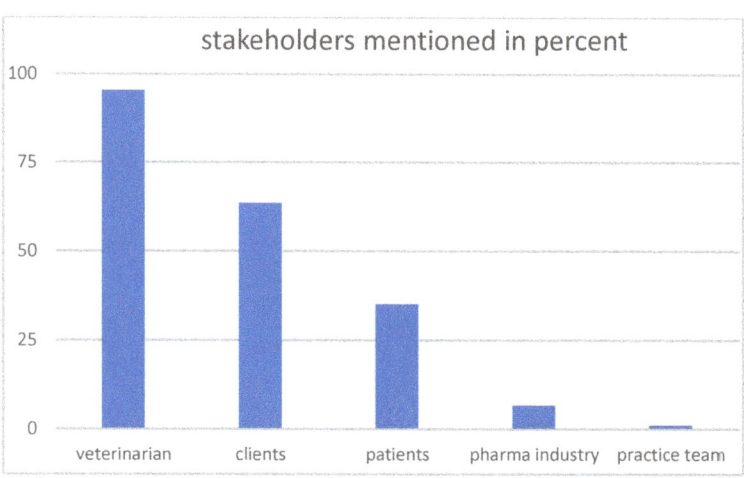

Figure 1. Answers to the second question, "Who is involved in the conflict (stakeholders)?" in percent.

3.3. What Information Is Important? Do You Need More Information?

Most students referred to the information that was already given in the vignette as necessary for their decision. They often mentioned the prognosis, which was roughly summarized in the scenario: "Without the medication, her/his condition would deteriorate rapidly and she might not survive the wait for the next delivery". However, the chances for complete healing were not given, nor were potential side effects, which the students also asked for. Additionally, they wanted to know more about the general health, stage of the cancer, and potential comorbidities of the two dogs, in particular of the nine-year-old dog who can be considered elderly. This also included characteristics of the dogs like their "will to live".

Besides, participants pointed out several ways to try to get the medication or alternative medication:

- Asking colleagues to help out or to take over the case,
- Looking for the same active agent in human medicine and ordering a medication for humans instead,
- Offering older/alternative and potentially less effective medication (given that in the vignette we wrote about a "new medication"),
- Searching for other ways of treatment like surgery or radiation therapy for one of the dogs,
- Trying to split the medication between the two dogs so every dog could receive a lower dosage,
- Thinking about palliative treatment.

Several students asked which dog had had the earlier appointment, had been higher on the waiting list or had entered the practice before the other, suggesting that, all other things being equal, this might be their final criterion when making a choice.

Furthermore, our participants needed more information on the animal owners that was not given in the vignette. For example,

- Who can afford the treatment?
- Can the family find a solution to take care of the dog while they are not at home?
- Does the elderly man have a support system he can activate?
- What is the animal owners' opinion regarding the problem?
- What is the animal owners' general attitude towards life?
- Who could better deal with the loss?/How close is the human-animal bond in both cases?

3.4. Which Dog Would You Give the Medication to? And Why?

As presented in Figure 2, almost 60% of the participants decided to give the medication to patient 1, the poodle. Circa 5% opted for the terrier, patient 2, and about a third suggested other solutions or refused to decide.

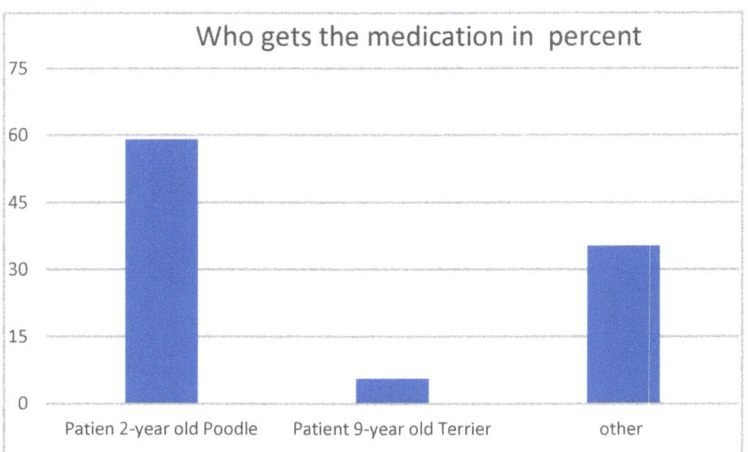

Figure 2. Answers to the third question "Which dog would you give the medication to? And why?" in percent. The answer "other" is further specified in the text below.

The students explained that their reasons for choosing the poodle had mainly to do with her higher life expectancy. Some additionally deduced a better general state of health and a lower risk for comorbidities compared to the older dog, or, even a better prognosis. A couple of participants argued that the older dog would be better taken care of which is why the younger animal was in greater need of the medication. In addition to these patient-related reasons, students justified their choices with a focus on the patient owners. A few respondents mentioned that more patient owners would grieve if the poodle died. One student argued that the elderly patient owner's second dog might "give him comfort in the time of trouble" if the sick dog died. Furthermore, a participant wondered if the elderly man might be overstrained with having to care for one sick animal and another dog. A different argument applied to the triage rules in times of COVID-19 when younger patients should be preferred in case of medication shortages.

The few students who chose to give the medication to the terrier referred to patient owner-related arguments as opposed to the patient's characteristics. They stated that the elderly man might be less flexible to look for the medication in another veterinarian's practice or even abroad. Moreover, the students argued that the patient owner's "own mental and psychological condition depends on the life of the dog" or that the dog was a more central friend for the elderly man than for the family. Similarly, one student assumed that "the family has enough distractions (work, school) and they have had the dog for two years or less, so the bond may not be as intense yet". Comparing the characteristics and well-being of the two dogs, some students concluded that it might be easier to bridge the time until the medication was available again with an alternative for the younger dog due to the potentially worse overall state of health of the older animal. In contrast to that, a few respondents pointed out that a young poodle getting cancer suggested an underlying condition or a worse general state of health in the two-year old dog, which is why the terrier should be preferred. One student even postulated that the terrier had a "more meaningful life" in their opinion.

Reasons for avoiding the decision were manifold. Several students explained that they would have sent one patient to a different practice/clinic and called the situation unrealistic. Most likely referring to their own experience in veterinary practice, they stated that the medication should be available somewhere else. To circumvent the problem, some participants suggested that dosage could be reduced, i.e., the medication could be split between the two patients.

Several participants would give the medication to the patient with the earlier appointment (one student referred to the criteria for organ donation). It was suggested a few times to discuss with the patient owners and see whether someone was prepared to voluntarily do without the medication. A few participants declared that they were not able to decide due to a lack of information. One participant emphasized that the shortage was not their fault so it was not up to them to find a "fair" solution in this impossible situation. A few times, the ability to afford the treatment was mentioned as an additional important point for clarification. Chance/tossing a coin was suggested by a few students.

3.5. How Would the Situation Change If Patient 2 (the Terrier) Was Your Own Dog?

The students' reactions to this question can be categorized in four groups.

The first emphasized the objective and rational argument that it must not make a difference if the dog was their own and any deviation due to a consideration of personal needs and feelings would be unprofessional. One student explicitly wrote, "I would try and make a rational decision as a VETERINARIAN (not as an owner)". A few participants stated that there was some "correct" decision in their view resulting from the balancing of arguments and this should be their conclusion in any case. A few tried to differentiate between what they knew they should do (give the medication to the dog with the better prognosis) and "if in reality I would actually sacrifice my own dog. I dare doubting that to be honest."

The second group of participants was inclined to admit that they would decide "egoistically", "subjectively", or "emotionally", and therefore give the medication to their own dog. They occasionally expressed awareness of this being a wrong or unprofessional decision, but, as one participant put it, "a veterinarian is human, too", or, in the words of another student "if it is my own dog, unfortunately, rationality no longer comes into play". One participant suggested that distance was an important factor in other moral decisions, too, and that it was, for example, considered morally acceptable to prefer relatives to strangers in forced decisions.

A third group, and that included several participants who had opted for giving the medication to the terrier in the previous question, would under these circumstances change their decision and give the medication to the younger dog (the poodle). They argued that, being vets, they would be able to take care of the suffering animal in a much better way than the family (or the elderly man) and could make him as comfortable as possible until the new medication arrived. In addition, some stated that they could cope better with the loss than the elderly man (in the original scenario) or the family (in direct comparison). Two participants brought up the unlikely idea that "due to my miscalculation of my medicine cabinet, my bad conscience would tempt me to treat the poodle".

A fourth group, again, tried to avoid the decision-making. Several participants suggested referring the other dog to a colleague. Some argued that they would not be in a position like that at all because they would have taken care of the dog and would have obtained the medication much earlier. Many students explained that they would nonetheless be unable to decide in this case due to a lack of information (on prognosis, the type of disease, comorbidity, etc.) and that would not change if it was their dog. Therefore, they would make the decision depending on further medical information like the first group. However, some admitted that in case of a "tie" they would opt for their own dog.

3.6. Judgement of Suggested Actions

The students judged the provided options to solve the conflict as follows on a scale from 1 (very poor) to 9 (very good) (see Figure 3): They agreed the most (median 7) on giving the medication to the poodle because of her higher life expectancy. The second best option (median 6) presented the option to give the medication to the terrier, as he would be better taken care of. A joint discussion involving the veterinarian and the two patient owners was judged to be somehow acceptable (median 4), whereas tossing a coin received a lower agreement (median 3). The students did rather not agree (median 2) to justify giving the medication to the poodle with the grieving family in contrast to the elderly man who would grieve for the terrier, and they depreciated the option to let the patient owners solve the issue in a discussion without the veterinarian (median 1).

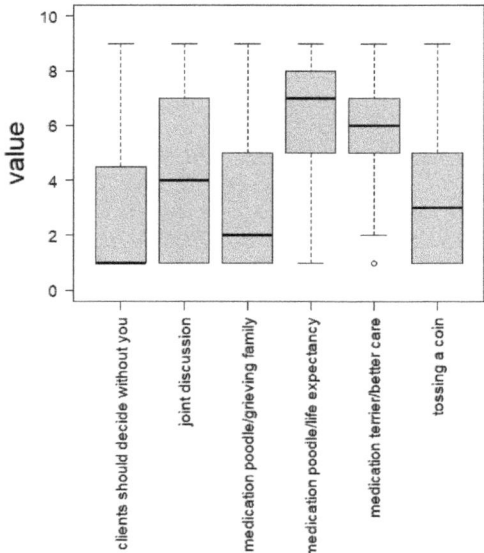

Figure 3. Answers for the six statements presenting different options for decisions, including medians. Judgement on a scale from 1 (very poor) to 9 (very good).

4. Discussion

The combination of being forced to decide, not having differentiating criteria to justify the decision, and the threatening deadly outcome for one of the patients made the decision explicitly challenging for the respondents. The free-text answers show that students found different strategies to cope with this problem.

- *Strategy 1: Patient-centered decision making*

Although quite a few students pointed out that they would need more details on the prognosis, the general health status of the patients, the progression of the disease, or the specifics of the medication, many justified their opting for the younger patient with the higher life expectancy and corresponding assumed better overall health status. Those opting for the older patient often argued similarly but came to a different conclusion: the younger dog was more likely to survive until the medication was available again, which was why the older one needed the dosage that was immediately available.

Focusing on the patients' interests, they might have internalized what Weich and Grimm [45] outlined as a role model: "clinical practice is guided by a normative dimension of the concept "animal patient" as an ethical ideal. In determining whether a veterinarian acts ethically, the norm of aiming at the health-related interests of the animal patient is decisive. Acting according to this norm constitutes good veterinary clinical care." (p. 262). This attitude or role is known as the "animals' advocate" [46].

While it should not be doubted that it is in the animal patient's interest to be cured of intestinal cancer, opting for the younger dog for the reason of her higher life expectancy points towards a more complicated assumption. When one participant referred to triage rules in human medicine and suggested preferring younger patients, they implied that animals, like humans, might expect a certain life expectancy or might prefer to live as long as possible (for a more exhaustive discussion of age in human and veterinary medical decision making, see [47]). If a lower age correlates with a better general state of health, this presents, however, a medically relevant difference that serves as an argument to prefer the younger dog. On comparing the free-text answers to the statements with suggested solutions, it is striking that the respondents to a greater extent agreed to the two patient-centered solutions (medians were 6 and 7 of 9; see Figure 3). This result again underlines the dominant role model of the veterinarian as the animal's advocate.

- *Strategy 2: Patient owner-centered decision-making*

Several arguments referred to the differences the veterinarian's decision would make for the patient owners rather than for the patients. By no means does this imply that the students providing these arguments consider themselves less as animals' advocates than those using strategy 1. It can be the case that the differences between the patients, especially regarding their interests and "claims" to obtain the medication, are perceived as insufficient for a decision. Turning to the patient owners is a comprehensible next step. Other than the prominent advocacy for the animal, weighing the interests of different patient owners is a rather uncommon or at least not an outspoken decision-making process in veterinary medicine. After all, the idea of a veterinarian telling the children of the poodle's family that the terrier's elderly owner would feel so lonely without him seems unusual. Given that the here presented case of resource allocation is also very rare in veterinary medicine, though, the patient owner-centered arguments cannot be excluded as less relevant per se. After all, the students' awareness of and sensitivity for the patient owners' needs and welfare are important goals of veterinary ethics teaching [30]. Similarly for the patient-centered strategy, several outcomes are possible. The fact that several people—some of them children—would grieve for the poodle compared to only one owner (and a partner dog, who is, however, rarely mentioned in this respect) for the terrier, is up against the fact that the family can be expected to have a fulfilled life full of activities even without their dog, whereas the elderly man might, for example, lose his daily routines and activities without a dog because he might be much more focused on the animal.

- *Strategy 3: Established ways of solving conflicts in veterinary practice*

About one third of the respondents were not willing to fully get involved in the scenario as a thought experiment. Many pointed towards usual procedures in veterinary practice that would circumvent the conflict we presented. Some highlighted the avoidable problem of scarcity. They suggested sending the patient to a colleague, calling several colleagues to still get the medication, or, if need be, to split the dosage so that both patients could be supplied for a short time. Additionally, the vignette framing the medication as "new" was understood in a way that an older medication could be available in the meantime. The alternative interpretation that the medication was an innovative approach in treating this type of cancer that way (i.e., without chemo- or radiation therapy) was not considered in those cases. The list of statements provided some suggestions that are not (or should not be) established in veterinary practice when it comes to involving patient owners. The idea of having a joint discussion with both patient owner groups was judged to be a comparatively good solution (4 of 9; see Figure 3). Buck passing, on the other hand, was not appreciated. Despite admitting that the decision was tough in this case, veterinary students obviously did not want to leave it to the patient owners to decide without themselves being involved.

- *Strategy 4: Arbitrary decision making*

Another way of reacting to the question can be attributed to an account of distributive justice. If the morally relevant properties of the two potential receivers of the scarce resource are equal, it might seem wrong to prefer one to the other. Following this argument, several participants suggested giving the medication to the dog who entered the practice first or was higher on the waiting list (a criterion practiced when allocating donated organs).

Others considered tossing a coin, which was also a suggestion in the provided list of statements (see Section 3.6), leaving the decision to chance. All of these decisions provided answers to the questions that other students raised to express their inability to come to a decision in the given situation (see Section 3.1).

The final question that would change if patient 2 was their own dog was meant to put the students in a position of merging professional and private arguments. This merging effect was reflected in the students' answers. Some reacted as (private) companion animal owners, stating that their own dog would obviously be preferred. That way, they fell back on a patient owner-centered argument. Others clearly judged the situation professionally, stating that it should not make a difference whom a patient belonged to and they would administer the medication according to objective criteria. A third way of reaction presented an attitude of a veterinarian as a special kind of dog owner. With their additional knowledge and skills, those participants felt a special responsibility in the given situation, taking the burden of caring for an animal without the proper medication on their shoulders because they could not impose it on a "non-professional" dog owner. This argument pattern presents a vivid illustration of a "unit of care" approach, considering both the interests of patients and patient owners, and the team effort they can contribute to the process together.

The overall reactions of the participants to this scenario suggest that resource shortages, a potentially manifest problem in European human and veterinary practice, have not been introduced thoroughly in veterinary ethics teaching. In human medicine, particularly in oncology, codes of conduct were developed by professional associations during the COVID-19 pandemic that can serve as guidelines when resources are scarce, especially for life-saving drugs. In this context, criteria were developed to enable physicians to make well-founded decisions in ethically extremely difficult situations. The American Society of Clinical Oncology recommendations [48], for example, implicitly mention factors that we similarly observed in veterinary students: "Ethical principles at the forefront of pandemic planning differ from patient-centered approaches that may be more familiar to oncologists." (p. 7). The students we interviewed based their assessment of the situation and their decision-making not only exclusively on the patient and his or her individual circumstances and criteria, such as age and chances of recovery, but also on the social environment in which the animal lived. Similarly, the guidelines address, for example, preference for one's animal in the context of "fairness": "Resources should be allocated based on ethically-relevant differences among individuals, free from unjustified favoritism and discrimination." (p. 10). It is possible that such guidelines and codes of conduct from human medicine could be adapted and modified for veterinary medicine, although such extreme cases of resource scarcity are fortunately very rare.

Given that the data collection took place in 2020, the consequences of the pandemic for the pharmaceutical market were not yet as explicit when the students filled out the survey. Not having a gold standard for this case, a clear guideline they could refer to when being confronted with a dilemma situation presented a discomforting challenge which individual students solved in different ways. Further research in this thematic field is needed to develop decision-making support for veterinarians in similar real-life situations.

Author Contributions: Conceptualization, K.P., W.-R.G., S.H. and P.K.; methodology, K.P. and S.H.; validation, W.-R.G.; formal analysis, K.P.; investigation, K.P. and W.-R.G.; writing—original draft preparation, K.P.; writing—review and editing, W.-R.G.; visualization, K.P. and S.H.; project administration, P.K.; funding acquisition, P.K. All authors have read and agreed to the published version of the manuscript.

Funding: This research was funded by the German Federal Ministry of Education and Research (BMBF), grant number 01PL16060. This Open Access publication was funded by the Deutsche Forschungsgemeinschaft (DFG, German Research Foundation)—491094227 "Open Access Publication Funding" and the University of Veterinary Medicine Hannover, Foundation.

Institutional Review Board Statement: Ethical review and approval were waived for this study because the animal welfare officer confirmed that the University's ethical requirements for student participation in studies in the form of surveys were met (see confirmation letter by Bernhard Hiebl, Animal Welfare Officer).

Informed Consent Statement: Informed consent was obtained from all subjects involved in the study.

Data Availability Statement: The data presented in this study are available on request from the corresponding author. The data are not publicly available in order to keep the anonymity of our (small number of) participants.

Acknowledgments: We would like to sincerely thank the students who participated and the university faculty who effectively shared our call for participation.

Conflicts of Interest: The authors declare no conflict of interest.

References

1. Von Gall, P. Agrarwende auch für Tiere. Gesellschaftliche Grundlagen und Herausforderungen. In *Haben Tiere Rechte? Aspekte und Dimensionen der Mensch-Tier-Beziehung*; Diehl, E., Tuider, J., Eds.; Bundeszentrale für Politische Bildung: Bonn, Germany, 2019; pp. 191–202.
2. Springer, S.; Sandøe, P.; Bøker Lund, T.; Grimm, H. "Patients' interests first, but . . . "–Austrian Veterinarians' Attitudes to Moral Challenges in Modern Small Animal Practice. *Animals* **2019**, *9*, 241. [CrossRef] [PubMed]
3. Voigt, L.C. Untersuchungen Zur Euthanasieentscheidung Von Tierbesitzern* Hinsichtlich Entscheidungsfindung. Umgang Und Trauerbewältigung. Ph.D. Thesis, Stiftung Tierärztliche Hochschule Hannover, Hannover, Germany, 2017.
4. Yeates, J.W. Response and responsibility: An analysis of veterinary ethical conflicts. *Vet. J.* **2009**, *182*, 3–6. [CrossRef] [PubMed]
5. Rollin, B. *An Introduction to Veterinary Medical Ethics: Theory and Cases*, 2nd ed.; Jon Wiley and Sons: Hoboken, NJ, USA, 2006.
6. Weich, K. Veterinärmedizinische Ethik. In *Handbuch Tierethik*; Ach, J.S., Borchers, D., Eds.; J.B. Metzler: Stuttgart, Germany, 2018; pp. 351–356.
7. Kipperman, B.; Morris, P.; Rollin, B. Ethical dilemmas encountered by small animal veterinarians: Characterisation, responses, consequences and beliefs regarding euthanasia. *Vet. Rec.* **2018**, *182*, 548. [CrossRef] [PubMed]
8. Moses, L.; Malowney, M.J.; Wesley Boyd, J. Ethical conflict and moral distress in veterinary practice: A survey of North American veterinarians. *J. Vet. Intern. Med.* **2018**, *32*, 2115–2122. [CrossRef]
9. Dürnberger, C. I Would like to, but I can't. An Online Survey on the Moral Challenges of German Farm Veterinarians. *J. Agric. Env. Ethics* **2020**, *33*, 447–460. [CrossRef]
10. Gardner, D.H.; Hini, D. Work-related stress in the veterinary profession in New Zealand. *N. Z. Vet. J.* **2006**, *54*, 119–124. [CrossRef]
11. Crane, M.F.; Bayl-Smith, P.; Cartmill, J. A Recommendation for Expanding the Definition of Moral Distress Experienced in the Workplace. *Australas J. Organ. Psychol.* **2013**, *6*, E1. [CrossRef]
12. Glaesmer, H.; Bahramsoltani, M.; Schwerdtfeger, K.; Spangenberg, L. Euthanasia Distress and Fearlessness About Death in German Veterinarians. *Crisis* **2021**, *42*, 71–77. [CrossRef]
13. Rollin, B.E. Euthanasia, moral stress, and chronic illness in veterinary medicine. *Vet. Clin. Small Anim. Pract.* **2011**, *41*, 651–659. [CrossRef]
14. Johnson, S.; Cooper, C.; Cartwright, S.; Donald, I.; Taylor, P.; Millet, C. The experience of work-related stress across occupations. *J. Manag. Psychol.* **2005**, *20*, 178–187. [CrossRef]
15. Arbe Montoya, A.I.; Hazel, S.; Matthew, S.M.; McArthur, M.L. Moral distress in veterinarians. *Vet. Rec.* **2019**, *185*, 631. [CrossRef] [PubMed]
16. Nett, R.J.; Witte, T.K.; Holzbauer, S.M.; Elchos, B.L.; Campagnolo, E.R.; Musgrave, K.J.; Carter, K.K.; Kurkjian, K.M.; Vanicek, C.F.; O'Leary, D.R.; et al. Risk factors for suicide, attitudes toward mental illness, and practice-related stressors among US veterinarians. *J. Am. Vet. Med. Assoc.* **2015**, *247*, 945–955. [CrossRef] [PubMed]
17. Killinger, S.L.; Flanagan, S.; Castine, E.; Howard, K.A. Stress and Depression among Veterinary Medical Students. *J. Vet. Med. Educ.* **2017**, *44*, 3–8. [CrossRef] [PubMed]
18. Batchelor, C.E.M.; McKeegan, D.E.F. Survey of the frequency and perceived stressfulness of ethical dilemmas encountered in UK veterinary practice. *Vet. Rec.* **2012**, *170*, 19. [CrossRef]
19. Ashall, V. Ethical dilemmas encountered by small animal veterinarians: Challenging the status quo? *Vet. Rec.* **2018**, *182*, 546–547. [CrossRef] [PubMed]
20. Bartram, D.J.; Baldwin, D.S. Veterinary surgeons and suicide: Influences, opportunities and research directions. *Vet. Rec.* **2008**, *162*, 36–40. [CrossRef]
21. Crane, M.F.; Phillips, J.K.; Karin, E. Trait perfectionism strengthens the negative effects of moral stressors occurring in veterinary practice. *Aust. Vet. J.* **2015**, *93*, 354–360. [CrossRef]
22. Schwerdtfeger, K.A.; Bahramsoltani, M.; Spangenberg, L.; Hallensleben, N.; Glaesmer, H. Depression, suicidal ideation and suicide risk in German veterinarians compared with the general German population. *Vet. Rec.* **2020**, *186*, e2. [CrossRef]

23. Tomasi, S.E.; Fechter-Leggett, E.D.; Edwards, N.T.; Reddish, A.D.; Crosby, A.E.; Nett, R.J. Suicide among veterinarians in the United States from 1979 through 2015. *JAVMA* **2019**, *254*, 104–112. [CrossRef]
24. Platt, B.; Hawton, K.; Simkin, S.; Mellanby, R.J. Systematic review of the prevalence of suicide in veterinary surgeons. *Occup. Med.* **2010**, *60*, 436–446. [CrossRef]
25. Kondrup, S.V.; Anhøj, K.P.; Rødsgaard-Rosenbeck, C.; Lund, T.B.; Nissen, M.H.; Sandøe, P. Veterinarian's dilemma: A study of how Danish small animal practitioners handle financially limited clients. *Vet. Rec.* **2016**, *179*, 596. [CrossRef] [PubMed]
26. Springer, S.; Grimm, H. Euthanasie als Thema der veterinärmedizinischen Ethik. *Wien. Tierärztliche Mon.* **2018**, *105*, 129–138.
27. Fawcett, A.; Mullan, S. Managing moral distress in practice. *InPractice* **2018**, *40*, 34–36. [CrossRef]
28. Morgan, C.A. *Stepping up to the Plate: Animal Welfare, Veterinarians, and Ethical Conflicts*; University of British Columbia: Vancouver, BC, Canada, 2009.
29. Kinnison, T. When veterinary teams are faced with clients who can't afford to pay. *Vet. Rec.* **2016**, *179*, 594–595. [CrossRef] [PubMed]
30. Morton, D.; Magalhaes Sant'Ana, M.; Ohl, F.; Ilieski, V.; Simonin, D.; Keeling, L.; Wöhr, A.-C.; Zemljic, B.; Neuhaus, D.; Pesie, S. *FVE, AWARE & EAEVE Report on European Veterinary Education in Animal Welfare Science, Ethics and Law*; Federation of Veterinarians of Europe, 2013. Available online: https://www.fve.org/cms/wp-content/uploads/full_report_aw_curriculum_adopted.pdf (accessed on 10 February 2023).
31. Kunzmann, P.; Schaper, E.; Tipold, A. *FERTHIK-Vermittlung Von Tiermedizinischen, Klinischen Fertigkeiten Unter Besonderer Berücksichtigung Ethischer Aspekte*; Stiftung Tierärztliche Hochschule Hannover: Hannover, Gernamy, 2017.
32. Persson, K.; Gerdts, W.-R.; Hartnack, S.; Kunzmann, P. Assessing Moral Judgements in Veterinary Students: An Exploratory Mixed-Methods Study from Germany. *Animals* **2022**, *12*, 586. [CrossRef] [PubMed]
33. Thöne-Reineke, C.; Hartnack, S.; Kunzmann, P.; Grimm, H.; Weich, K. Veterinärmedizinische Ethik in der universitären Lehre im deutschsprachigen Raum. *Berl. Münch. Tierärztl. Wochenschr.* **2020**, *133*. [CrossRef]
34. *Einführung in Die Angewandte Ethik*; Knoepffler, N.; Kunzmann, P.; Pies, I.; Siegetsleitner, A. (Eds.) Verlag Karl Alber: Freiburg, Germany, 2016; ISBN 9783495860816.
35. Kunzmann, P. Wenn Tierärzte töten–Angewandte Ethik in ihrem Verhältnis zu Moral und Recht. *Berl. Und Münchener Tierärztliche Wochenschr.* **2020**, *133*.
36. Vettical, B.S. An Overview on Ethics and Ethical Decision-Making Process in Veterinary Practice. *J. Agric. Env. Ethics* **2018**, *31*, 739–749. [CrossRef]
37. McCulloch, S. What if it was your dog? *InPractice* **2012**, *34*, 494–495. [CrossRef]
38. Melchers, V. Engpässe bei Impfstoffen und Arzneimitteln: In Ganz Europa Sind Lieferschwierigkeiten bei Veterinärmedizinischen Produkten Häufiger Geworden. Praktizierende Tierärzte Fühlen sich Nicht Selten nur Unzureichend Informiert. Available online: https://www.vetline.de/engpaesse-bei-impfstoffen-und-arzneimitteln (accessed on 4 January 2022).
39. Vereecke, N.; Carnet, F.; Pronost, S.; Vanschandevijl, K.; Theuns, S.; Nauwynck, H. Genome Sequences of Equine Herpesvirus 1 Strains from a European Outbreak of Neurological Disorders Linked to a Horse Gathering in Valencia, Spain, in 2021. *Microbiol. Resour. Announc.* **2021**, *10*, e00333-21. [CrossRef]
40. Fn, D. Herpes-Impfung bei Pferden: Equines Herpesvirus: Ausbrüchen Vorbeugen. Available online: https://www.pferd-aktuell.de/ausbildung/pferdehaltung/impfung/herpes-impfung (accessed on 4 January 2023).
41. FDA. Current Animal Drug Shortages: Medically Necessary Veterinary Products. Available online: https://www.fda.gov/animal-veterinary/product-safety-information/current-animal-drug-shortages (accessed on 4 January 2023).
42. Maille, V.; Hoffmann, J. Compliance with veterinary prescriptions: The role of physical and social risk revisited. *J. Bus. Res.* **2013**, *66*, 141–144. [CrossRef]
43. Huth, M.; Weich, K.; Grimm, H. Veterinarians between the Frontlines?! The Concept of One Health and Three Frames of Health in Veterinary Medicine. *Food Ethics* **2019**, *3*, 91–108. [CrossRef]
44. Hobson-West, P.; Jutel, A. Animals, veterinarians and the sociology of diagnosis. *Sociol. Health Illn.* **2020**, *42*, 393–406. [CrossRef] [PubMed]
45. Weich, K.; Grimm, H. Meeting the Patient's Interest in Veterinary Clinics. Ethical Dimensions of the 21st Century Animal Patient. *Food Ethics* **2018**, *1*, 259–272. [CrossRef]
46. Coghlan, S. Strong Patient Advocacy and the Fundamental Ethical Role of Veterinarians. *J. Agric. Env. Ethics* **2018**, *31*, 349–367. [CrossRef]
47. Persson, K.; Selter, F.; Kunzmann, P.; Neitzke, G. Killing Kira, Letting Tom Go?-An Empirical Study on Intuitions Regarding End-of-Life Decisions in Companion Animals and Humans. *Animals* **2022**, *12*, 2494. [CrossRef] [PubMed]
48. Marron, J.M.; Joffe, S.; Jagsi, R.; Spence, R.A.; Hlubocky, F.J. Ethics and Resource Scarcity: ASCO Recommendations for the Oncology Community During the COVID-19 Pandemic. *J. Clin. Oncol.* **2020**, *38*, 2201–2205. [CrossRef] [PubMed]

Disclaimer/Publisher's Note: The statements, opinions and data contained in all publications are solely those of the individual author(s) and contributor(s) and not of MDPI and/or the editor(s). MDPI and/or the editor(s) disclaim responsibility for any injury to people or property resulting from any ideas, methods, instructions or products referred to in the content.

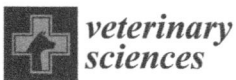

Article

Nurturing a Respectful Connection: Exploring the Relationship between University Educators and Students in a Spanish Veterinary Faculty

Ana S. Ramírez [1,2], José Raduan Jaber [1,2,*], Rubén S. Rosales [1], Magnolia Conde-Felipe [1,2], Francisco Rodríguez [1], Juan Alberto Corbera [1], Alejandro Suárez-Pérez [1], Mario Encinoso [3] and Ana Muniesa [4]

1. Faculty of Veterinary Medicine, University of Las Palmas de Gran Canaria, Trasmontaña, 35413 Arucas, Las Palmas, Spain; anasofia.ramirez@ulpgc.es (A.S.R.); ruben.rosales@ulpgc.es (R.S.R.); magnolia.conde@ulpgc.es (M.C.-F.); francisco.guisado@ulpgc.es (F.R.); juan.corbera@ulpgc.es (J.A.C.); alejandro.suarezperez@ulpgc.es (A.S.-P.)
2. VETFUN, Educational Innovation Group, University of Las Palmas de Gran Canaria, Trasmontaña, 35413 Arucas, Las Palmas, Spain
3. Veterinary Clinical Hospital, Faculty of Veterinary Medicine, University of Las Palmas de Gran Canaria, Trasmontaña, 35413 Arucas, Las Palmas, Spain; mencinoso@gmail.com
4. Faculty of Veterinary, University of Zaragoza-CITA, Miguel Servet, 177, 50013 Zaragoza, Zaragoza, Spain; animuni@unizar.es
* Correspondence: joseraduan.jaber@ulpgc.es; Tel.: +34-928-457428

Simple Summary: Though knowledge and the communication capacity of teachers play a crucial role in the student learning process, adequate teaching also relies on the respect of teachers for their students. We initiated this research after a conversation with a group of university students, who expressed their discontent regarding the lack of respect shown towards them by some teachers. The results obtained in online surveys highlighted the need for faculty members to analyze and question their attitudes towards their students.

Abstract: The respect of the teacher for the student is essential for effective teaching from the perspective of the students, even in comparison to the knowledge and communication capacity of the teacher. Consequently, the optimal development of this characteristic fosters a more effective and efficient student–teacher relationship. We initiated this research following a conversation with a group of university students, who expressed their discontent regarding the lack of respect shown towards them by some teachers. Therefore, we conducted a descriptive study using online surveys, focusing on the central axis in the teacher–student relationship. The results highlighted the need for faculty members to analyze and question their attitudes towards their students. This paper presents initial results of the data collected at the Veterinary Faculty of the University of Las Palmas de Gran Canaria.

Keywords: respect; teacher–student relationship; veterinary students

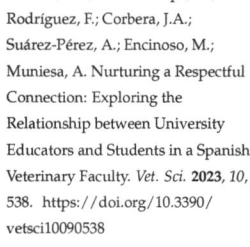

Citation: Ramírez, A.S.; Jaber, J.R.; Rosales, R.S.; Conde-Felipe, M.; Rodríguez, F.; Corbera, J.A.; Suárez-Pérez, A.; Encinoso, M.; Muniesa, A. Nurturing a Respectful Connection: Exploring the Relationship between University Educators and Students in a Spanish Veterinary Faculty. *Vet. Sci.* **2023**, *10*, 538. https://doi.org/10.3390/vetsci10090538

Academic Editor: Lieta Marinelli

Received: 12 July 2023
Revised: 13 August 2023
Accepted: 22 August 2023
Published: 24 August 2023

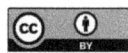

Copyright: © 2023 by the authors. Licensee MDPI, Basel, Switzerland. This article is an open access article distributed under the terms and conditions of the Creative Commons Attribution (CC BY) license (https://creativecommons.org/licenses/by/4.0/).

1. Introduction

Nowadays, having a university education is one of the more relevant tools enabling considerable changes in society to be made. However, the university environment is very challenging due to the increasing demands, standards, and expectations of the population. Lecturers feel overwhelmed with multiple functions and tasks, such as teaching, conducting promotional research, attending meetings and congresses, requesting projects, participating in community service activities, and helping students in various university activities. Due to these requirements, the characteristics and skills of university teachers are considered to be foremost factors in avoiding negative emotions such as tension, hostility, depression, anger, nervousness, frustration, and even burnout [1–3]. Therefore, it is essential for university teachers to possess not only the appropriate knowledge, but also to develop an adequate attitude that would benefit the development of a positive relationship between the student and themselves, as this relationship is one of the fundamental elements in the teaching–learning process [4]. The communication between educators and learners can impact each other either negatively or positively [5]. Hence, teachers must respect the student as a person and be friendly and communicative [6].

The personal characteristics of teachers can help to understand and accept diverse student perspectives, which reinforces the teacher–student relationship [7]. It is known that an effective education process may depend on the teacher's characteristics [8]. Anderson [9] summarized the characteristics associated with effective teachers, such as confidence, reliability, commitment, analytical and conceptual thinking, information search, initiative, flexibility, responsibility, passion for learning, and respect. This last attribute is particularly valuable, as treating students with respect and expecting the same in return enhances the students' learning progress [10] and is a motivating factor for students [11].

Delaney et al. [12] analyzed the latter characteristic and concluded that effective teachers had a sense of respect for their students; this was found to be the most essential attribute, even more so than knowledge. Similar results were reported by Bahador et al. and Al-Mohaimeed [13,14]. According to the American philosopher and essayist Ralph Waldo Emerson (1803–1882), "The secret of education lies in respect for the disciple". However, respect is a controversial concept, and its implications can vary from one culture to another, especially in Western cultures, where respect is considered a mutual and fundamental obligation [15]. It raises the question: how does a professor show respect to their students? Osborne [16] suggested that the common denominator of all answers is the rule of ethical conduct: Do unto others as you would have them do unto you. The relationship between a teacher and a student is more productive when there is mutual respect, and an environment of respect, caring, and trust increases teaching effectiveness [17].

The impetus for this study arose because of the complaints of first-year veterinary college students at the University of Las Palmas de Gran Canaria (ULPGC) regarding disrespectful behavior from some teachers. Thus, this study aimed to assess student perceptions of teacher respect towards students for different academic years within the same faculty.

2. Materials and Methods

2.1. Study Design and Questionnaire

We conducted a descriptive survey from May to June 2018. The study population (n = 434) comprised students from the Veterinary Faculty of Las Palmas de Gran Canaria University (Canary Islands, Spain), who were in their first to fifth year of study. The inclusion criteria were that students were enrolled in an academic year and had willingness to participate in the study. Answers were collected anonymously via convenience sampling. The minimum sample size was calculated (given a total of 79 answers for a confidence level of 95% and an absolute accepted error of 10%.) using Win Episcope 2.0 [18]. A total of 142 surveys was obtained, and Google Forms (forms.google.com) was used to create and collect answers from the questionnaires.

Before enabling data collection for the questionnaire, we verified the time required for its completion, and communicated this to the student cohort. The survey link was sent through the Moodle platform corresponding to each relevant academic subject, accompanied by explicit elucidation that participation denoted a deliberate bestowal of informed consent. Prior to answering the questionnaire, the students were provided with an informed consent statement that explained the survey's purpose, estimated completion time, and assured confidentiality. As the survey targeted the students of the Veterinary Faculty, the response rate could be calculated despite conducting the study using an anonymous online Google Form.

The researchers of the survey designed a questionnaire to measure student perceptions of respect at the university. It comprised 25 questions grouped into three domains: student demographic profile (gender, date of birth, and year of study), positive attitudes of the teacher, and negative attitudes of the teacher. Table 1 shows questions 1 to 14, which are concerned with the attitude of teachers from a positive point of view, and questions 15 to 22, which are concerned with the attitude of teachers from a negative point of view.

Table 1. Questionnaire used to measure student perceptions of respect at the university. Questions in Spanish, the original language of the study, are shown in parenthesis and in grey.

Domain	Question	Abbreviation
Positive attitudes of the teachers	1. My teachers treat all the students equally (Mis profesores tratan a todos los alumnos por igual)	Treat_Equal
	2. My teachers usually smile (Mis profesores suelen sonreír)	Smile
	3. My teachers are polite with the students (Mis profesores son educados con los estudiantes)	Polite
	4. My teachers have a positive attitude towards the students (Mis profesores tienen actitud positiva hacia los alumnos)	Pos_Attit
	5. My teachers motivate me in my studies and professional future (Mis profesores me motivan en mis estudios y futuro profesional)	Motive
	6. My teachers have patience (Mis profesores tienen paciencia)	Patient
	7. My teachers are willing to help students who have difficulties (Mis profesores se muestran dispuestos a ayudar a los estudiantes que tienen dificultades)	Helpful
	8. My teachers show a receptive and respectful attitude in their relationship with the students (Mis profesores manifiestan una actitud receptiva y respetuosa en su relación con el alumnado)	Rec_Resp
	9. My teachers are accessible to the students (Mis profesores se muestran accesibles a los estudiantes)	Accessible
	10. My teachers respect the student diversity (Mis profesores respetan la diversidad)	Resp_Div
	11. The personal behavior I have received from my teachers has been correct (El trato personal que he recibido por parte de mis profesores ha sido correcto)	Correct
	12. My teachers apologize when they make a mistake (Mis profesores se disculpan cuando cometen un error)	Apol_Mist
	13. My teachers have a sense of humor (Mis profesores tienen sentido del humor)	Sen_Hum
	14. My teachers show enthusiasm (Mis profesores muestran entusiasmo)	Enthusiastic
Negative attitudes of the teachers	15. My teachers abuse their authority (Mis profesores abusan de su autoridad)	Abu_auth
	16. My teachers present sexist attitudes (Mis profesores presentan actitudes sexistas)	Sexist
	17. My teachers are rude to the students (Mis profesores son maleducados con los alumnos)	Rude
	18. My teachers shout at the students (Mis profesores gritan a los alumnos)	Shout
	19. My teachers present a vengeful attitude toward the students (Mis profesores presentan una actitud vengativa hacia los alumnos)	Veng_Attit
	20. My teachers humiliate the students (Mis profesores humillan a los alumnos)	Hum
	21. My teachers threaten/coerce the students (Mis profesores amenazan/coaccionan a los alumnos)	Thr_Coer
	22. My teachers are sarcastic when dealing with the students (Mis profesores son sarcásticos en el trato con los alumnos)	Sarcastic

2.2. Statistical Analysis

The questionnaire responses were collected in an Excel spreadsheet, and the same program (Excel 2016) was used to perform descriptive statistical analysis and create graphical representations. Data were entered, and statistical analysis was carried out using SPSS 19 (Statistical Package for the Social Sciences). The demographic attributes, including gender, age, and the year of study, were analyzed using descriptive statistical methods. We assessed the rest of the questions using a five-point Likert scale, where students indicated the extent to which they agreed with each statement (1—None, 2—Almost none, 3—About half, 4—The majority, 5—All). Regarding the responses on the Likert scale, in a subsequent analysis, the answers were simplified into two options. Responses of "All" and "Most" relating to positive attitudes were considered as "Most", while the remaining responses were categorized as "Some". On the contrary, for responses concerning negative attitudes, the 'Some' option included "None" or "Some", and the rest were considered as "Most".

The responses were ordinal variables, so descriptive analysis was based on the median, interquartile range, and mode calculation. For inferential analysis, the chi-squared test was used to analyze the gender effect. Somers' D statistics were calculated to measure the correlation between ordinal variables (Likert scale and academic year), and Cronbach's alpha was used to assess the reliability and consistency of each domain in the questionnaires. The alpha error was set at 0.05.

3. Results

In this study, a total of 142 students completed an online questionnaire. The response rate was 29.89%, and the absolute error of the sample size was 6.75%. Incorrect responses to the birth date question were given by 11 students (7.7%), indicating that their age was missing. The age range was 18–42 years old, with an average age of 22.75, a median of 21, and a mode of 19 years old. Most participants were female (99, 69.72%), with 43 males (30.28%). The distribution of answers related to the academic year in descending order was first year (45%), fifth year (19%), second year (16%), fourth year (11%), and third year (9%). The distribution of answers with taking into account year of study and gender is shown in Figure 1.

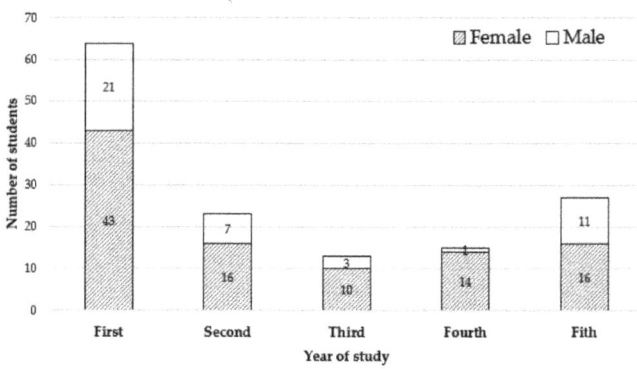

Figure 1. Distribution and gender of the students related to the year of study.

Regarding reliability and consistency, we obtained a Cronbach's alpha of 0.935 for the second domain (positive attitude of the teacher) and 0.865 for the third domain (negative attitude of the teacher). Cronbach's alpha is a measure of internal consistency, which is closely related to the homogeneity of a set of items. A high value suggests that the items within the scale or questionnaire are strongly correlated with each other, indicating a high degree of interrelatedness and coherence in measuring the targeted construct.

The results of the frequency, percentage, median, interquartile range, and mode of the levels of the Likert scale are presented in Table 2. These questions pertain to two domains: positive attitudes of teachers (Questions 1–14) and negative attitudes of teachers (Questions 15–22). Focusing on the results of the first 14 questions (first domain), we can see that the questions with a median answer of "The majority" were Questions 1 (My teachers treat all the students equally), 3 (My teachers are polite with the students), 8 (My teachers show a receptive and respectful attitude in their relationship with the students), 10 (My teachers respect the students' diversity) and 11 (The personal behavior I have received from my teachers has been correct). In these questions, more than 85 students (approximately 60% of the sample) reported that "The majority" or "All" of the teachers complied with these premises. In this domain, Question 5 (My teachers motivate me in my studies and professional future) had the worst rating, with 51 students reporting that "None" (7) or "Some" (44) of the teachers motivated the students. Moreover, it is fundamental to highlight that concerning the questions such as whether the teachers tend to smile (Question 2), are willing to help students who have difficulties (Question 7), apologize when they make a mistake (Question 12), have a sense of humor (Question 13) and show enthusiasm (Question 14) (see Table 2), more than 25 students responded with "None" or "Some".

Table 2. Descriptive statistics, the responses for the five levels of the Likert scale (1–None 2–Some 3–About half 4–The majority 5–All) are expressed as frequencies and percentages of total student responses.

Domain	Question [1]	None	Some	About Half	The Majority	All	Median (Q3–Q1 #)	Mode	Somers' d
Positive attitudes of the teachers	1. Treat_Equal	2 / 1.41%	11 / 7.75%	36 / 25.35%	80 / 56.34%	13 / 9.15%	The majority / 1	The majority	0.545
	2. Smile	1 / 0.7%	27 / 19.01%	45 / 31.69%	62 / 43.66%	7 / 4.93%	About half / 1	The majority	0.059
	3. Polite	0 / 0.00%	11 / 7.75%	40 / 28.17%	78 / 54.93%	13 / 54.93%	The majority / 1	The majority	0.169
	4. Pos_Attit	0 / 0.00%	22 / 15.49%	55 / 38.73%	59 / 41.55%	6 / 4.23%	About half / 1	The majority	0.345
	5. Motivate	7 / 4.93%	44 / 30.99%	53 / 37.32%	33 / 23.24%	5 / 3.52%	About half / 2	About half	0.481
	6. Patient	2 / 1.41%	22 / 15.49%	53 / 37.32%	58 / 40.85%	7 / 4.93%	About half / 1	The majority	0.558
	7. Helpful	3 / 2.11%	31 / 21.83%	54 / 38.03%	45 / 31.69%	9 / 6.34%	About half / 1	About half	0.909
	8. Rec_Resp	1 / 0.7%	15 / 10.56%	41 / 28.87%	78 / 54.93%	7 / 4.93%	The majority / 1	The majority	0.082
	9. Accessible	1 / 0.7%	17 / 11.97%	54 / 38.03%	61 / 42.96%	9 / 6.34%	About half / 1	The majority	0.900
	10. Resp_Div	0 / 0.00%	12 / 8.45%	33 / 23.24%	58 / 40.85%	39 / 27.46%	The majority / 2	The majority	0.135
	11. Correct	0 / 0.00%	4 / 2.82%	36 / 25.35%	75 / 52.82%	27 / 19.01%	The majority / 1	The majority	0.950
	12. Apol_Mist	11 / 7.75%	34 / 23.94%	47 / 33.1%	37 / 26.06%	13 / 9.15%	About half / 2	About half	0.208
	13. Sen_hum	1 / 0.7%	25 / 17.61%	74 / 52.11%	35 / 24.65%	7 / 4.93%	About half / 1	About half	0.811
	14. Enthusiastic	3 / 2.11%	35 / 24.65%	63 / 44.37%	38 / 26.76%	3 / 2.11%	About half / 2	About half	0.386
Negative attitudes of the teachers	15. Abu_auth	21 / 14.79%	37 / 26.06%	54 / 38.03%	29 / 20.42%	1 / 0.7%	About half / 1	About half	0.740
	16. Sexist	30 / 21.13%	30 / 21.13%	63 / 44.37%	18 / 12.68%	1 / 0.7%	About half / 1	About half	0.276
	17. Rude	26 / 18.31%	49 / 34.51%	60 / 42.25%	7 / 4.93%	0 / 0.00%	Some / 1	About half	0.728
	18. Shout	52 / 36.62%	53 / 37.32%	37 / 26.06%	0 / 0.00%	0 / 0.00%	Some / 2	Some	0.538
	19. Veng_Attit	36 / 25.35%	65 / 45.77%	37 / 26.06%	4 / 2.82%	0 / 0.00%	Some / 2	Some	0.005
	20. Hum	22 / 15.49%	66 / 46.48%	52 / 36.62%	1 / 0.7%	1 / 0.7%	Some / 1	Some	0.572
	21. Thr_Coer	90 / 63.38%	32 / 22.54%	19 / 13.38%	0 / 0%	1 / 0.7%	None / 1	None	0.547
	22. Sarcastic	18 / 12.68%	42 / 29.58%	65 / 45.77%	15 / 10.56%	2 / 1.41%	About half / 1	About half	0.708

Quartile 3 minus quartile 1 in Likert scale. [1] Abbreviations are shown in Table 1.

Figure 2 presents a simplification of the results for the questions regarding positive attitudes of the teachers towards the students, while in Figure 3, we can see the results related to negative attitudes. Both figures present outcomes analogous to those found in Table 2, but they are dichotomized to enhance the interpretation of the results. In Figure 2, we observed that the majority of the teachers treat the students fairly, are polite, are receptive/respectful, respect diversity, and are courteous in their manner, while only a few smile, have a positive attitude, and are patient, motivate, assist students, are approachable, apologize for a mistake, have a sense of humor, or show enthusiasm. Statistical analysis revealed statistically significant disparities across most traits between the two groups.

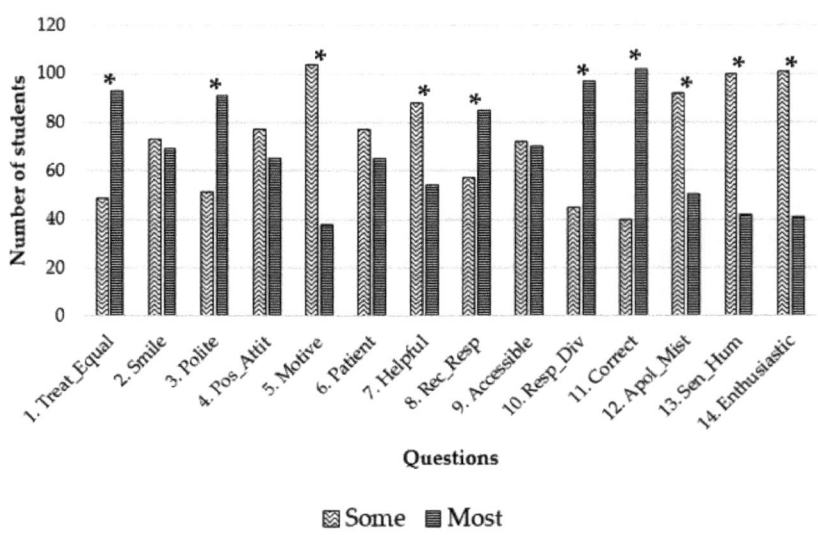

Figure 2. Dichotomized answers to the questions about positive attitudes of the teachers. Statistically significant differences in proportions are marked with an asterisk.

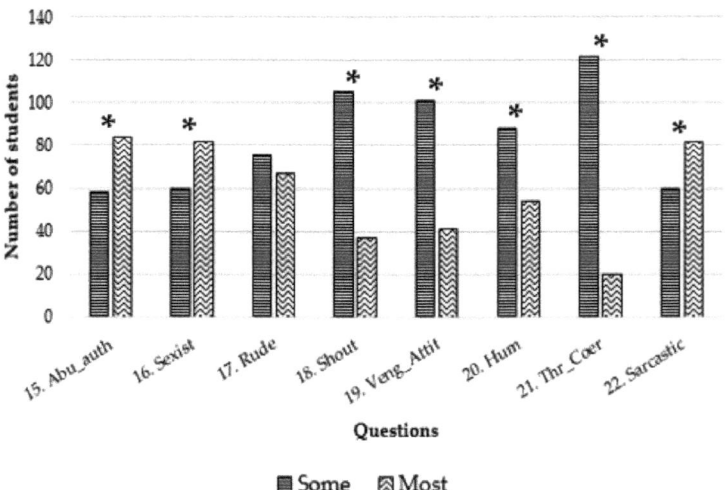

Figure 3. Dichotomized answers to the questions about negative attitudes of the teachers. Statistically significant differences in proportions are marked with an asterisk.

Table 2 shows the results of questions 15 to 22, which addressed the negative attitudes of the teachers. Five of these questions had a median of "Some" or "None". At least 75 students (>52% of the sample) considered that "None" or "Some" of the teachers were rude (Question 17), shouted at the students (Question 18), were vengeful (Question 19), humiliated the students (Question 20), or threatened or coerced them (Question 21). The latter question was rejected by nearly 86% of the students. Additionally, 17 students considered that most or all teachers were sarcastic (Question 22), 19 considered that they presented sexist attitudes (Question 16), and 30 reported authority abuse (Question 15). Notable attention should be given to this last result, as more than 21% of the students had a negative perception of the teaching staff. In Figure 3, we observed that behaviors such as being rude, shouting, presenting vengeful attitudes, humiliating, and threatening the students are not commonly observed. However, students feel that a majority of the teachers abuse their authority, exhibit sexist attitudes, and employ sarcasm. Statistically significant differences were found in all of these questions, except for being rude.

Another variable used for stratifying the data was the academic year. Questions corresponding to the positive attitudes of the teachers (7, 9, 11, and 13) were correlated with the academic year using Somers' D statistic with a value >0.8, and questions 15, 17, and 22 about the negative attitude of teachers had a value >0.7 (Table 2). Somers' D is a measure of association used to assess the strength and direction of the relationship between two ordinal variables. It ranges from −1 to 1, where 0 indicates no association, positive values suggest a positive association.

4. Discussion

The present study investigated the student perceptions of teachers' respect towards students of different academic years of the Veterinary College of ULPGC. Interestingly, most of the respondents to the survey were in their first year of study. It was unsurprising, as these were the ones who initiated the work and thus became more engaged in the study. Moreover, the fact that more female students than males responded to the questionnaire was due to the increased presence of female students in Spanish universities [19], particularly in veterinary faculties, where feminization is a statistical reality [20], which is in line with other international veterinary faculties [21]. It is particularly pertinent in the ULPGC, where the percentage of female students is very high (72.9%), and a similar percentage was found at our veterinary faculty. However, no association was found between student gender and the other variables, as previously found by Mortazavi et al. [22]. We did not ask if the students were nationals or foreigners because the latter represent less than 3% of the total, and asking this question could have jeopardized their anonymity.

The fact of asking questions about the attitudes of the professors from a positive or negative point of view was conducted to avoid the drawbacks of the Likert scale, since the positive answers always exceeded the negative ones. In our study, we wanted to obtain results more reflective of reality than the manipulation of both types of questions, as recommended by Barnette [23]. Furthermore, by analyzing the consistency of the question within the domains, gave a Cronbach alpha value of 0.935 for the second domain (positive attitude of the teacher) and 0.865 for the third domain (negative attitude of the teacher). According to George and Mallery [24], who provided widely referenced guidelines for interpreting Cronbach's alpha, the values above 0.9 provide excellent internal consistency, while values between 0.8 and 0.9 show good internal consistency. Therefore, a Cronbach's alpha of 0.935 and 0.865 falls within the "excellent and good internal consistency" range, indicating that the items in the scale are reliably measuring the same underlying construct. This level of internal consistency lends support to the validity and reliability of the measurement instrument [25]. This result was in contrast with other authors who pointed out issues such as internal consistency when negatively worded questions were used [23,25,26].

Regarding the academic year, Somers' D analysis showed that appreciation for the teacher's attitude increased only in seven of the 22 questions. However, we must consider that questions 7, 9, 11, and 13 are included in the domain of positive teacher attitude, while questions 15, 17, and 22 deal with the negative teacher attitude (Table 1). Interpreting a Somers' D value higher than 0.7 indicates a strong positive association between two ordinal variables and suggests a substantial degree of correlation between the two variables, implying that as one variable increases, the other tends to increase as well [27].

In this study, the results of the Likert scale questions were presented in two ways: the complete information provided in Table 2, and the dichotomized results depicted in Figures 2 and 3. Dichotomizing the results of a five-degree Likert scale offers potential benefits, such as simplifying the analysis, facilitating communication, highlighting extreme values, allowing direct comparison of proportions in the two groups. However, it is essential to note that dichotomizing Likert scale data also entails limitations, including information loss, misinterpretation, and oversimplification of participant responses [25].

Regarding the positive attitudes expected from the teachers, it seems that most of the students found that most of the teachers treat them in a correct manner. Question 10 inquired about whether the teachers respect student diversity. Nearly 70% of the students responded that most of the teachers do so. At the veterinary faculty of ULPGC, diversity is more closely linked to gender diversity, given the homogeneity of the student body. In fact, ULPGC promotes initiatives for raising awareness and providing training, along with measures to support research, aimed at the university community to promote respect and ensure the protection of the right to freely self-determine gender identity and expression. Cornell et al. [28] studied the significance of inclusive learning environments and found that respectful teacher–student relationships positively affected students from diverse backgrounds. These relationships created a sense of belonging and engagement among students, ultimately contributing to improved academic performance and retention. The question most assessed by the students was Question 11, which referred to the correct treatment received from them, with 102 out of 142 (71.8%) agreeing.

In the modern educational landscape, the role of university teachers extends beyond the mere transmission of knowledge. Teachers are entrusted with the crucial task of creating an inclusive environment that ensures effective and engaging instruction. However, a paradox emerges when some educators succeed in cultivating an inclusive atmosphere yet fall short in delivering captivating and effective teaching methodologies. In this study, we detected a failure in most of the teachers in the affective–motivational dimension, which refers to the emotional and motivational aspects of the teaching and learning process. It encompasses the teacher's ability to create a positive emotional climate, foster motivation, and establish a supportive relationship with students. It recognizes that emotions, attitudes, and motivation play a significant role in shaping students' learning experiences and outcomes. Thus, Question 5, in which students felt that the teachers did not motivate them in their studies and professional future, was the least rated, with only 38 out of 142 (26.8%) indicating that teachers motivated them.

While the promotion of a positive and inclusive environment is essential for nurturing a supportive learning community, it is equally crucial for teachers to complement this effort with engaging and effective teaching practices. By recognizing the divergence in skill sets, addressing pedagogical barriers, and embracing a willingness to evolve, educators can bridge the gap between inclusivity and engagement. Through a balanced approach, teachers can empower their students with not only a sense of belonging but also a passion for learning that extends far beyond the classroom. Ryan and Deci's self-determination theory [29] emphasizes the importance of fostering intrinsic motivation and autonomy in students' learning, arguing that respectful and supportive teacher–student relationships satisfy students' psychological needs, promoting intrinsic motivation and active engagement in the learning process.

Previous evidence indicates that students believe that a positive teacher–student relationship is essential to improve the educational environment [30]. Other studies reported that the quality of the teacher–student relationship has a strong impact on learning, performance, and students' satisfaction [31]. Furthermore, the teachers' behavior has a notable role in the teacher–student relationship, while other variables such as gender, age, and physical appearance of the teacher have lesser influence [3,22,32]. Another characteristic of outstanding teachers is the demonstration of enthusiasm in their classroom, despite having taught the same subject for many years [17]. Delaney et al. [12] analyzed positive attitudes of educators and considered that effective teachers had a sense of respect for their students. This is because students were more likely to consider teachers who were compassionate and understanding, treated them with respect, and made them feel comfortable asking questions. The same authors asked their students what characteristics were essential for effective teaching from the student's perspective, and respect turned out to be the most important, even more so than knowledge and the ability to communicate. In addition, we should consider that a sense of humor in university teaching could play a significant role in creating a positive and engaging learning environment by promoting a sense of warmth and approachability. Humor has the potential to reduce stress and anxiety among students. This reduction can enhance cognitive functioning and information retention and help to capture students' attention and maintain their engagement with the material [33].

The relationship between educators and students is a critical factor that significantly influences students' academic performance, emotional well-being, and overall learning experience. Numerous studies emphasize the role of positive teacher–student relationships in academic achievement. Roorda et al. [34] conducted a meta-analysis involving 99 studies and found that supportive teacher–student relationships positively correlated with higher academic motivation and engagement. While a longitudinal study by Hamre and Pianta [35] revealed that positive teacher–student interactions were associated with greater academic progress over time. Effective communication is a crucial component of a respectful connection between educators and students. Martin and Dowson [36] investigated the role of communication in teacher–student relationships and highlighted that open and transparent communication enhances the quality of the relationship and student satisfaction with the learning experience. Also, the emotional well-being of students is deeply influenced by their relationship with educators. Jennings and Greenberg [37] explored the impact of teacher–student relationships on student mental health and found that supportive relationships contributed to reduced stress and anxiety levels. Conversely, negative relationships were associated with emotional distress and academic disengagement.

Concerning the negative attitudes of the teachers observed in our study, thirty out of 142 students (21.1%) reported that most of the teachers had abused their authority, whereas 82 (57.7%) answered that about half or more had exhibited sexist attitudes or been sarcastic. Gender bias is a prevalent issue within the medical field, often taking the form of microaggressions that begin to surface during medical school. This study highlights that female medical students consistently experience significant microaggressions, resulting in heightened stress levels. Among the various microaggression domains, the concept of "leaving gender at the door" emerges as the predominant and particularly distressing category. It may potentially signify the existence of societal pressure to downplay feminine attributes in the pursuit of success. [38]. In the context of veterinarians practicing in rural areas, it has been observed that the prevalence of sexist attitudes among certain farmers and colleagues constitutes a significant disadvantage [39]. Sometimes, sarcasm is considered a sort of offensive humor, but it is considered inappropriate in the classroom. Research has shown that the use of sarcasm by educators can have negative consequences. Sarcasm, when not well-received, can lead to misunderstandings, create a hostile classroom environment, and hinder effective communication. It might impede students' comprehension, discourage participation, and adversely affect teacher–student relationships [40].

Fortunately, most students did not feel threatened/coerced by the teachers (122/142, 85.9%). Additionally, most of them thought that most teachers did not shout at them (105/142, 73.9%) nor display a vengeful attitude (101/142, 71.1%). Different authors focus on the teacher's respect towards students in order to maintain an appropriate learning environment, while others agree that mutual respect is essential for student–teacher communication [17,41–43]. Therefore, avoiding negative attitudes and constructing a respectful association and interaction between students and teachers is essential to stimulate and encourage the learning of a subject, as the impact of educator relational behaviors on educational responsibility, favorable outcome, and enthusiasm of beginners is the basis of most studies [44,45]. Furthermore, a quality teacher–student relationship has been linked to more enjoyment and less anxiety and anger [46]. It is important to remember that teaching is not only about imparting knowledge; it should also concern the development of an interest and love for learning. Teachers must inspire and motivate students [47].

5. Conclusions

The results of this study emphasize the importance of nurturing a respectful connection between educators and students. Positive teacher–student relationships have been linked to improved academic achievement, enhanced emotional well-being, increased intrinsic motivation, and the creation of an inclusive learning environment. Therefore, educational institutions should implement strategies and initiatives to promote a culture of respect and support, ultimately to enrich the educational experience for all students. To evaluate further this perspective, studies involving more veterinary colleges should be conducted. In addition, although the teachers received positive assessments across most surveyed aspects, the absence of affective–motivational dimensions towards students warrants an active review. These attitudes can impact students' development and future professional endeavors. Similarly, the presence of sexist attitudes and instances of authority abuse identified through this survey should be critically examined and controlled to eliminate such behavior toward students within the university.

Author Contributions: Conceptualization, A.S.R., R.S.R., A.M. and M.C-F.; methodology, A.S.R., R.S.R., J.R.J., F.R. and A.M.; formal analysis, A.S.R., R.S.R., A.S.-P. and A.M.; investigation, F.R., J.A.C. and M.E.; writing—original draft preparation, F.R., J.A.C., J.R.J., A.S.-P. and M.E.; writing—review and editing, M.C-F.; visualization, M.C-F.; supervision, A.S.R., A.M. and J.R.J. All authors have read and agreed to the published version of the manuscript.

Funding: This research received no external funding.

Institutional Review Board Statement: Not applicable.

Informed Consent Statement: Informed consent was obtained from all subjects involved in the study.

Data Availability Statement: Not applicable.

Conflicts of Interest: The authors declare no conflict of interest.

References

1. Ismail, A.; Suh-Suh, Y.; Ajis, M.N.; Dollah, N.F. Relationship between Occupational Stress, Emotional Intelligence and Job Performance: An Empirical Study in Malaysia. *J. Theor. Appl. Eng.* **2009**, *10*, 3–16.
2. Chatani, Y.; Nomura, K.; Horie, S.; Takemoto, K.; Takeuchi, M.; Sasamori, Y.; Takenoshita, S.; Murakami, A.; Hiraike, H.; Okinaga, H.; et al. Effects of Gaps in Priorities between Ideal and Real Lives on Psychological Burnout among Academic Faculty Members at a Medical University in Japan: A Cross-Sectional Study. *Environ. Health Prev. Med.* **2017**, *22*, 32. [CrossRef]
3. Maleki, F.; Talaei, M.H.; Moghadam, S.R.M.; Shadigo, S.; Taghinejad, H.; Mirzaei, A. Investigating the Influence of Teachers' Characteristics on the Teacher-Student Relations from Students' Perspective at Ilam University of Medical Sciences. *J. Clin. Diagn. Res.* **2017**, *11*, JC04–JC08. [CrossRef] [PubMed]
4. Demirkaya, P.N.; Bakkaloglu, H. Examining the Student-Teacher Relationships of Children Both with and without Special Needs in Preschool Classrooms. *J. Educ. Sci. Theory Pract.* **2015**, *15*, 159–175. [CrossRef]
5. Luo, Y.; Deng, Y.; Zhang, H. The Influences of Parental Emotional Warmth on the Association between Perceived Teacher–Student Relationships and Academic Stress among Middle School Students in China. *Child Youth Serv. Rev.* **2020**, *114*, 105014. [CrossRef]
6. Hassan, N.; Jani, S.H.M.; Som, R.M.; Hamid, N.Z.A.; Azizam, N.A. The Relationship between Emotional Intelligence and Teaching Effectiveness among Lecturers at Universiti Teknologi MARA, Puncak Alam, Malaysia. *Int. J. Soc. Sci. Humanit.* **2015**, *5*, 1–5. [CrossRef]
7. Nelson, D.B.; Low, G.R. *Emotional Intelligence: Achieving Academic and Career Excellence*, 2nd ed.; Prentice Hall: Boston, MA, USA, 2011; pp. 9–13, ISBN 978-0-13-502299-3.
8. Rahmatullah, M. The Relationship between Learning Effectiveness, Teacher Competence and Teachers Performance Madrasah Tsanawiyah at Serang, Banten, Indonesia. *High Educ. Stud.* **2016**, *6*, 169. [CrossRef]

9. Anderson, L.W. Increasing Teacher Effectiveness. In *Fundamentals of Educational Planning*, 2nd ed.; UNESCO: Paris, France, 2004; pp. 21–24, ISBN 978-92-803-1258-4.
10. Moreno Rubio, C. Efective Teachers-Profesional and Personal Skills. *Ensayos* **2009**, *24*, 35–46.
11. Bidabadi, N.S.; Isfahani, A.N.; Rouhollahi, A.; Khalili, R. Effective Teaching Methods in Higher Education: Requirements and Barriers. *J. Adv. Med. Educ. Prof.* **2016**, *4*, 170–178.
12. Delaney, J.G.; Johnson, A.; Johnson, T.D.; Treslan, D. Students' Perceptions of Effective Teaching in Higher Education. In *Project Report*; Memorial University of Newfoundland: St. John's, NL, Canada, 2010; Available online: https://research.library.mun.ca/8370/ (accessed on 31 May 2023).
13. Bahador, H.; Faraji Armaki, A.; Ghorbani, R.; Dehghani, E. Effective Factors on Communication between Teacher and Student Medical Students of Basic Sciences Level View. *Educ. Strategy Med. Sci.* **2014**, *6*, 195–200.
14. Al-Mohaimeed, A.A. Comparison between Faculty and Students Perspectives on the Qualities of a Good Medical Teacher: A Cross-Sectional Study. *Int. J. Health Sci.* **2018**, *12*, 15–20.
15. Celkan, G.; Green, L.; Hussain, K. Student Perceptions of Teacher Respect toward College Students. *Procedia Soc. Behav. Sci.* **2015**, *191*, 2174–2178. [CrossRef]
16. Osborne, C.A. Teaching Our Students as We Want to Be Taught. *J. Vet. Med. Educ.* **2003**, *30*, 297–300. [CrossRef] [PubMed]
17. Rossetti, J.; Fox, P.G. Factors Related to Successful Teaching by Outstanding Professors: An Interpretive Study. *J. Nurs. Educ.* **2009**, *48*, 11–16. [CrossRef] [PubMed]
18. Thrusfield, M.; Ortega, C.; De Blas, I.; Noordhuizen, J.P.; Frankena, K. WIN EPISCOPE 2.0: Improved Epidemiological Software for Veterinary Medicine. *Vet. Rec.* **2001**, *148*, 567–572. [CrossRef] [PubMed]
19. Gómez Marcos, M.T.; Vicente Galindo, M.P.; Martín Rodero, H. Mujeres en la universidad española: Diferencias de género en el alumnado de grado. *Int. J. Educ. Psychol.* **2019**, *2*, 443–454. [CrossRef]
20. Sistema Universitario Español. Available online: https://www.universidades.gob.es/portal/site/universidades/ (accessed on 30 June 2020).
21. Giuffrida, M.A.; Burton, J.H.; Dechant, J.E.; Winter, A. Gender Imbalance in Authorship of Veterinary Literature: 1995 versus 2015. *J. Vet. Med. Educ.* **2019**, *46*, 429–437. [CrossRef]
22. Mortazavi, S.S.; Heidari, A.; Mortazavi, Z.; Seyedtabib, M. Factors Affecting Teacher-Student Relationship from the Perspective of Students in School of Rehabilitation, Hamadan University of Medical Sciences. *J. Med. Educ. Dev.* **2019**, *12*, 41–48. [CrossRef]
23. Barnette, J.J. Effects of Stem and Likert Response Option Reversals on Survey Internal Consistency: If You Feel the Need, There Is a Better Alternative to Using Those Negatively Worded Stems. *Educ. Psychol. Meas.* **2000**, *60*, 361–370. [CrossRef]
24. George, D.; Mallery, P. *SPSS for Windows Step by Step: A Simple Guide and Reference, 11.0 Update*, 4th ed.; Allyn & Bacon: Boston, MA, USA, 2003.
25. DeVellis, R.F. *Scale Development: Theory and Applications*, 4th ed.; SAGE Publications: Thousand Oaks, CA, USA, 2017.
26. Sauro, J.; Lewis, J.R. When Designing Usability Questionnaires, Does It Hurt to Be Positive? In Proceedings of the SIGCHI Conference on Human Factors in Computing Systems, Vancouver, BC, Canada, 7–12 May 2011; pp. 2215–2224.
27. Agresti, A. *Categorical Data Analysis*, 3rd ed.; Wiley: New York, NY, USA, 2018.
28. Cornell, D.; Huang, F. Authoritative School Climate and High School Student Risk Behavior: A Cross-sectional Multi-level Analysis of Student Self-Reports. *J. Youth Adolesc.* **2016**, *45*, 2246–2259. [CrossRef]
29. Ryan, R.M.; Deci, E.L. Intrinsic and extrinsic motivations: Classic definitions and new directions. *Contemp. Educ. Psychol.* **2000**, *25*, 54–67. [CrossRef]
30. Chan, Z.C.; Tong, C.W.; Henderson, S. Power Dynamics in the Student-Teacher Relationship in Clinical Settings. *Nurse Educ. Today* **2017**, *49*, 174–179. [CrossRef]
31. Mobashery, M.; Deris, F.; Taji, F.; Taheri, Z.; Mardanpour, E. Characteristics of a Good Teacher in Terms of Students of Health School in Shahrekord University of Medical Sciences. *J. Res. Med. Sci.* **2011**, *3*, 1–8.
32. Song, Z. Teacher Stroke as a Positive Interpersonal Behavior on English as a Foreign Language Learners' Success and Enthusiasm. *Front. Psychol.* **2021**, *12*, 761658. [CrossRef] [PubMed]
33. Şahin, A. Humor Use in School Settings: The Perceptions of Teachers. *SAGE Open* **2021**, *11*, 21582440211022691. [CrossRef]
34. Roorda, D.L.; Koomen, H.M.; Spilt, J.L.; Oort, F.J. The Influence of Affective Teacher–Student Relationships on Students' School Engagement and Achievement: A Meta-Analytic Approach. *Rev. Educ. Res.* **2011**, *81*, 493–529. [CrossRef]
35. Hamre, B.K.; Pianta, R.C. Early teacher-child relationships and the trajectory of children's school outcomes through eighth grade. *Child Dev.* **2001**, *72*, 625–638. [CrossRef] [PubMed]
36. Martin, A.J.; Dowson, M. Interpersonal relationships, motivation, engagement, and achievement: Yields for theory, current issues, and educational practice. *Rev. Educ. Res.* **2009**, *79*, 327–365. [CrossRef]
37. Jennings, P.A.; Greenberg, M.T. The prosocial classroom: Teacher social and emotional competence in relation to student and classroom outcomes. *Rev. Educ. Res.* **2009**, *79*, 491–525. [CrossRef]
38. Struble, S.L.; Ohno, A.; Barthelmass, M.; Ogunyemi, D. Prevalence and Nature of Sexist Microaggressions against Female Medical Students. *Acad. Med.* **2022**, *97*, S178. [CrossRef]
39. Heath, T.J.; Niethe, G.E. Veterinary practitioners in rural Australia: A national survey. *Aust. Vet. J.* **2001**, *79*, 464–469. [CrossRef] [PubMed]

40. Linh, P.T.T. Teacher's Humor Use in the Classroom and Students' Perceptions of Its Effectiveness and Appropriateness. Ph.D. Thesis, Vietnam National University, Hanoi University of Languages and International Studies Faculty of English Language Teacher Education, Hanoi, Vietnam, 2011.
41. Ekperi, P.; Onwuka, U.; Nyejirime, W. Teachers' attitude as a correlate of students' academic performance. *Int. J. Res. Sci. Innov. Appl. Sci.* **2019**, *3*, 205–209.
42. Rani, N. The Secret in Education Lies in Respecting the Student. BrainBuxa. 2014. Available online: https://www.brainbuxa.com/blog/the-secret-in-education-lies-in-respecting-the-student (accessed on 10 October 2022).
43. Gillespie, M. Student-Teacher Connection: A Place of Possibility. *J. Adv. Nurs.* **2005**, *52*, 211–219. [CrossRef] [PubMed]
44. Gao, Y. Toward the Role of Language Teacher Confirmation and Stroke in EFL/ESL Students' Motivation and Academic Engagement: A Theoretical Review. *Front. Psychol.* **2021**, *12*, 723432. [CrossRef] [PubMed]
45. Xie, F.; Derakhshan, A. A Conceptual Review of Positive Teacher Interpersonal Communication Behaviors in the Instructional Context. *Front. Psychol.* **2021**, *12*, 708490. [CrossRef]
46. Frenzel, A.C.; Fiedler, D.; Marx, A.K.G.; Reck, C.; Pekrun, R. Who Enjoys Teaching, and When? Between- and Within-Person Evidence on Teachers' Appraisal-Emotion Links. *Front. Psychol.* **2020**, *11*, 1092. [CrossRef]
47. Lujan, H.L.; DiCarlo, S.E. A Personal Connection: Promoting Positive Attitudes towards Teaching and Learning. *Anat. Sci. Educ.* **2017**, *10*, 503–507. [CrossRef]

Disclaimer/Publisher's Note: The statements, opinions and data contained in all publications are solely those of the individual author(s) and contributor(s) and not of MDPI and/or the editor(s). MDPI and/or the editor(s) disclaim responsibility for any injury to people or property resulting from any ideas, methods, instructions or products referred to in the content.

MDPI
St. Alban-Anlage 66
4052 Basel
Switzerland
www.mdpi.com

Veterinary Sciences Editorial Office
E-mail: vetsci@mdpi.com
www.mdpi.com/journal/vetsci

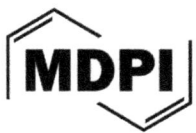

Disclaimer/Publisher's Note: The statements, opinions and data contained in all publications are solely those of the individual author(s) and contributor(s) and not of MDPI and/or the editor(s). MDPI and/or the editor(s) disclaim responsibility for any injury to people or property resulting from any ideas, methods, instructions or products referred to in the content.

www.ingramcontent.com/pod-product-compliance
Lightning Source LLC
LaVergne TN
LVHW070409100526
838202LV00014B/1420